The Bioarchaeology of Individuals

Bioarchaeological Interpretations of the Human Past:
Local, Regional, and Global Perspectives

UNIVERSITY PRESS OF FLORIDA

Florida A&M University, Tallahassee

Florida Atlantic University, Boca Raton

Florida Gulf Coast University, Ft. Myers

Florida International University, Miami

Florida State University, Tallahassee

New College of Florida, Sarasota

University of Central Florida, Orlando

University of Florida, Gainesville

University of North Florida, Jacksonville

University of South Florida, Tampa

University of West Florida, Pensacola

The Bioarchaeology of Individuals

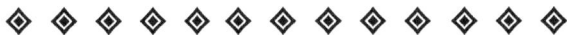

❖ ❖ ❖ ❖ ❖ ❖ ❖ ❖ ❖ ❖ ❖ ❖ ❖

Edited by Ann L. W. Stodder and Ann M. Palkovich

Foreword by Clark Spencer Larsen

University Press of Florida

Gainesville/Tallahassee/Tampa/Boca Raton

Pensacola/Orlando/Miami/Jacksonville/Ft. Myers/Sarasota

We dedicate this book to three remarkable young women who inspire us every day. Our daughters:

Emma Ellen Stodder

Meredith S. S. Shaw

Anna M. Shaw

Copyright 2012 by Ann L. W. Stodder and Ann M. Palkovich

All rights reserved

Printed in the United States of America on acid-free paper

First cloth printing, 2012
First paperback printing, 2014

Library of Congress Cataloging-in-Publication Data

The bioarchaeology of individuals / edited by Ann L.W. Stodder and Ann M. Palkovich ; foreword by Clark Spencer Larsen.
p. cm. -- (Bioarchaeological interpretations of the human past : local, regional, and global perspectives)
Includes bibliographical references and index.
ISBN 978-0-8130-3807-0 (cloth: acid-free paper)
ISBN 978-0-8130-6027-9 (pbk.)
1. Human remains (Archaeology) 2. Persons--History. 3. Biography. 4. Bones--Social aspects--History. 5. Excavations (Archaeology) 6. Historic sites. 7. Social archaeology. I. Stodder, Ann Lucy Wiener. II. Palkovich, Ann M.
CC79.5.H85B56 2012
930.1--dc23
2012001109

The University Press of Florida is the scholarly publishing agency for the State University System of Florida, comprising Florida A&M University, Florida Atlantic University, Florida Gulf Coast University, Florida International University, Florida State University, New College of Florida, University of Central Florida, University of Florida, University of North Florida, University of South Florida, and University of West Florida.

University Press of Florida
15 Northwest 15th Street
Gainesville, FL 32611-2079
http://www.upf.com

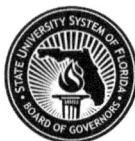

Contents

Figures

Tables

Foreword

The record of the history of the human condition is provided by a range of sources. This book series focuses on the remarkable fund of data recovered from the contextualized study of ancient human remains. Previous books in the series highlight key trends and circumstances, ranging from global patterns of health and the agricultural transition (Cohen and Crane-Kramer 2007) to the identity and construction of social persona (Knudson and Stojanowski 2009). One of the clear strengths of bioarchaeology is our ability to extend the understanding of human adaptations and population biology into the past based on the study of collections of skeletons. In this volume, Stodder and Palkovich convincingly argue that populations are comprised of individuals and that individuals provide a potentially rich source for developing an informed understanding of the lives, lifeways, and lifestyles of ancestors. Simply, an individual skeleton presents information about identity, life history, circumstances of birth (and death), and the particular roles that person played in a society. The osteobiographic approach (sensu Saul 1972) acknowledges and underscores the importance of individual people and their lives to the history of our species. Importantly, this approach adds considerable richness and meaning to the social and behavioral context for the study of an individual's bones and teeth.

The editors were inspired by their own research in the American Southwest, realizing especially the significant gap in relating the bioarchaeological record to the lives of individual persons. They present here a collection of essays encompassing a diversity of settings and personages from around the world. After reading these accounts, I came away feeling that I had met each of the people and knew something of their role in society and their life challenges and the highlights of their lives from birth to death. These essays tell us that bioarchaeologists are in a unique position to relate a prehistoric or historic person's story in a well-informed way.

One of the most amazing of the essays pertains to the "Axed Man" from Mosfell, Iceland. Near a Viking longhouse, a building occupied by important chieftains and their families, bioarchaeologist Phillip Walker and his colleagues recovered the remains of an older adult male Viking. Having survived multiple challenges affecting his health, this middle-age man died suddenly and violently. Dramatic cuts on the side and back of his head, produced by an ax and by a sword, respectively, tell a vivid story of violence and death. As is so well documented in the Icelandic sagas, this man died under circumstances that may have simply amounted to being in the wrong place at the wrong time. The combined use of archival, archaeological, and skeletal evidence gives us a snapshot of one man's life and death in the context of Scandinavian colonization heretofore known mostly from tales and stories.

The interdisciplinary study of the Axed Man and the other osteobiographies in this book are not just descriptions of individual skeletons. Rather, they are scientific accounts that place the individuals within the context of their respective populations.

This important book provides a crucial perspective on our shared human condition. Beyond summary statistics and population tendencies, it reminds the reader that each person in a population is part of the larger record, a part of the larger story that is a crucial for understanding variation and evolution, and for reconstructing and interpreting the human experience.

Clark Spencer Larsen
Series Editor

References Cited

Cohen, Mark Nathan, and Gillian M. M. Crane-Kramer (editors)
2007   *Ancient Health: Skeletal Indicators of Agricultural and Political Intensification.* University Press of Florida, Gainesville.
Knudson, Kelly J., and Christopher M. Stojanowski (editors)
2009   *Bioarchaeology and Identity in the Americas.* University Press of Florida, Gainesville.
Saul, Frank
1972   *The Human Skeletal Remains of Altar de Sacrificios: An Osteobiographic Analysis.* Papers of the Peabody Museum of Archaeology and Ethnology Vol. 63, No. 2. Harvard University, Cambridge.

The Bioarchaeology of Individuals

1 ◆ Osteobiography and Bioarchaeology

Ann L. W. Stodder and Ann M. Palkovich

This book is a compilation of osteobiographies—interpretations of the lives of people whose remains were excavated from archaeological sites. The foundation of each chapter is the study of an individual beginning with the skeleton and then expanding the analytical and interpretive scale from the grave outward to understand this person's context in life and in death. We asked the contributors to tell the story of one individual: someone they had encountered as a burial during excavation, or as a skeleton in a larger collection; someone whose life touched theirs, whom they identified with, whose investigation posed an intellectual challenge. We provided the template for the individual profiles that appear at the beginning of each chapter and issued the deceptively simple instruction that contributors present the individual and their investigation in a manner accessible to students and nonexperts, without glossing the scientific aspect of their methods, or oversimplifying the problems and limitations inherent in the research.

The resulting essays tell the stories of people who lived at vastly different times (ranging from 3200 B.C. to A.D. 1848) and in vastly different contexts: Bronze Age Thailand, a remote oasis in Egypt, an island in the western Pacific, a family farm in nineteenth-century Canada, ancient Turkey, Viking Iceland, Cypress, ancient Peru, a small farming village in Maya Belize, medieval Portugal, the American Southwest, Teotihuacán. These are the biographies of people who lived in urban and rural settings, in the tropics and the desert and the northern forests. This volume is about people, not just bones: they were parents, children, farmers, masons, artisans, immigrants, nomads, warriors, healers. The contributors use oral history and legends, ancient texts and imagery, ethnographic and ethnohistoric sources, death records and tombstones, analysis of bone chemistry and ancient DNA, evidence of habitual activity patterns inscribed on the skeleton, genetic traits recorded in the teeth and bones, and indicators of health and disease in childhood and beyond. The wide range of information and methods brought to the research exemplifies the creative, interdisciplinary nature of bioarchaeology.

As students of the explicitly scientific, adaptation-oriented "new physical anthropology" and "new archaeology," we learned that our purpose was to analyze skeletal populations to document major biocultural trends in human adaptation; individuals were seldom the subject of research, and case studies were rarely published. Justification of the study of human remains is most often framed as the contribution to understanding big questions about the evolution of our species, such as the impact of agriculture or the emergence and reemergence of diseases (e.g., Armelagos 2003). But over several decades of adaptation-oriented work with an emphasis on statistical analysis of large assemblages of (typically well-preserved) skeletons, we set aside the opportunity to ask many other kinds of questions about the lives of people in the past. Unusual individuals were deleted as outliers or "abstracted" in the drive to generate higher-level data characterizing age and sex groups, social classes, and populations (Joyce 2005: 149). The increasingly sophisticated analytical methods that we bring to skeletal and archaeological analysis continue to expand our understanding of our past (Hunt 2001; Larsen 2006), but distance the study of skeletal remains from the lives of the people we study (Goldstein 2006). None of the work reported in these essays was done in isolation; the populational data provides the context for interpreting the skeletal morphology and life history of these individuals as much as the archaeological data. We see the study of individuals as a complementary domain to the populational framework of bioarchaeology. Both approaches are essential to the relevance of the field. As written by the late Phillip Walker, "The information about historical events encoded in the skeletons of our ancestors can be thought of as a complex message from the past that we can decode through bioarchaeological research. Each individual skeleton has a unique story to tell about that individual's life as well as the evolutionary events that constitute the history of our species" (2008: 26).

With roots in the work of Krogman and Angel (Buikstra 2006: 348), the term "osteobiography" was coined by Saul in 1961 (Saul 1972; Saul and Saul 1989). The life-history approach in analysis of human remains is not new, but it is more welcome in the current research climate. The emerging realm of socially oriented bioarchaeology (Sofaer 2006; Gowland and Knüsel 2006; Knudson and Stojanowski 2008, 2009; Agarwal and Glencross 2010), with an emphasis on identity and life history, takes bioarchaeological research from the population scale to the much more intimate scale of human life in social context. This more inclusive paradigm stems from the archaeology of gender, which admitted women and children into interpretations of the archaeological record (e.g., Moore and Scott 1997; Arnold and Wicker 2001; Kamp 2002; Baxter 2008), and from the impact of practice theory and the notion of agency. Osteobiography is a uniquely valuable component to the study of prehistory that considers individuals, their intentions, and their socially contextualized identities as fundamental to understanding the past.

In these chapters archaeological and skeletal data are used together to examine various stages of the life course of specific individuals in specific societies, an approach that is crucial to archaeology with "a human scope" (Gilchrist 2000). Unlike many other studies that use material culture and mortuary data, sometimes without addressing human remains at all, the skeleton is in the forefront here. In the approach advocated by Sofaer, "the plasticity of the body means that the body is never presocial and is contextually dependent" (2006: 74). Isotope studies illuminate the place of origin of individuals and enhance our understanding of migration and residence patterns. Burials in houses and cemeteries illustrate the role of mortuary ritual in the creation of social memory in the personal and collective spheres (Cannon 2002). The consideration of the body in the grave is informed by the incorporation of taphonomy in tracing the interaction of human actions and postdepositional processes that create the bioarchaeological record (Nawrocki 1995; Haglund and Sorg 2002; Stodder 2008), and the analysis of traumatic injuries exemplifies the increasingly prominent role of forensic anthropology and its overlap with bioarchaeology (Walker 2001; Ubelaker 2008).

The chapters also touch on many facets of the work of bioarchaeology: the imperative to make conservative and well-grounded interpretations, to find balance between facts and the unknowable dimensions of the past; the range of experiences we have in working with archaeologists; and the experience of interacting with living descendants and with the dead. Another theme here is that understanding archaeological features, including burials and skeletal remains, is a long process of gathering many different kinds of data and generating a synthetic interpretation that may change as other pieces of the puzzle of the past are brought to bear. The burials discussed in this book were excavated as long ago as 1925 and 1939, and as recently as 2005. Archaeology can be terrifically exciting, but most revelations do not happen in the field; we gain our insights later (sometimes much later) after careful, detailed study.

The volume is organized into four thematic groups: Ancestors and Descendants, Ancient Travelers and "Others," Craftsmen and Artisans, and Farm and Village. The first of four essays in part 1, Ancestors and Descendants, Neitzel's account of the so-called Magician of Ridge Ruin in northern Arizona, is about the individual who was the original inspiration for this book. After writing about the bioarchaeology of the U.S. Southwest for many years, we realized that the literature on this region is almost completely devoid of descriptions and interpretations of individual people. Renewed interest in this individual and his intriguing array of grave goods attests to the importance of human remains to living descendants, and their role in archaeology today. Chapters 3 and 4, by Walker and colleagues, and Heathcote and colleagues, respectively, present archaeological and skeletal data and contextualize them in Viking and Chamorro legends and culture histories. The Axed Man of Mosfell, Iceland, and Taotao Tagga' of Tinian embody the legendary ancestors, and their remains provide new details to the enduring stories of these iconic culture heroes whose importance today reflects postcolonial trends in revisiting and reclaiming the past. In the fourth chapter in this group, Wrobel describes the burial of two young men within an abandoned elite residence in an example of the role of mortuary ritual as personal and political statement, and the blending of Christian and indigenous traditions as resistance in the Spanish Colonial era.

The essays in part 2, Ancient Travelers and "Others," are about individuals whose morphology and contexts signal them as "others." Morphological analysis, ancient DNA, and strontium isotope studies are used to explore the identities of these individuals. The individual from El Yaral, Peru, not born locally and buried with objects of nonlocal manufacture, is interpreted by Lozada and coauthors as a *curandero*, an itinerant healer, his treatment in death reflecting the fear and respect with which these individuals were viewed. The Neolithic Nomad found at Dakhleh Oasis with just a few contemporaries represents a small nomadic population living in a watered refugium, their economy neither agricultural nor pastoral. Thompson's study documents a little-known component of Egyptian history and the bioarchaeology of Dakhleh, dominated by burial populations from the Dynastic and Roman periods. Martin and Potts describe a young woman from the site of Tell Abraq in the United Arab Emirates with a progressive neurodegenerative condition, perhaps from poliomyelitis, whose body was carefully wrapped and placed in a tomb with some 300 others whose remains were jumbled and mixed. Hers is the only intact body in the tomb, raising questions about the meaning of her special treatment in death. In the final chapter about "others," Powell and colleagues use a variety of data to investigate the identity of a morphologically and genetically distinct woman buried in a place of honor in the Chapel at Torre de Palma. An African in medieval Portugal, was she a freed slave?

Part 3, Craftsmen and Artisans, focuses on individuals who worked in special roles. Everyday, well-used artifacts found in association with a body are interpreted as personal items belonging to the deceased and often lead us to imagine what they meant to the deceased in life. The bone needle discovered with a woman from medieval Polis, Cyprus, led Baker and coauthors to consider whether she was a seamstress in life. The detailed and well-illustrated analysis supports their interpretation, revealing skeletal markers associated with the habitual activity patterns one would find in someone who regularly works with fibers. Dubbed "Vulcan" by workers at the Bronze Age Ban Chiang archaeological site in Thailand, the individual reported by Douglas and Pietrusewsky was buried with the tools of his trade. His skill as a metallurgist is evident from the fine quality of the implement he made; his body reflects the physical demands of his craft.

The burial of a pre-Columbian patriarch at Tlajinga in Teotihuacán, Mexico, is interpreted by Storey and Widmer. The variety and richness of the items found in this man's grave as well as its prominent location suggest he was the founder of a local residential compound and a master artisan, perhaps the head of a guild of skilled workers to whom homage was paid upon his death. The detailed history of the remodeling of the compound in the process of commemoration of this person exemplifies the multiple scales at which mortuary activity operates to create social memory. The biography of the plazas in the compound reveals one of these scales of the material correlates of ritual practice (Gosden and Marshall 1999; Gillespie 2008). Boutin offers the osteobiography of a Bronze Age craftsman from Tell Atchana (ancient Alalakh) in southern Turkey. The physically demanding work associated with harvesting and preparing reeds for baskets and tapestries leaves its mark on the mouth, arms, and even legs, and distinguishes this craftsman from others in his group. This chapter demonstrates the power of the carefully crafted fictive narrative as a means of acquainting the reader with people in antiquity.

Part 4, Farm and Village, highlights the lives of ordinary people whose stories bring us empathic understanding of life and death in small communities in the distant and recent past. Katzenberg and Saunders introduce us to a nineteenth-century Scottish immigrant to the Ontario region of Canada. Their careful assessment of the archaeological data allows them to match individual interments to their original gravestones, and their use of stable isotope analysis provides us with insights into breastfeeding practices among these families. This meticulous analysis allows us to see the impact of epidemic disease on fragile family life, as the loss of a husband and father presages by a year the deaths of his child followed a few days later by his wife. This study reminds us that villagers in many other times and places in the past faced health hazards.

Merbs's discussion of the infant death at Nuvakwewtaqa, a Sinaguan Pueblo village from A.D. 1350, poignantly highlights the hazards of early life and childbirth. He notes that the pattern of partially healed fractures suggests this infant managed to survive for a short period, but ultimately succumbed to the trauma of a difficult birth. Using ethnographic accounts of Puebloan burial practices,

Merbs offers a picture of the harsh realities of childbirth in fourteenth-century Arizona, one where infants often died early in life and where women also at times succumbed to the hazards of childbirth. Palkovich likewise considers health issues among ancestral Puebloans in the fourteenth-century village of Arroyo Hondo in New Mexico. While the bone deformities of rickets are acquired early in life, the physical impairments are lasting. Palkovich poses the question of assessing "disabilities" among those long ago, and whether our perceptions of physical limitations were necessarily experienced or understood in the same ways by those living in the past. She notes that while these physical limitations were very real, the implications for shaping the social lives of these individuals is not necessarily revealed in the archaeological record.

Rural life is reflected in Geller's analysis of a young man from a Classic period Maya community dating to circa A.D. 750. Drawing on ethnographic accounts and a detailed analysis of this individual's funerary goods, Geller suggests this man likely played a special role in his community as a medico-religious specialist. Close attention to archaeological detail allows Geller to demonstrate that veneration was not exclusive to central figures in Maya society. Those who played special roles in their local communities were also venerated ancestors in death. Geller explicitly addresses the importance of biography in peopling the past. She traces the roots of her research in feminist archaeology, and elegantly argues for the importance of putting faces on people in the past.

Bioarchaeology faces many challenges today, not least of which is the perception that bioarchaeologists are concerned only with death and disease or with the spectacular funerary remains of earlier civilizations, and that sophisticated laboratory analyses provide simple answers to complex questions. We hope this contribution to bioarchaeology conveys the level of detail and care with which we approach the study of human remains. And finally, we hope that these essays will inspire students and all readers to wonder and learn about the breadth of human experience as told by all of our ancestors.

Acknowledgments

We thank the contributors for their work on this project, series editor Clark Spencer Larsen for his support of this somewhat unorthodox publication, and the participants in the original symposium, including Christopher Knüsel, Judith Littleton, George Milner, Barra O'Donnabhain, and John Verano. Kate Babbitt assisted us with the manuscript preparation, and Christine Sulok improved the quality of several of the images included in the volume. We would also like to thank the volume's reviewers for their thoughtful comments.

References Cited

Agarwal, Sabrina, and Bonnie Glencross (editors)
2010   *Social Bioarchaeology.* Wiley-Blackwell, New York.
Armelagos, George J.
2003   Bioarchaeology as Anthropology. *Archaeological Papers of the American Anthropological Association* 13: 27–41.
Arnold, Bettina, and Nancy Wicker (editors)
2001   *Gender and the Archaeology of Death.* AltaMira Press, Walnut Creek, Calif.
Baxter, Jane E.
2008   The Archaeology of Childhood. *Annual Review of Anthropology* 37: 159–75.
Buikstra, Jane E.
2006   On to the 21st Century, Introduction. In *Bioarchaeology: The Contextual Analysis of Human Remains*, edited by J. E. Buikstra and L. A. Beck, pp. 347–57. Elsevier, New York.
Cannon, Aubrey
2002   Spatial Narratives of Death, Memory, and Transcendence. *Archaeological Papers of the American Anthropological Association* 11(1): 191–99.
Gilchrist, Roberta
2000   Archaeological Biographies: Realizing Human Lifecycles, Courses and Histories. *World Archaeology* 31(1): 325–28.
Gillespie, Susan D.
2008   History in Practice: Ritual Deposition at La Venta Complex A. In *Memory Work: Archaeologies of Material Practices*, edited by B. J. Mills and W. H. Walker, pp. 109–36. School of Advanced Research Press, Santa Fe, N.Mex.
Goldstein, Lynne
2006   Mortuary Analysis and Bioarchaeology. In *Bioarchaeology: The Contextual Analysis of Human Remains*, edited by J. E. Buikstra and L. A. Beck, pp. 375–87. Elsevier, New York.
Gosden, Chris, and Yvonne Marshall
1999   The Cultural Biography of Objects. *World Archaeology* 31(2): 169–78.
Gowland, Rebecca, and Christopher Knüsel (editors)
2006   *The Social Archaeology of Funerary Remains.* Oxbow Press, Oxford.
Haglund, William D., and Marcella H. Sorg (editors)
2002   *Advances in Forensic Taphonomy: Method, Theory, and Archaeological Perspectives.* CRC Press, Boca Raton, Fla.
Hunt, David R.
2001   The Value of Human Remains for Research and Education. In *Human Remains: Conservation, Retrieval and Analysis*, edited by E. Williams, pp. 129–34. Archaeopress, Oxford.
Joyce, Rosemary
2005   Archaeology of the Body. *Annual Review of Anthropology* 34: 139–58.
Kamp, Kathryn Ann (editor)
2002   *Children in the Prehistoric Puebloan Southwest.* University of Utah Press, Salt Lake City.

Knudson, Kelly, and Christopher Stojanowski

2008   New Directions in Bioarchaeology: Recent Contributions to the Study of Human Social Identities. *Journal of Archaeological Research* 16: 397–432.

Knudson, Kelly, and Christopher Stojanowski (editors)

2009   *Bioarchaeology and Identity in the Americas.* University Press of Florida, Gainesville.

Larsen, Clark S.

2006   The Changing Face of Bioarchaeology: An Interdisciplinary Science. In *Bioarchaeology: The Contextual Analysis of Human Remains*, edited by J. E. Buikstra and L. A. Beck, pp. 359–74. Elsevier, New York.

Moore, Jenny, and Eleanor Scott (editors)

1997   *Invisible People and Processes: Writing Gender and Childhood into European Archaeology.* Leicester University Press, London.

Nawrocki, Stephen P.

1995   Taphonomic Processes in Historic Cemeteries. In *Bodies of Evidence: Reconstructing History through Historical Analysis*, edited by A. L. Grauer, pp. 49–68. Wiley-Liss, New York.

Saul, Frank P.

1972   *The Human Skeletal Remains of Altar de Sacrificios: An Osteobiographic Analysis.* Papers of the Peabody Museum of Archaeology and Ethnology Vol. 63, No. 2. Harvard University, Cambridge.

Saul, Frank P., and Julie M. Saul

1989   Osteobiography: A Maya Example. In *Reconstructing Life from the Skeleton*, edited by M. Y. Iscan and K. A. R. Kennedy, pp. 287–302. Alan R. Liss, New York.

Sofaer, Joanna R.

2006   *The Body as Material Culture: A Theoretical Osteoarchaeology.* Cambridge University Press, New York.

Stodder, Ann L. W.

2008   Taphonomy and the Nature of Archaeological Assemblages. In *The Biological Anthropology of the Human Skeleton*, edited by M. A. Katzenberg and S. R. Saunders, pp. 71–114. Wiley-Liss, New York.

Ubelaker, Douglas H.

2008   Forensic Anthropology: Methodology and Diversity of Applications. In *The Biological Anthropology of the Human Skeleton*, edited by M. A. Katzenberg and S. R. Saunders, pp. 41–69. Wiley-Liss, New York.

Walker, Phillip L.

2001   A Bioarchaeological Perspective on the History of Violence. *Annual Review of Anthropology* 30: 573–96.

2008   Bioarchaeological Ethics: A Historical Perspective on the Value of Human Remains. In *The Biological Anthropology of the Human Skeleton*, edited by M. A. Katzenberg and S. R. Saunders, pp. 3–40. Wiley-Liss, New York.

ONE ◆ Ancestors and Descendants

2 ❖ The Magician

AN ANCESTRAL HOPI LEADER

Jill E. Neitzel

Individual Profile

Site: Ridge Ruin (AR-03-04-02-885; also NA 1785)
Location: Approximately 30 km east of Flagstaff, Arizona
Cultural Affiliation: Elden phase Sinagua, ancestral Hopi, early Pueblo III
Date: A.D. 1150–1175, based on decorated ceramics and tree-ring dates
Feature: Burial 16
Location of Grave: Room 13, subfloor
Burial and Grave Type: A single primary inhumation extended in an approximately 1 m deep oval pit covered with log roof
Associated Materials: 613 cataloged objects
Preservation and Completeness: Skeleton—almost complete, fair preservation with most elements fragmentary; Teeth—4 missing, good preservation
Age at Death and Basis of Estimate: Approximately 35 years, based on dentition
Sex and Basis of Determination: Male, probably based on pelvis morphology
Conditions Observed: Very tall, cradleboard modification of skull, enamel hypoplasia, antemortem tooth loss, periodontal disease, healed forearm fracture, arthritis of jaw and ankles
Specialized Analysis: None
Excavated: 1939, Museum of Northern Arizona; project directed by John C. McGregor
Archaeological Report: McGregor 1941, 1943
Current Disposition: Curated at Museum of Northern Arizona; repatriation and reburial being negotiated by representatives of the Hopi tribe, the Coconino National Forest, and the Museum of Northern Arizona

A burial from the site of Ridge Ruin in northern Arizona is renowned among archaeologists who work in the U.S. Southwest. When excavated in 1939, the grave was found to be one of the richest ever documented in the region. Because the mortuary offerings included ritual artifacts similar to those used by the Hopi in a sleight-of-hand ceremony, the interred man was named "the Magician." Physical anthropologists have studied the Magician's skeleton, and both archaeologists and Hopi cultural advisers have analyzed his associated grave goods. These numerous and unusual artifacts are the primary reason why Ridge Ruin and its surrounding sites were nominated to the U.S. National Register of Historic Places. The nomination described Ridge Ruin as being associated with the Magician, who met the National Register criterion of being a significant individual in the nation's past.

Ridge Ruin and the Magician's Discovery

Ridge Ruin is a small pueblo located in the Coconino National Forest, approximately 30 km east of Flagstaff, Arizona (figure 2.1). Built on a low hill, the site offers a panoramic view of the surrounding region, with the most visible landmark being the San Francisco Peaks, which are sacred to the Hopi. Dating to the Elden phase (A.D. 1100–1200) of the Sinagua cultural tradition, Ridge Ruin consists of roughly 20 ground-floor rooms, some of which once had a second story (figure 2.1). Other notable features include a raised platform; two rock enclosures; several small plazas; rooms with fancy masonry similar to that found in Chaco Canyon, New Mexico; and two earlier ball courts at the base of the hill.

Ridge Ruin was excavated in the spring of 1939 by the Museum of Northern Arizona under a grant from the Works Projects Administration (WPA) (McGregor 1941). Project personnel included director John C. McGregor, field foreman Milton Wetherill, and a WPA crew of roughly 50 men. They completely excavated three rooms, tested along the walls of several more down to their floors, and exposed the tops of the remaining rooms' walls. The project also tested the two ball courts and several trash mounds.

The Magician's burial was uncovered beneath the floor of a trash-filled room located just off the north side of the pueblo (figure 2.1). The room's excavation began with the removal of the trash and the discovery of a ventilator and two parrot skeletons, possibly of Mesoamerican origin (Creel and McKusick 1994). Thinking that the work was done, McGregor (1941) tentatively identified the room as a ceremonial chamber or kiva. Luckily, when Wetherill was cleaning up, he noticed that the middle of the floor seemed disturbed (McGregor 1987, n.d.). Closer examination revealed several painted sticks just below the surface,

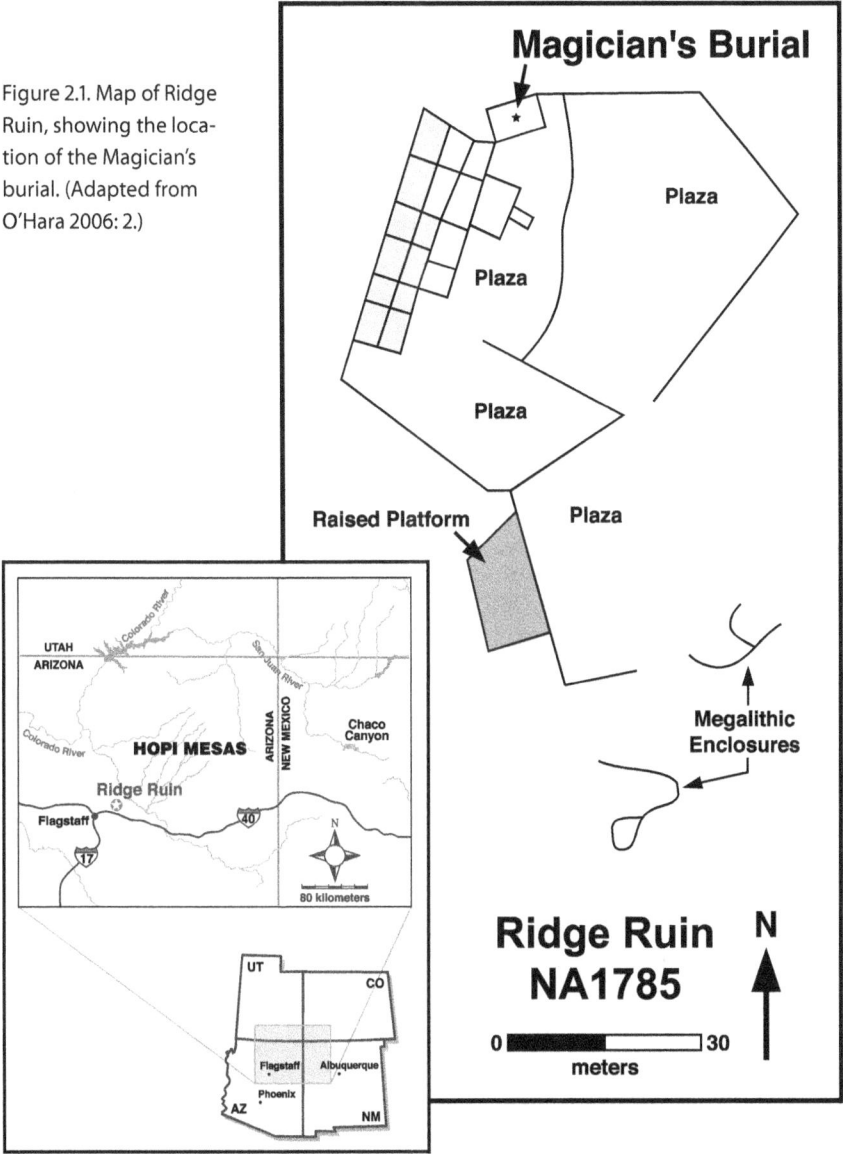

Figure 2.1. Map of Ridge Ruin, showing the location of the Magician's burial. (Adapted from O'Hara 2006: 2.)

and further testing uncovered a collapsed log roof above an oval pit. Inside the approximately 1 m deep pit was an extended skeleton accompanied by lavish grave goods.

The burial was carefully excavated the next day by Wetherill and James Kewanwytewa, a Hopi Indian employed by the Museum of Northern Arizona (McGregor 1987, n.d.). After being mapped, photographed, and inventoried

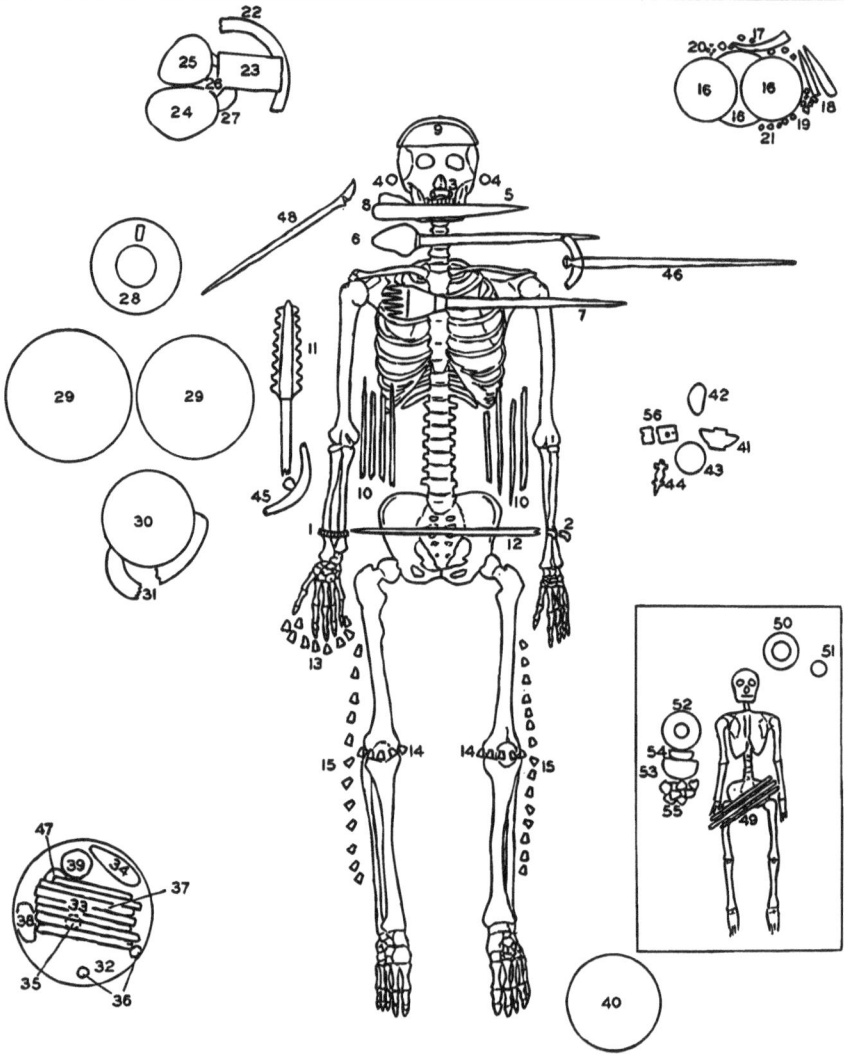

Figure 2.2. Maps of the Magician's burial, showing the artifacts whose locations were recorded. The large map shows the lower level; the inset shows the upper level (McGregor 1943: diagram, 272; numbered list of artifacts, 273).

Table 2.1. Burial map key

1. Turquoise bead bracelet
2. Turquoise animal heads
3. Nose plug
4. Ear pendants
5. Large inlaid* bone awl
6. Shell on stick
7. Painted** wood hand on stick
8. Obsidian knife blade
9. Beaded cap
10. Painted sticks
11. Carved painted stick
12. Painted stick
13. Loops of conus tinklers
14. Loops of conus tinklers
15. Strings of conus tinklers
16. Three black-on-white bowls
17. Rim of large shell
18. Two large knife blades
19. Two shell pendants
20. Mass of specular iron crystals on shell fragments
21. Scattered mass of copper ore
22. Painted basket fragments
23. Inlaid basket arm band
24. Abalone shell
25. Three marine shells
26. Inlaid bird bracelet ornament
27. Inlaid pendant
28. Red pitcher
29. Two polychrome bowls
30. Black-on-white bowl
31. Painted basket fragments
32. Coiled basket
33. Reeds filled with paint
34. Gourd with paint inside
35. Skin sacks with paint
36. Hematite paint fragments
37. Mountain lion claws and teeth
38. Mass of hair
39. Mass of string
40. Black-on-white bowl
41. Inlaid bird shape
42. Inlaid ear shape
43. Inlaid circle
44. Shell lizard
45. Inlaid stick ornament
46. Stick with inlay
47. Lignite button
48. Painted wood deer foot on stick
49. Three sticks, one with deer foot and one with human hand (both painted wood)
50. Black-on-white jar
51. Black-on-white bowl
52. Red jar
53. Black-on-white bowl
54. Black-on-white bowl
55. Crushed black-on-white bowl
56. Two painted green stone pendants

Source: Adapted from McGregor 1943: 273.

*Inlaid mosaic is usually turquoise or turquoise and shell.

**Paint colors on various sticks are blue, red, and green.

(figure 2.2, table 2.1), the grave's contents were taken to the museum for cataloging, analysis, and storage, a responsibility that the museum has continued to fulfill since that time.

Osteobiography

The Magician's skeleton was almost complete, but its overall condition was only fair, with virtually all elements fragmentary. Apart from four missing teeth, dental preservation was good. Shortly after excavation, the Magician's remains were analyzed by Katharine Bartlett of the Museum of Northern Arizona and Wilton Krogman of the University of Chicago (Bartlett 1941; McGregor 1941, 1943). In 1973 the remains were restudied by Dana Hartman and C. Hess of the Museum of Northern Arizona. Since then, several other physical anthropologists have conducted more cursory examinations.

The Magician was an adult male who died when he was approximately 35 years old—Bartlett's estimate was 35–40 years, and Hartman and Hess's (1973) was 30–35 years. With a height between 5 feet 7 inches and 5 feet 9 inches, the Magician was 4–6 inches taller than his average-size male peers (Bartlett 1941; McGregor 1943; Hartman and Hess 1973). His face and slender nose were long; his cheek bones were unusually flat; his jaw was broad and protruding; and typical of Native American populations, the inside surfaces of his incisors were markedly concave (shovel-shaped) (McGregor 1943; Hartman and Hess 1973; figure 2.3). One anomaly was severe flattening of the back of his skull (Bartlett 1941; McGregor 1943). According to Krogman, 75 percent of this deformation

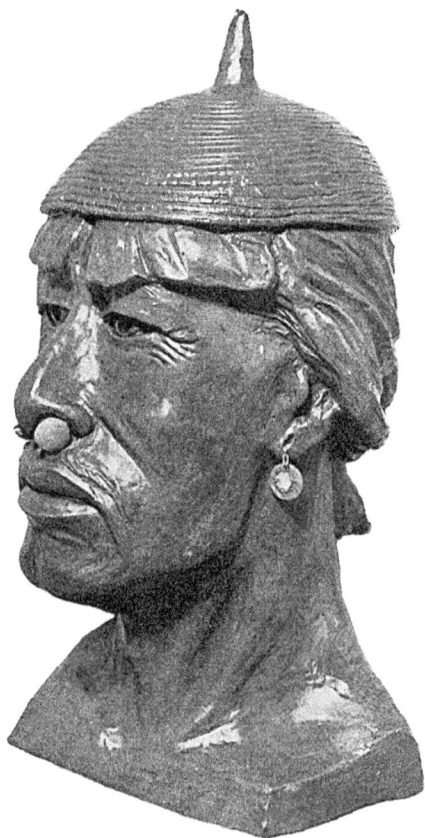

Figure 2.3. Virgil Hubert's reconstruction of the Magician's head, showing his facial features, the turquoise ornament decorating one end of his large nose plug, one of his turquoise earrings inlaid with shell, and his pointed cap made of 3,600 extremely small black stone beads strung together with several hundred shell beads (McGregor 1943: 293).

was postmortem (McGregor 1943). McGregor (1943) attributed the remaining 25 percent to the effects of being bound to a cradleboard when young, and indeed this was standard among the very great majority of prehistoric people of the northern Southwest. An unusual inherited trait was the presence of double foramina on his fourth and fifth cervical vertebrae (Hartman and Hess 1973).

The Magician's health conditions included a healed fracture of his two right forearm bones, slight arthritis of the jaw, and a more severe case of arthritis in the ankles (McGregor 1943; Hartman and Hess 1983; Pilles 1990). He also lost four molars prior to death due to unknown causes and suffered from gum disease around his upper incisors (Hartman and Hess 1973). Horizontal grooves (enamel hypoplasia) on his lower left canine and premolar indicate that his early growth was disrupted by either inadequate nutrition or disease (Hartman and Hess 1973).

Archaeologist Jonathan Reyman (1978) has cited the Magician's height and flattened skull as evidence that he was from Mesoamerica. This idea has been uniformly rejected by physical anthropologists who have examined the skeleton. The Magician certainly was tall—his stature is more typical of high-status adult males from Pueblo Bonito in Chaco Canyon and from Chacoan outliers in the San Juan Basin (Akins 1986; Malville 2008). But his various physical characteristics fall within ranges documented for the Sinagua. Furthermore, cradleboard modification of the back of the skull was the norm in this region. Based on comparisons with skeletons from several prehistoric and historic groups, physical anthropologist Mahmoud El-Najjar concluded that the Magician was a local Sinaguan, not an outsider from Mesoamerica, and that the Sinagua were physically most similar to the historic Hopi (Pilles 1976, 1996).

The Artifacts and Their Distribution

The Magician's grave goods are famous for their quantity, unique forms, and fine workmanship. Milton Wetherill and James Kewanwytewa mapped two distinct levels of these offerings (figure 2.2, table 2.1) and noted a third (McGregor 1943). The size of the assemblage is much greater than the 613 catalog numbers assigned to it, because some individual numbers were applied to multiple pieces (for example, beads comprising a bracelet).

The richest level was on the pit's floor where the Magician's body was laid. The body was dressed with a cap, jewelry, and the remains of leggings (figures 2.2–2.4, table 2.1). The cap was made of roughly 4,000 small beads, mostly stone and some shell. His jewelry included turquoise earrings with inlaid shell; a large nose plug of argillite and turquoise; and two bracelets, one with 73 turquoise

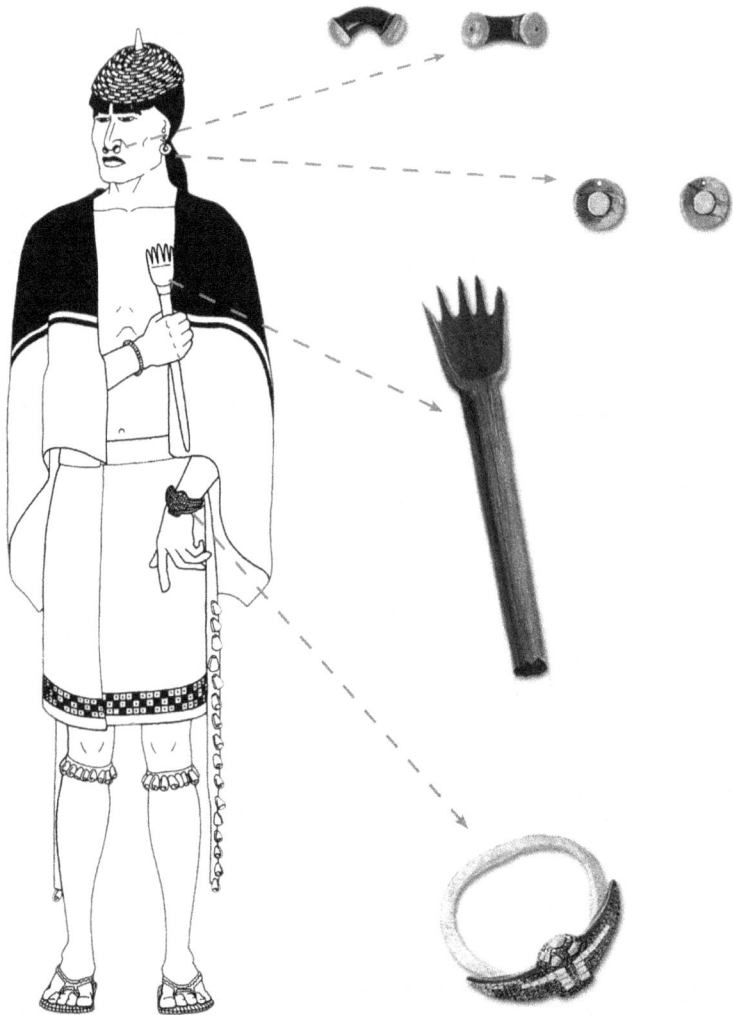

Figure 2.4. Wesley Jernigan's drawing of a Sinagua man ca. A.D. 1200, together with Eleanor Bareiss's drawings of artifacts recovered from the Magician's burial (McGregor 1943: plates 2–3). Jernigan's drawing accurately shows the Magician's beaded cap, nose plug, earring, bracelet of turquoise beads on his right wrist, and loops of shell tinklers around his knees. The carved stick in the figure's right hand is similar to that found laid across the Magician's chest. The bracelet on the figure's left wrist was recovered from one of the lower-level grave good clusters. In contrast to what is depicted in this drawing, no cloak, kilt, sash, or sandals were found with the Magician, and the strings of shell tinklers were probably attached to leggings. Note that the illustrations of individual artifacts are not to scale. (Jernigan's drawing reprinted by permission of University of New Mexico Press from *Jewelry of the Prehistoric Southwest*, 1978: 132.)

beads and the other with two mosaic grasshopper heads. The Magician also had several sets of shell tinklers—a loop in one hand, two more loops around each of his knees, and two lines along each of his legs. The tinklers were probably once attached to leg coverings. Contrary to the illustration in figure 2.4, no textile garments were preserved.

In addition to being wrapped in a large, woven mat, the Magician's body had 13 artifacts placed directly on or next to it (figure 2.2, table 2.1). They included an obsidian knife; a large bone awl with inlaid turquoise; two groups of four short sticks, which were carved and painted; and three longer sticks, two of which were topped with ornaments—a large shell on one and a painted wooden hand on the other (figures 2.4, 2.5e). Near the body were two more ornamented sticks and two ornaments without sticks. A painted, wooden deer foot (figure 2.5h) and an antler shape inlaid with turquoise and shell (figure 2.5g) decorated the complete specimens. The stickless ornaments included another inlaid antler shape (figure 2.5d) and a serrated sword made of painted wood (figure 2.5f).

The other grave goods from this level were found at six locations around the body, three on the left matched by three on the right (figure 2.2, table 2.1). With the exception of a single ceramic bowl by the Magician's left foot, the artifacts occurred in clusters of varying kinds. The cluster by his right foot consisted of the contents of a large coiled basket—a lignite button; mountain lion claws and teeth; a mass of hair; a clump of string; hematite paint fragments; and reeds, small skin sacks, and a gourd, all containing paints.

Two more clusters were found on opposite sides of the Magician's torso. Next to the wooden staffs by his right side were a fragmentary painted basket, three ceramic bowls, and a ceramic pitcher. The cluster by his left side included a lizard-shaped shell pendant, two painted stone pendants, and three examples of intricate turquoise and shell mosaic in the shapes of a circle (figure 2.5c), a bird (figure 2.5b), and an ear.

The last two clusters were placed above the Magician's head. To his right were three more examples of turquoise and shell mosaic—a pendant, a bird attached to a shell bracelet (figure 2.4), and a 12 cm tall basketry tube, possibly an armband, covered with more than 1,500 pieces of turquoise and additional orange, red, and black inlays (figure 2.5a). Accompanying these items were an abalone shell, three other marine shells, and another fragmentary painted basket. The left cluster included three ceramic bowls, two shell pendants, two large knife blades, the rim of a large shell, shell fragments covered with specular iron crystals, and a scattered mass of copper ore.

The second level of grave goods was 25 cm above the first. Three carved and

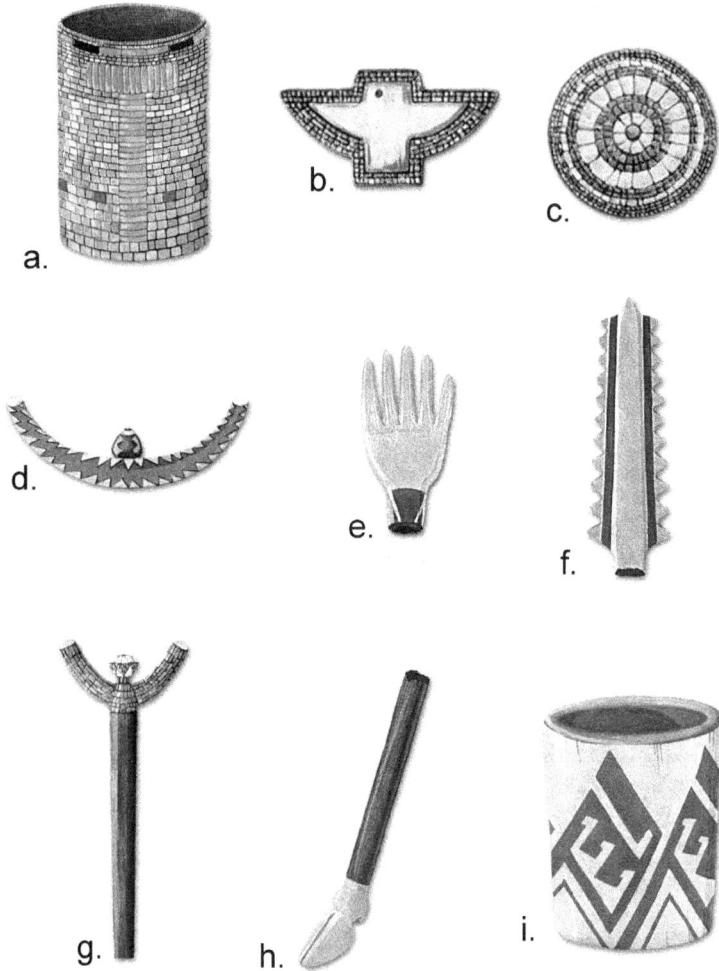

Figure 2.5. Examples of the Magician's mosaic and wooden artifacts drawn by Eleanor Bareiss (McGregor 1943: plates 1–3): (a) turquoise inlaid basketry armband with beaver teeth, red argillite, and black stone; (b) bird-shaped shell ornament with turquoise inlay; (c) circular brooch inlaid with turquoise and shell; (d) turquoise and shell inlaid ceremonial stick ornament in the form of antlers; (e) wooden hand-shaped stick ornament painted blue and red; (f) wooden stick ornament in the shape of serrated sword (agave plant?) painted green and red; (g) carved wooden stick painted red with turquoise and shell inlaid ornament in the shape of antlers; (h) carved wooden stick painted red with wooden, hoof-shaped ornament painted blue and green; (i) carved wooden cup painted blue and red. Illustrations are not to scale.

painted sticks were laid diagonally above the Magician's pelvis. One was topped with a wooden human hand and another with a deer foot. A ceramic jar, two bowls, and a crushed bowl were placed above the artifact cluster by the Magician's right arm; another bowl and jar were deposited above the cluster on the left side of his head.

The third level of artifacts, which lay immediately above the second level, coincided with the pit's .35 m thick collapsed wooden roof. Wetherill and Kewanwytewa inventoried but did not map hundreds of miniature wooden bows and reed arrow shafts along with 420 projectile points. The points were found in clusters of 8–12, which were probably from bundles of arrows that had been placed on the burial pit's wooden roof.

Between the three levels, the excavators found hundreds of other objects whose locations were not recorded. These artifacts included several more carved wooden sticks, including one decorated with a deer foot and another with a hand; two turquoise ear pendants; a string of 107 turquoise beads; shell pendants and earrings; 11 ceramic vessels; a painted wooden cup (figure 2.5i); fragments of painted wooden bowls; and bone awls, spatulas, and tube fragments. Also found were several quartz crystals, a calcite rod, a stone cube, worked slate, grooved volcanic tuff, and a variety of minerals and pigments. Some plant (for example, cornstalk fragment, pumpkin seeds, squash rind) and animal remains (cocoons, egg shell fragments, spider nests, lac balls) were also recovered.

Artifact Interpretations

The Magician's grave goods have been studied by both Hopi cultural advisers and archaeologists with the goal of determining the Magician's role in Sinagua society. Soon after the assemblage was brought to the Museum of Northern Arizona, John McGregor (1943) showed a few of the items to Hopi employees and visitors. They consistently identified the artifacts as ritual objects and successfully predicted what else should have also been found. This exercise represents one of the only independently verified concordances between archaeological remains and native oral tradition (Mason 2000).

Analyses of the Magician's grave goods have revealed continuity in religious society and clan organization between the ancestral and contemporary Hopi (for detailed discussion of Hopi, see Eggan 1950; Levy 1992; Parsons 1939; Titiev 1944). According to McGregor's cultural advisers, as well as other Hopi who have assisted subsequent archaeologists, the Magician was a powerful and important person, possibly a chief priest or medicine man, in both the warrior and the Motswimi religious societies (McGregor 1943; Hohman 1982; Ferguson and Lomaomvaya in press). The latter's performance includes the sleight-of-hand ceremony of swallowing sticks that inspired McGregor to call the burial's occupant "the Magician." The Magician may have also been a member of the Spider or Bluebird clans, which provide members to the Motswimi society. Hopi cultural advisers posited that so many ritual items were interred with the Magician because he died without having passed his ritual knowledge on to someone else. Thus a ceremony may have been retired with his burial.

Archaeologist Michael O'Hara (2006) recently compared the contents of each of the Magician's grave good clusters to ethnographic data for the Hopi as well as to a series of other Puebloan and non-Puebloan groups throughout the Southwest. He concluded that in addition to being a member of two religious associations, the Antelope and Bow sodalities, the Magician was a weather control shaman, a shamanic diviner and/or curer, a hunt/war shaman, a political arbitrator/negotiator, and a community leader who controlled local craft production and interregional trade. O'Hara also identified two groups of mourners, members of the One Horn and Two Horn sodalities. Their offerings of sword-swallowing sticks together with those belonging to the Magician effectively retired the complete set of ritual items used in winter solstice weather control ceremonies. O'Hara (2007) has suggested that other groups of mourners may also be reflected in the grave good clusters. If so, then some of the roles that researchers have assigned to the Magician may have actually belonged to others, prompting the question of what circumstances would have caused survivors to bury their valuables with him.

Taking a broader view to reconstruct how the Sinagua as a whole were organized, archaeologist John Hohman (1982) included the Magician in his analyses of all Sinagua burials. He concluded that Elden phase society was divided into a three-tier hierarchy within which status was ascribed. The Magician belonged to the top tier of this hierarchy.

Other researchers have used the Magician's grave goods to investigate the topics of chronology and outside connections. The most recent ceramic and tree-ring analyses suggest that the Magician was buried between A.D. 1150 and 1175 (Downum 1988; O'Hara 2006). O'Hara (2006) believes that the burning and abandonment of Ridge Ruin and the founding of a nearby ritual site were connected to the Magician's burial.

Several kinds of outside connections have been identified in both the Magician's burial and at Ridge Ruin. The first is trade. Most of the Magician's grave goods were imported, including all 22 of his decorated vessels from non-Sinagua groups to the north and east; shells from the Pacific Coast and the Gulf of

California; and turquoise, obsidian, minerals, and pigments from a variety of sources (McGregor 1943). Another outside connection was with the powerful and complex society centered at Chaco Canyon, New Mexico. Its influence can be seen in the hatched, Dogoszhi-style design on one of the Magician's ceramic jars (Neitzel 1995) and the Chacoan-style masonry used in building portions of Ridge Ruin (O'Hara 2000). The two ball courts next to Ridge Ruin indicate earlier contacts with Hohokam society, which was centered in the Phoenix Basin of south-central Arizona (Wilcox and Sternberg 1983). Finally, interaction with Mesoamerican groups, either direct or through intermediaries, may be evidenced by the two parrot skeletons recovered from the Magician's burial room (Creel and McKusick 1994).

The Magician's Future

The passage of the Native American Graves Protection and Repatriation Act (NAGPRA) in 1990 gave the Hopi tribe the legal right to repatriate and rebury the excavated skeletons and grave goods of its ancestors. When and how this will occur for the Magician's burial is being negotiated by representatives of the tribe, the Museum of Northern Arizona, and the Coconino National Forest. Until an agreement is reached, the Hopi's paramount concern is that the grave's contents be treated with sensitivity and respect. But the tribe also has questions about its past cultural affiliations that might be answered by further analyses of the Magician's skeleton and grave goods.

Given that the last comprehensive report on the burial was published almost 70 years ago, both physical anthropologists and archaeologists advocate thorough documentation and additional study prior to repatriation. They would like to investigate new research questions and apply new analytical techniques that have emerged in their disciplines in recent years. Since some of these questions and techniques can be used to address the Hopi's interest in cultural affiliation, the collaboration between scientists and living descendants that marked the Magician's excavation and initial interpretation could continue in his future as well.

Acknowledgments

Our current understanding of the Magician's burial is indebted to its careful excavation and documentation by John McGregor, Milton Wetherill, and James Kewanwytewa, and to the insights of James Kewanwytewa, Edmund Nequatewa, and other Hopi cultural advisers. The information presented in this essay was gathered with the assistance of Christian Downum, T. J. Ferguson, Leigh Kuwanwisiwma, Michael O'Hara, Peter Pilles, and David Wilcox. The figures were produced by Don McElroy based on images published previously by Wesley Jernigan and John McGregor. I alone am responsible for any errors.

References Cited

Akins, Nancy J.
1986   *A Biocultural Approach to Human Burials from Chaco Canyon, New Mexico.* National Park Service, Santa Fe, N.Mex.

Bartlett, Katharine
1941   Appendix No. 3: Skeletal Material from Winona and the Ridge Ruin. In *Winona and Ridge Ruin*, Part I, *Architecture and Material Culture*, by John C. McGregor, pp. 300–305. Bulletin No. 18. Museum of Northern Arizona, Flagstaff.

Creel, Darrell, and Charmion McKusick
1994   Prehistoric Macaws and Parrots in the Mimbres Area, New Mexico. *American Antiquity* 59: 510–24.

Downum, Christian E.
1988   "One Grand History": A Critical Review of Flagstaff Archaeology, 1851–1988. Ph.D. dissertation, Department of Anthropology, University of Arizona, Tucson.

Eggan, Fred
1950   *Social Organization of the Western Pueblos.* University of Chicago Press, Chicago.

Ferguson, T. J., and Micah Loma'omvaya
In press   Nuvatukya'ovi, Palatsmo, Niqw Wupatki: Hopi History, Culture, and Landscape. In *Sunset Crater Archaeology: Prehistoric Settlement in the Shadow of a Volcano*, edited by Mark Elson. Anthropological Papers No. 37. Center for Desert Archaeology, Tucson.

Hartman, Dana, and C. Hess
1973   Skeletal Analysis Sheet. On file, Museum of Northern Arizona, Flagstaff.

Hohman, John W.
1982   Sinagua Social Differentiation: Inferences Based on Prehistoric Mortuary Practices. Ph.D. dissertation, Department of Anthropology, Arizona State University, Tempe.

Jernigan, E. Wesley
1978   *Jewelry of the Prehistoric Southwest.* University of New Mexico Press, Albuquerque.

Levy, Jerrold E.
1992   *Old Orayvi Revisited: Social Stratification in an "Egalitarian" Society.* School of American Research Press, Santa Fe, N.Mex.

Malville, Nancy J.
2008   Stature of Ancestral Puebloan Populations: Population Density, Social Stratification, and Dietary Protein. In *Reanalysis and Reinterpretation in Southwestern Bioarchaeology*, ed. Ann L. W. Stodder, pp. 105–26. Arizona State University Anthropological Research Papers No. 59. Arizona State University, Tempe.

Mason, Ronald J.
2000   Archaeology and Native Oral Traditions. *American Antiquity* 65: 239–66.

McGregor, John C.

1941   *Winona and Ridge Ruin*, Part I, *Architecture and Material Culture*. Bulletin No. 18. Museum of Northern Arizona, Flagstaff.

1943   Burial of an Early American Magician. *Proceedings of the American Philosophical Society* 86(2): 270–98.

1987   Taped interview conducted on April 3, 1987, by S. Thysony. On file, Coconino National Forest, Flagstaff, Ariz.

n.d.   Archaeological Reminiscences. Manuscript on file, Museum of Northern Arizona, Flagstaff.

Neitzel, Jill E.

1995   Elite Styles in Hierarchically Organized Societies: The Chacoan Regional System. In *Style, Society, and Person: Archaeological and Ethnological Perspectives*, edited by Christopher Carr and Jill E. Neitzel, pp. 393–417. Plenum Press, New York.

O'Hara, Michael

2000   Plazas, Platforms, and Terraces: Communal Architecture of the Flagstaff Area. Paper presented at the Katharine Bartlett Symposium, Museum of Northern Arizona, Flagstaff.

2006   The Magician of Ridge Ruin: An Interpretation of His Social, Political, and Ritual Roles, and His Context in the Development of Hopi Religious Institutions. Manuscript on file, Department of Anthropology, Arizona State University, Tempe.

2007   The Magician of Ridge Ruin—Research in Progress. Manuscript on file, Department of Anthropology, Arizona State University, Tempe.

Parsons, Elsie Clews

1939   *Pueblo Indian Religion*. University of Chicago Press, Chicago.

Pilles, Peter

1976   Correspondence. On file, Coconino National Forest, Flagstaff, Ariz.

1990   Correspondence. On file, Coconino National Forest, Flagstaff, Ariz.

1996   Cultural Affiliation Assessment: Sinagua. In *Cultural Affiliations: Prehistoric Cultural Affiliations of Southwestern Indian Tribes*, compiled by Frank E. Wozniak, pp. 189–97. U.S. Forest Service, Southwestern Region, Albuquerque, N.Mex.

Reyman, Jonathan E.

1978   Pochteca Burials at Anasazi Sites? In *Across the Chichimec Sea: Papers in Honor of J. Charles Kelley*, edited by Carroll L. Riley and Basil C. Hedrick, pp. 242–59. Southern Illinois University Press, Carbondale.

Titiev, Mischa

1944   *Old Oraibi: A Study of the Hopi Indians of Third Mesa*. Peabody Museum of American Archaeology and Ethnology, Cambridge, Mass.

Wilcox, David R., and Charles Sternberg

1983   *Hohokam Ballcourts and Their Interpretation*. Archaeological Series 160. Arizona State Museum, Tucson.

3 ❖ The Axed Man of Mosfell

Skeletal Evidence of a Viking Age Homicide,
the Icelandic Sagas, and Feud

*Phillip L. Walker, Jesse Byock, Jacqueline T. Eng, Jon M. Erlandson,
Per Holck, Henry P. Schwarcz, and Davide Zori*

Individual Profile

Site: Kirkjuhóll
Location: Hrísbrú farm, Mosfell Valley (Mosfellsdalur), western Iceland
Cultural Affiliation: Icelandic Viking
Date: A.D. 855–1015 based on calibrated radiocarbon dates and tephrochronology
Feature: Trench CK-2001-3 (F2/2001)
Location of Grave: About 1 m east of the eastern end (chancel) of the church at Hrísbrú
Burial and Grave Type: A single primary inhumation extended with the head to the west; the body was resting on, partially dug into, a stratum of organic material that appears to be decayed hay or animal dung
Associated Materials: Stones were found under the thoracic area and at the top of the cranium; a poorly preserved lozenge-shaped object was found near the knee
Preservation and Completeness: Cranium is well preserved; many of the long bones have been affected by the acidic conditions at the site and are partially decalcified
Age at Death and Basis of Estimate: 40–45 years, based on age-related changes of pelvic morphology, tooth wear, and fusion of cranial vault sutures
Sex and Basis of Determination: Male, based on cranial and pelvic morphology
Conditions Observed: Massive cranial trauma with a gaping wound in the right parietal and a slice of bone removed from the occipital
Specialized Analysis: Accelerator Mass Spectrometry radiocarbon dating, thermal ionization mass spectrometry
Excavated: 2001, Mosfell Archaeological Project, directed by Jesse Byock and Phillip L. Walker
Archaeological Report: Byock et al. 2002
Current Disposition: National Museum of Iceland (þjóðminjasafn)

When Christianity was adopted by law in Iceland (1000 A.D. [*sic*]) Grim of Mosfell was baptized and built a church there. . . . When a church was built at Mosfell, the one Grim built at Hrísbrú was demolished and a new graveyard was laid out. Under the altar some human bones were found, much bigger than ordinary human bones, and people are confident that these were Egil's because of stories told by old men.

—*Egils saga Skalla-Grímsonar*, ca. A.D. 1230

The discovery of the skeletal remains of the person described in this chapter is one of many scientific results of the Mosfell Archaeological Project, an ongoing international research effort we began in 1995. The project's goal is to produce a comprehensive reconstruction of human adaptation and environmental change in Iceland's Mosfell Valley from Viking times until the present. To do this, we have used a multidisciplinary approach that integrates information from archaeology, physical anthropology, saga studies, and the environmental sciences (Byock et al. 2005; Holck 2005).

One facet of our work has been the use of archaeological evidence to test the historicity of the Icelandic sagas. These prose histories, which were mostly written down in the thirteenth century, describe life several hundred years earlier during the Viking Age. Some historians view the period of saga oral transmission as a yawning gap across which very little historically accurate information is likely to have been transmitted (Jones 1968: 11). Others take the position that the proportion of fact to fiction varies from saga to saga, and the quantities of each can best be decided through the minute examination and comparison of individual texts (Ciklamini 1971: 100). A third view, which does not negate the second, is that the sagas provide information analogous to that collected by ethnographers; these stories are a vehicle of social memory combining social, historical, and literary functions. When carefully evaluated in conjunction with independent evidence sources, they can reveal much about cultural patterns, normative codes, and historical events (Byock 2001: 21).

In our research, we have extended and refined the last approach by using archaeological excavations to "ground truth" saga passages, such as the one at the beginning of this chapter, that make specific statements about historical events that are supposed to have occurred in the Mosfell Valley (figure 3.1). The most rewarding efforts along these lines have been our archaeological explorations at the Hrísbrú farm. According to *Egil's Saga* (Nordal 1933: 298–99), Hrísbrú is the place where the bones of the saga's protagonist, Egil Skallagrímsson, were temporarily laid to rest before removal to the cemetery of a new church built at Mosfell (Byock 1993, 1994, 1995). After several field seasons of fruitlessly testing

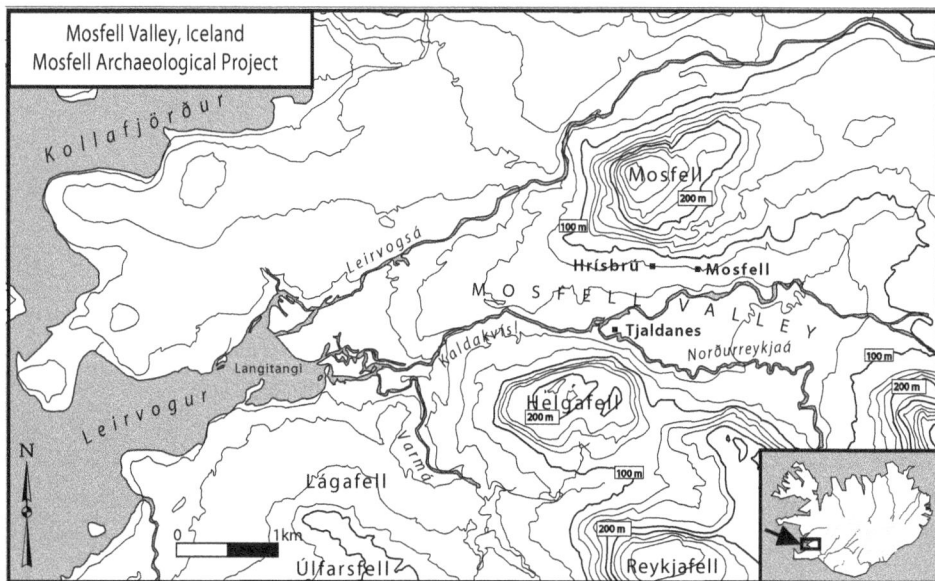

Figure 3.1. Map of the Hrísbrú site in the Mosfell Valley, Iceland.

areas at Hrísbrú that phosphate and remote sensing data suggested might contain ancient structures, we decided in 2001 to take Icelandic oral tradition at face value. For many generations a small knoll behind the modern horse barn at Hrísbrú had been known by local farmers as Kirkjuhóll, or "Church Knoll." Although our earlier magnetometer and resistivity maps of the area did not suggest the presence of subterranean architectural features, we decided it was worth testing the site because of its place name. In rapid succession in 2001 and 2002, the Kirkjuhóll excavations revealed concentrations of burned animal bone and other domestic refuse from a settlement period (*landnám*) farm, graves with an east–west orientation indicating the presence of a Christian cemetery, and finally the foundations of buildings that our subsequent excavations have shown to be the Hrísbrú church mentioned in the sagas (Byock 2009a). Also uncovered was a large adjacent Viking Age longhouse (Byock 2009b) suitable for habitation by important chieftains such as Egil Skallagrímsson (the son of Bald Grim) and Grim Svertingsson, a prominent chieftain who was Egil's son-in-law and Iceland's law-speaker (A.D. 1002–1004) at the annual Icelandic national assembly, the Althing.

At the end of our third Kirkjuhóll trench, we uncovered the skeleton of the person we have come to know as the "Axed Man" (figures 3.2, 3.3). The skeleton of this middle-age man and its archaeological context speak eloquently about the circumstances of his life, death, and burial in Viking Age Iceland. Through our efforts to reconstruct his life, we have learned much about the living conditions and social world of early Icelanders.

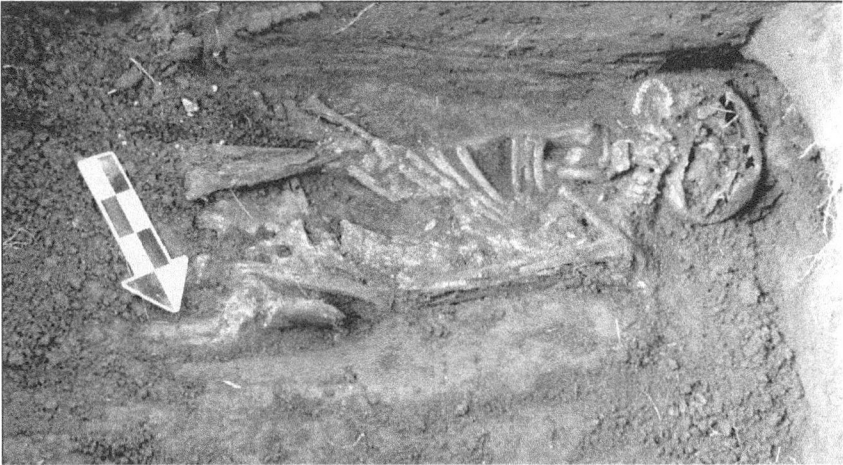

Figure 3.2. Photograph of the Axed Man, Feature 2, Trench CK-2001-3.

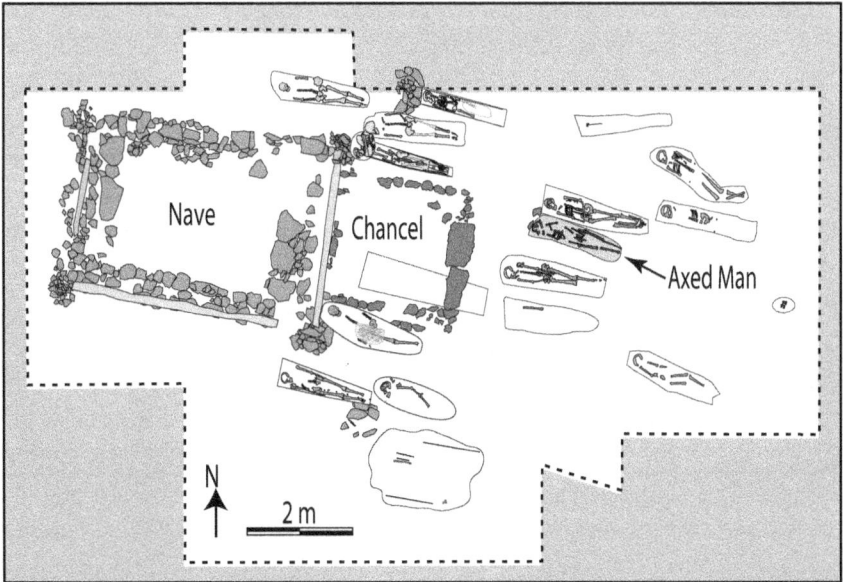

Figure 3.3. Map of the Kirkjuhóll cemetery at Hrísbrú showing the location of the Axed Man's grave in the small stave church.

Childhood

Although we know less about the Axed Man's childhood than we do about his adulthood, his remains are far from mute concerning the events of his early life. One strategy we have followed to learn more about the childhood lives of the people buried in the Kirkjuhóll cemetery at Hrísbrú is to use the elemental composition of their teeth to make inferences about the food they ate and the water they drank as children. This research exploits the truth in the adage "you are what you eat." For example, the concentrations of isotopes in the collagen of your bones echo the concentrations in the protein sources ingested during the last years of your life. For the enamel of your teeth, it would be more precise to say, "you are what you ate." Enamel is composed of the chemicals you ingested during the childhood period of dental development that become locked into the metabolically inactive crystalline structure of your teeth.

We use isotope data to learn more about what the Viking Age inhabitants of Hrísbrú ate and drank as children and adults, and to test theories about where they were born. The ratio of two strontium isotopes ($^{87}Sr/^{86}Sr$) in rocks, soil, and drinking water varies geographically in northern Europe. These differences are especially large between Iceland's much younger volcanic rocks and the ancient geological formations of western Norway, believed to be the place of origin of many Viking immigrants to Iceland.

Individuals with the best preservation in tooth enamel were selected for isotopic analysis. Owing to the destructive nature of the analysis upon the sampled teeth, as well as the importance of preserving Axed Man's remains for further analysis, his teeth have not been tested. Isotopic studies of the well-preserved teeth of six other people buried in the Kirkjuhóll cemetery, however, suggest that they all grew up in Iceland, not in Scandinavia or the British Isles. Based upon our work so far, it appears that most, if not all, of the people in the Hrísbrú cemetery (a minimum of 21 individuals) were native Icelanders removed by a generation or two from the first wave of Viking settlers who, according to the sagas and archaeological evidence, began colonizing the island late in the mid-ninth century.

The conclusion that the Axed Man was born in Iceland is consistent with a radiocarbon date on collagen extracted from one of his bones. This sample produced an uncorrected age of 1360±40 radiocarbon years before the present (RYBP) and a $^{13}C/^{12}C$ ratio of -17.4°/$_{oo}$. The carbon isotope ratio ($^{13}C/^{12}C$) resulting from this test suggests that, in the decade or so before his death, he obtained about 25–30 percent of the protein in his diet from marine sources. Since the carbon in marine foods is often considerably older than the carbon in terrestrial food sources (Kennett et al. 1997), a special correction procedure was used to estimate the age of the sample in conventional calendar years. The resulting estimates for the year the Axed Man died range between A.D. 890 and 990, with the curve intercept at A.D. 960. Given our estimated age at death for the Axed Man of about 40–45 years, these tests give a 97 percent probability that he was born sometime between A.D. 805 and 970. Other archaeological evidence strongly suggests that he was born near the end of this range. Thus, although the Axed Man could have traveled to Iceland with the initial wave of immigrants, he probably was a descendant of one of these early settlers. He most likely lived during the late pagan period, and died shortly after the Icelandic population had begun converting to Christianity (officially in A.D. 1000).

The *Book of Settlements* (*Landnámabók*) speaks of Thord Skeggi, a settler, or *landnámsmaðr*, as the first to colonize the area around Hrísbrú in the year 900 (Benediktsson 1968; Byock et al. 2005), and it is conceivable that the Axed Man was a descendant or kinsman of Thord. In the decades before and after the year 1000 when Mosfell was the home of the chieftain, or *goði*, Grim Svertings-son (Thorsson 2000: 729), the sagas tell us that the elderly Egil Skallagrímsson also lived there and died at Grim's farm (ca. 990). The Axed Man is thus very likely to have had personal encounters with both of these historically important figures.

The Axed Man's teeth bear the stigmata of childhood sicknesses (figure 3.4). If illnesses occur that disrupt development during the period of permanent tooth crown formation (around the time of birth to ~15 years), transverse grooves (hypoplastic lesions) reflecting that growth disruption permanently scar the teeth. Because tooth crowns develop in a regular sequence, the location of these hypoplastic lesions on the crown can be used to estimate when during a person's childhood the disrupted development occurred (Martin et al. 2008; Sarnat and Schour 1941; Schour and Massler 1941). Several hypoplastic lesions are visible in the teeth of the Axed Man: in the upper jaw, both canine teeth have lines that reflect a health problem between the ages of four and five. The right canine tooth has an additional line from growth disruption between the ages of five and six. In the lower jaw, the right canine has lesions reflecting health problems between the ages of three and four, the ages of four and five, and the ages of five and six (figure 3.4). It seems clear that the Axed Man's childhood was a stressful period punctuated by a series of severe illnesses.

Our estimated adult height of the Axed Man may also suggest less than opti-mal health during childhood. These stature estimates are based upon equations that allow a person's height to be estimated from long bone lengths (Trotter and Gleser 1958). Using the measures of several long bones, including the femur, tibia, humerus, and radius, the average height estimates suggest that the Axed Man was about 5 feet 6 inches (~168 cm) tall. He is among the shortest of the five adult men whose remains we have recovered from the Hrísbrú cemetery, who range from 5 feet 4 inches to 5 feet 9 inches, with a group average of 5 feet 7 inches (170 cm). This average height of the Hrísbrú males is shorter than that of other Icelandic male burial collections dating to the Viking Age and medieval period (Prizer et al. 2004). The Axed Man's relatively short stature (and possibly those of the other Hrísbrú males) may be explained by the association between disrupted childhood growth (suggested by his teeth) and reduced adult height (Silventoinen 2003).

Adulthood

Our confidence that this person is a man and not a woman is based on evidence from the pelvis and the skull, two of the most highly sexually dimorphic areas of the human skeleton. One feature, the greater sciatic notch of the hip bone, has a masculine shape that is found in less than 5 percent of women of European ancestry (Walker 2005). The skull has an array of hypermasculine features that, using sex prediction equations developed for people of European ancestry (Walker 2008), yield a 99.99 percent probability that the Axed Man is a male.

Most of his teeth were accounted for and give indications of the Axed Man's oral health. In addition to the wear of enamel that might be expected of a middle-age adult, his lower jaw showed signs of general inflammation (periodontitis). Calculus, deposits of mineralized plaque, is also found on the lower incisors and canines, and there is a small carious defect on the lingual side of an upper molar. These findings suggest that the Axed Man suffered slight dental disease before death.

As an adult (and likely before), the Axed Man experienced a life of strenuous physical activity. Signs of degenerative joint disease are evident throughout his skeleton. Osteoarthritis is present at the base of his left thumb. This may be an indication of handedness or habitual work-related activities, or perhaps it was the result of an injury that traumatized this joint. There are arthritic changes in the elbow joints of both arms, and, in the lower back, the second and third lumbar vertebrae exhibit arthritic lipping. The bones of the shoulder girdle bear signs of heavy lifting (figure 3.5). The right and left clavicles display lesions associated with trauma to the costoclavicular ligament during activities in which a person's shoulders are bent forward while the arms are used to move heavy loads. Ethnographic and ethnohistorical accounts of occupational activities causing this type of injury include plowing, stone house building, hunting,

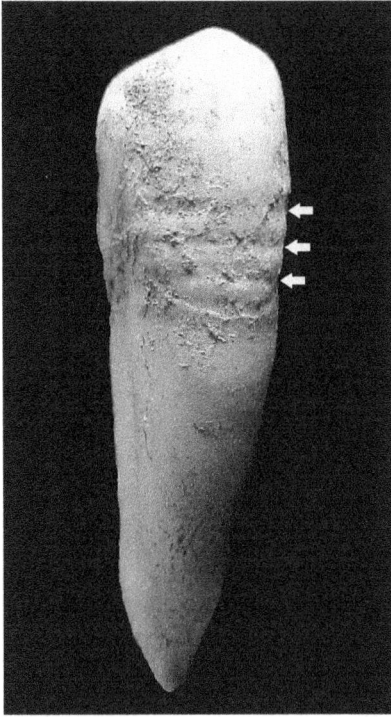

Figure 3.4. The lower right canine tooth of the Axed Man. Arrows point to three hypoplastic lesions that reflect a series of childhood growth disruptions.

Figure 3.5. Inferior view of the sternal end of the Axed Man's left clavicle showing irregular bone in the area of the costal tuberosity produced by heavy lifting. The boxed area in the top drawing of a clavicle delimits the area seen in the photograph below.

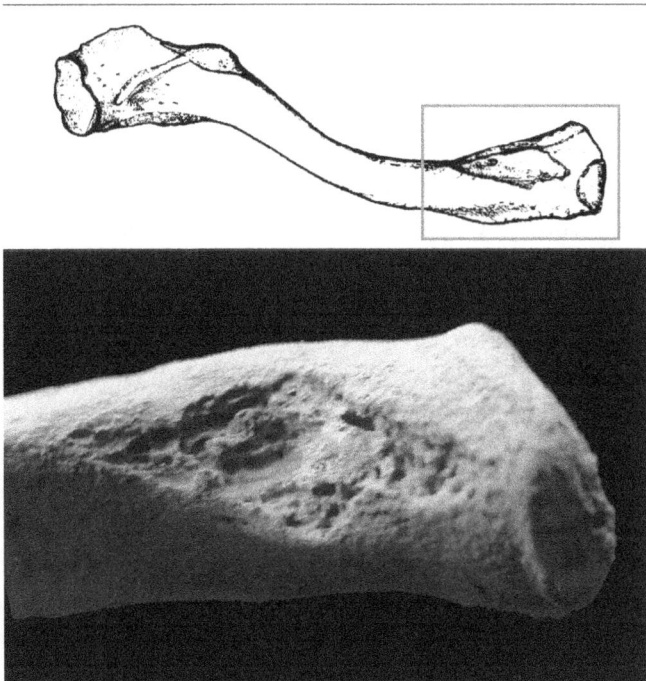

and ship maintenance (Capasso et al. 1999: 52). These degenerative changes in the Axed Man's skeleton suggest a life of heavy labor and are consistent with saga descriptions of Viking Age Icelandic farming and seafaring activities (Steffensen 1975: 109–32).

Death

The Axed Man died in middle age. We know this because the sutures between the bones of his cranial vault had begun to fuse. Following the recommendations outlined in Buikstra and Ubelaker (1994: 21–38), an estimated age at death of 38 years is derived from the sutural data, which is also consistent with age-related changes in his pubic bones: 45–49 years old using the Todd scoring system, 35–45 years old using the Suchey-Brooks system; and the auricular surface of his sacroiliac joint: 40–49 years old using the Meindl and Lovejoy system. Based on all of these aging criteria, our best guess is that he was about 40–45 years old when he died.

In forensic work, a distinction is made between the manner of death (that is, natural, accidental, suicide, homicide, or undetermined) and the cause of death, which refers to the specific conditions leading to death such as hanging, sharp-force trauma, blunt-force trauma, asphyxiation, and so on. The cause of the Axed Man's death is clear: his braincase shows two gaping wounds, each produced by the blade of a heavy weapon (figure 3.6). Both of these wounds would have severed major endocranial blood vessels. The massive brain damage and blood loss resulting from them would have rendered him almost immediately unconscious as his blood pressure plummeted. Within a minute or so, this exsanguination would have resulted in irreversible shock followed by death. The manner of death was homicide, as these wounds were certainly inflicted by another person (or persons) wielding a bladed weapon.

One of these injuries is a deep cut in the right side of his braincase that extends from the frontal bone to the back of the skull. The weapon that produced it would have severed many major cerebral vessels and penetrated deeply into his brain. The second injury removed a large round slice of bone from the back of the head. In doing so, the weapon would have cut through the transverse sinus, a large blood vessel that drains venous blood from the head. The Axed Man's death would have been a ghastly sight. If the blow to the back of the skull occurred first, large quantities of venous blood would immediately have gushed from the back of his head. If the blow to the side of his head occurred first, a spray of arterial blood under high pressure would most likely have showered his assailant and anyone else who was standing nearby.

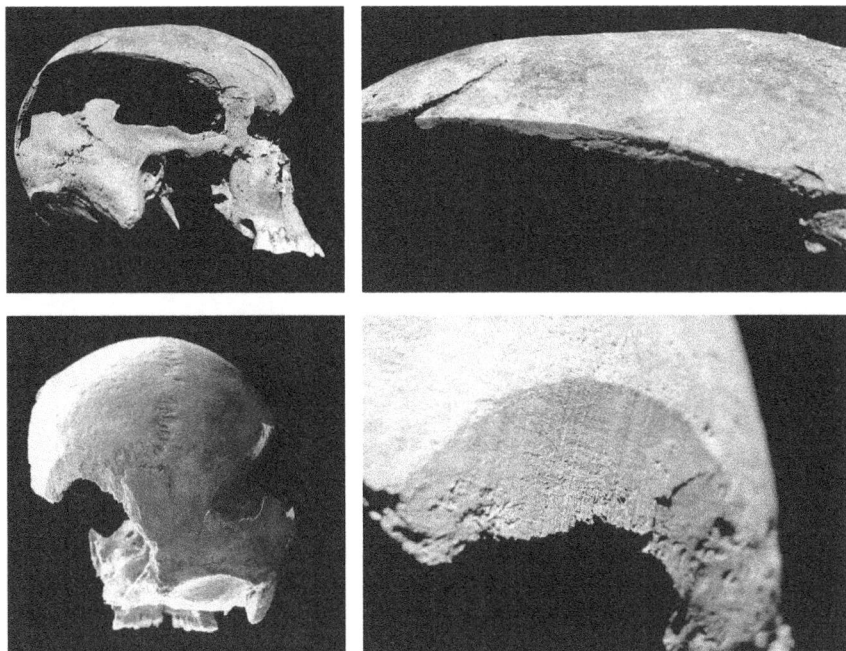

Figure 3.6. The Axed Man's cranium showing parietal (*top*) and occipital (*bottom*) injuries made by a bladed weapon such as an ax.

Different kinds of bladed weapons leave distinctive marks in bone, and the distinctions can be used in determining the details concerning the manner of death (Walker and Long 1977; Spitz and Fisher 1993: 252–310; Walker 2001). We gave the Axed Man his name because the gaping defect in the right side of his head exhibits all of the diagnostic features of an ax wound. Especially important is the abrupt termination of the injury at one end. This feature and the straight, clean-cut edge of the wound are both characteristics of the injuries produced by the heavy blades of sharp, short-bladed, chopping weapons such as Viking battle-axes (figures 3.6, 3.7).

We are less certain about the weapon used to slice the piece of bone from the back of the Axed Man's head. Instead of embedding in the skull, the weapon producing this wound sliced through it. Although both of these injuries may have been made by two blows in rapid succession from the same ax, it is also conceivable that the wound in the back of his head was produced by a slashing blow from the sword of a second assailant. Arguing for this is the width of the injury (90 mm or more) to the back of the skull, which implies a weapon with an even wider cutting edge. Viking Age axes were of all kinds, but the common ax used for everyday tasks often had blades narrower than this. An interesting

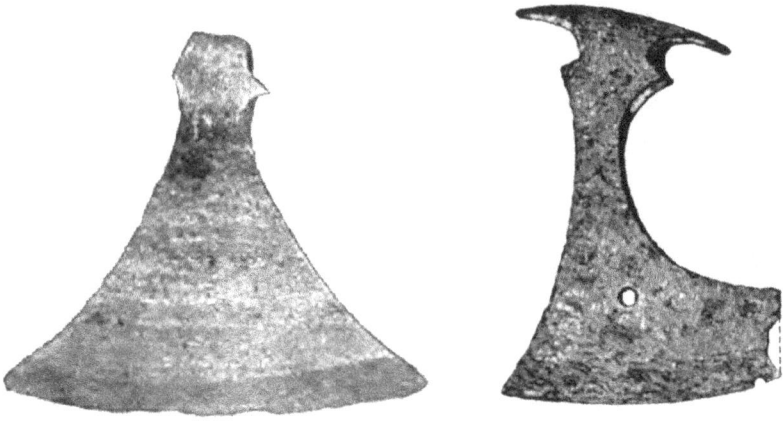

Figure 3.7. Examples of axes akin to the type likely responsible for the Axed Man's cranial injuries. *Left:* Ax found with two other axes, a horse bit, and a bell in a Norwegian tumulus; *right:* iron ax, Hemse, Götland. (Drawings after Du Chaillu 1890: 89, 231. For Viking Age axes found in Iceland, see Eldjárn 2000: 345–48.)

feature of this wound is the striated surface it produced while passing through the bone (figure 3.6). This reflects irregularities in the edge of the blade that produced it: a blade that evidently had been damaged through heavy use.

That the Axed Man is aptly named is reinforced by the prominent role of axes in saga accounts of interpersonal violence. War axes were highly prized and given poetic names such as "witch of the helmet," "wolf of the wound," "fiend of the shield," "wound-biter," and so on (Du Chaillu 1890: 89; Thorsson 2000: 61). When used in fights, the opponent's head was typically targeted. For instance, when Egil was seven years old, he is said in his saga to have driven an ax through the head of a playmate because of an earlier humiliation after losing a game. Elsewhere in *Egil's Saga*, a shipboard incident is described in which an ax is embedded up to its shaft in the helmeted head of a Viking warrior. In attempting to retrieve his weapon from his victim's head, the assailant retracted the ax with such force that his victim's body was swung into the air and over the side of the ship (Thorsson 2000: 45).

Consistent cross-cultural findings have shown that men are much more likely than women to be both the perpetrators and victims of homicidal violence (Walker 2001), so it is probable that the Axed Man's killer was another man. Nevertheless, the killer could have been a woman, and murders committed by ax-wielding Viking women are occasionally mentioned in sagas. For instance, Freydis, the infamous daughter of Erik the Red, reportedly ordered the killing of several of her fellow Greenland explorers and is also known for personally taking an ax to five women whom the men on her expedition refused to kill (Thorsson 2000: 650).

The unequivocal evidence of violence provided by the Axed Man's remains is consistent, at least in a general way, with a description in the *Saga of Gunnlaug Serpent-Tongue (Gunnlaugs saga ormstungu)* of a killing at Mosfell around A.D. 1010, as part of a feud between the families of the chieftain Onund of Mosfell and the chieftain Illugi the Black from Gilsbakki. Illugi, who has lost his son Gunnlaug in a fight with Onund's son Hrafn, attacks seeking vengeance (Thorsson 2000: 593). "People say that during the autumn, Illugi rode off from Gilsbakki with about thirty men, and arrived at Mosfell early in the morning. Onund and his sons rushed into the church, but Illugi captured two of Onund's kinsmen. One of them was named Bjorn and the other Thorgrim. Illugi had Bjorn killed and Thorgrim's foot cut off. After that, Illugi rode home, and Onund sought no reprisals for this act" (Thorsson 2000: 59). This account leads us to focus on Icelandic feuding, one of the most likely social circumstances leading to the Axed Man's death. He may have been killed because of some relatively minor interpersonal dispute such as the one that enraged the young Egil enough to kill his playmate. One cannot be certain that factual information from the sagas is correct, but *Gunnlaug's Saga* gives us a plausible understanding, as mentioned, that the chieftain at Mosfell was involved in a deadly blood feud, and the archaeology does not refute this possibility. Among the settlers of Iceland, such killings rarely went unavenged: the sagas suggest that family feuds were rampant and frequently led to cycles of retaliatory killing that lasted for generations (Byock 1982, 1988, 2001, 2007; Miller 1990). The Axed Man's death may thus have been part of a larger cycle of violence.

Another, less likely possibility is that the Axed Man was killed as an outlaw. In Viking Age Iceland, a person convicted and sentenced to outlawry in the law courts was condemned to banishment abroad or to the unpopulated areas of Iceland. The latter was in fact a death sentence. Although not imprisoned or subject to judicial execution, outlaws were extremely vulnerable because they could be hunted down and killed with impunity by anyone, including people hired for the task (Byock 2001: 231–32). But, as we shall see, the prominent location of the Axed Man's burial just outside the eastern end of the chancel at the Hrísbrú church argues against the idea that he was a social outcast (figure 3.3).

Burial

The location of the Axed Man's burial in the Hrísbrú church cemetery is full of symbolic significance (figure 3.3). Pagan Viking Age burials typically include grave goods and sometimes also sacrificed animals intended for use by the deceased in the afterlife (Williams 1920: 411–29; Eldjárn 2000). Early Christians, in contrast, tended to shun grave goods, in keeping with Christian teachings but also presumably in part because of their pagan connotations. The Axed Man and all of the other primary inhumations in the Hrísbrú cemetery are oriented with the feet to the east, a symbolic reference to the direction of Jerusalem and the rising sun on judgment day (Gordon 1971: 215). Another aspect of Christian burial practices is the exclusion of pagans, suicides, and other social outcasts from the consecrated ground of Christian cemeteries (Herbermann et al. 1914). The east–west orientation of the Axed Man's burial and its location in a symbolically significant location near the church's chancel indicate that he was considered a Christian and a person of some social standing in his community, possibly a relative of the chieftain who owned such private churches or chapels. It is doubtful that an outlaw would have received such respectful treatment.

We first thought the Axed Man was buried inside a wooden casket because we initially believed that the traces of organic material under the Axed Man's skeleton were decomposed wood (Byock et al. 2002). This now seems unlikely. Subsequent excavations in the immediately surrounding areas of the graveyard and laboratory analysis showed that this layer was instead a living surface of livestock dung and remnants of hay, that is, a floor or surface of a livestock holding area deposited inside or outside a small turf structure that predates and lies under the church and the burial. The grave appears to have been dug down to this livestock surface level, and it is also possible that the Axed Man may have been buried near the surface of the ground with earth piled on top of him to form a low mound. In keeping with our reassessment of the organic material on which the Axed Man was resting, some of the subsequent burials that we have excavated at the Hrísbrú cemetery did show clear evidence of wooden planks, and many of these graves also contained traces of iron nails and clench bolts, while no iron fasteners were found in the grave with the Axed Man. The iron fasteners found in many of the other Hrísbrú graves were easily recognizable since they were typically arranged linearly, reflecting their use in rows to hold together planks forming a casket or planks from part of a ship. Ship planks were common in the Hrísbrú graves, suggesting a syncretization of the pagan and Christian ritual systems that incorporated Viking Age ship symbolism into this early Christian graveyard (Zori 2007).

Outside the context of the cemetery, rocks are present elsewhere on the living surface upon which the Axed Man's body rested. This may explain two flat stones we found during excavation of the Axed Man's burial. One, measuring 5 × 20 × 17 cm, was under his chest, and the other, measuring 4 × 18 × 8 cm, was resting against the top of his skull. We also found a very fragile 4 cm long, dark brown, lozenge-shaped object near his left knee. This object, the use of which we were unable to determine, may have been made of leather or some other organic material.

We found a Viking Age iron ring pin of the West Norse variety (showing Celtic influence) in the soil just above and west of the Axed Man's skull (Byock et al. 2003). Such pins were used to fasten the cloaks of men over the right shoulder, so their sword arm was free. Perhaps the dead man's clothes were placed in the grave, with the pin becoming part of that grave offering.

Conclusion

The skeletons of the Axed Man and the other people buried at Hrísbrú provide important new evidence about the health status and living conditions of Iceland's earliest inhabitants (Walker et al. 2004). Skeletal lesions associated with a life of heavy labor are common among these early Icelandic settlers. Unfavorable conditions for growth and development are also suggested by the comparatively short stature of these people compared to contemporaneous populations elsewhere in northern Europe. Hypoplastic lesions in the teeth of several individuals from the Hrísbrú cemetery show that, among these people, childhood growth disruption like that suffered by the Axed Man was not a unique phenomenon. Skeletal evidence suggestive of tuberculosis is present in several of the Hrísbrú burials (Walker et al. 2004). Given the epidemiological characteristics of this contagious disease, it seems likely that most, if not all, of the people living at Hrísbrú were infected with the tuberculosis bacterium. These bioarchaeological findings imply that some of Iceland's earliest inhabitants experienced poor living conditions soon after they colonized the island, and our evidence from Hrísbrú contrasts with the picture of health that has often been assumed for early Icelandic life. Sickness and ill heath are mentioned in the sagas, but the texts tend not to dwell on illness (Steffensen 1975; Kaiser 1998). Perhaps, as our bioarchaeological findings suggest, health problems were so common that they were viewed as a condition of life that was unworthy of note. Further research is clearly needed to resolve these and other health-related issues (Byock 1993, 1994, 1995).

The sagas are full of accounts of violence, killing, fighting, and feuds. When the Mosfell Archaeological Project began archaeological research in Iceland more than a decade ago, we started with the working hypothesis that the rampant violence described in the sagas referred to rare events that storytellers focused upon for dramatic purposes. The discovery of the Axed Man's skeleton at the beginning of our Hrísbrú excavations made it clear that extremely violent interpersonal encounters did occur in Viking Age Iceland. While none of the 20 or so burials we have subsequently excavated at Hrísbrú show signs of violent death, many of these skeletons are so poorly preserved that the presence of lethal injuries would be difficult or impossible to detect. Although the presence of someone who clearly was a homicide victim in such a small sample is suggestive, more archaeological work will be necessary before we can say with any certainty how common violent deaths like that of the Axed Man's were in Viking Age Iceland.

Acknowledgments

The Mosfell Archaeological Project is an international effort done in collaboration with the town of Mosfellsbær and the National Museum of Iceland (þjóðminjasafn). We have received valuable logistic and financial support from the Icelandic Ministry of Education, Science, and Culture (Menntamálaráðuneyti), the Norwegian Kulturdepartementet, Icelandair, Landsvirkun, the National Geographic Society, the John Simon Guggenheim Foundation, the Fulbright Foundation, the National Science Foundation, the National Endowment for the Humanities, the Arcadia Trust, Norvik, the Norwegian government, the University of Oslo, the University of Oregon, the Social Sciences and Humanities Research Council of Canada, Árngrímur Jóhannesson, the academic senates of the University of California at Los Angeles (UCLA) and Santa Barbara, and the Cotsen Institute of Archaeology at UCLA.

Many organizations and individuals made this excavation possible. We very much appreciate the archaeological expertise and support given us by Margrét Hallgrímsdóttir, Guðmundr Ólafsson, Lilja Árnadóttir, and Halldóra Ásgeirsdóttir of þjóðminjasafn. Bjarki Bjarnson, Magnús Guðmundsson, and Helgi Þorláksson shared with us their great knowledge and worked with us on the project as consultants on historical issues. We remain especially indebted for the help we have received from the people of Mosfellsbær. Over the years, Björn Þráinn Þórðarson at the Mosfellsbær town office has consistently worked with us and been of enormous help, and Davið Sigurðsson and the people at Áhaldahús are always ready to help. Jóhann Sigurðsson, Ragnheiður Ríkarðsdóttir, and Haraldur Sverisson have worked closely with us, incorporating archaeology into their vision of the town's history. In Mossfellsdalur, we have been welcomed by the inhabitants, and Valur Þorvaldsson has given freely of his time. We especially thank Ólafur Ingimundarson and Andréas Ólafsson, the bændur at Hrísbrú, on whose farm we excavate. The kindness, steady friendship, and interest shown from the start by Ólafur; his wife, Ásgerður; and their sons and daughter, Andrés, Ingimundur, and Ingibjörg, have been an important part of the project.

The final version of our chapter is dedicated to the memory of Phil Walker, who played a central role in the discovery, recovery, and analysis of the Axed Man of Mosfell, but died before this book was published.

Authors' note

The selection from *Egils saga* cited in the epigraph to this chapter is translated by Jesse Byock from Sigurður Nordal's 1933 edition, chapter 86, pp. 298–99.

References Cited

Benediktsson, Jakob
1968   *Landnámabók (The Book of Settlements). Íslenzk fornrit.* I. Hið íslenzka fornritafélag, Reykjavík.
Buikstra, Jane E., and Douglas H. Ubelaker (editors)
1994   *Standards for Data Collection from Human Skeletal Remains.* Arkansas Archaeological Survey Research Series No. 44. Arkansas Archaeological Survey, Fayetteville.
Byock, Jesse L.
1982   *Feud in the Icelandic Saga.* University of California Press, Berkeley.
1988   *Medieval Iceland: Society, Sagas, and Power.* University of California Press, Berkeley.
1993   The Skull and Bones in *Egils saga*: A Viking, a Grave, and Paget's Disease. *Viator: Medieval and Renaissance Studies* 24: 23–50.
1994   Hauskúpan og beinin í Egils sögu. *Skírnir (Vor)*: 73–109.
1995   Egil's Bones. *Scientific American* 272(1): 82–87.
2001   *Viking-Age Iceland.* Penguin, New York/London.
2007   Defining Feud: Talking Points and Iceland's Saga Women. In *Feud in Medieval and Early Modern Europe*, edited by J. B. Netterstrøm and B. Poulsen, pp. 69–94. Aarhus University Press, Aarhus.
2009a   Sagas and Archaeology in the Mosfell Valley, Iceland. In *Á austrvega: Saga and East Scandinavia: Preprint Papers of the 14th International Saga Conference, Uppsala, 9th–15th August 2009*, edited by A. Ney, H. Williams, and F. C. Ljungqvist, pp. 167–75. Gävle University Press, Gävle.
2009b   Findings from the Mosfell Archaeological Project's Seminal 2002 Excavations. In *Heimtur: Ritgerðir til heidurs Gunnari Karlssyni sjötugum*, edited by G. Jónsson, H. S. Kjartansson, and V. Ólason, pp. 94–109. Mál og menning, Reykjavík.
Byock, Jesse L., Phillip L. Walker, Jon Erlandson, Per Holck, Jacqueline Eng, and Magnús A. Sigurgeirsson
2002   Excavation Report: Hrísbrú, Mosfellssveit, Iceland, August 20–28, 2001. Fornleifavernd Ríkisins, Reykjavík.
Byock, Jesse L., Phillip L. Walker, Jon Erlandson, Per Holck, Davide Zori, Guðmundsson Magnús, and Mark Tveskov
2005   Viking-Age Valley in Iceland: The Mosfell Archaeological Project. *Medieval Archaeology: Journal for the Society for Medieval Archaeology* 49: 195–218.

Byock, Jesse L., Phillip L. Walker, Jon Erlandson, Mark Tveskov, Alan Dicken, Jacqueline T. Eng, Magnús Guðmundsson, Per Holck, Kaethin Prizer, Melissa Reid, Henry Schwarcz, David Scott, Magnús A. Sigurgeirsson, and Davide Zori

2003   Excavation Report: Hrísbrú, Mosfellssveit, Iceland, July 31–August 20, 2002. Fornleifavernd Ríkisins, Reykjavík.

Capasso, Luigi, Kenneth A. R. Kennedy, and Cynthia A. Wilczak

1999   *Atlas of Occupational Markers on Human Remains.* Journal of Paleopathology Monographic Publication 3. Edigrafital S.p.A., Teramo, Italy.

Ciklamini, Marlene

1971   Old Norse Epic and Historical Tradition. *Journal of the Folklore Institute* 8(2/3): 93–100.

Du Chaillu, Paul B.

1890   *The Viking Age: The Early History, Manners, and Customs of the Ancestors of the English-Speaking Nations.* Vol. 2. C. Scribner's Sons, New York.

Eldjárn, Kristján

2000   *Kuml og haugfé.* Mál og menning, Reykjavík.

Gordon, B. L.

1971   Sacred Directions, Orientation, and the Top of the Map. *History of Religions* 10(3): 211–27.

Herbermann, Charles George, Edward A. Pace, Condé Benoist Pallen, Thomas Joseph Shahan, and John J. Wynne

1914   *The Catholic Encyclopedia.* Encyclopedia Press, New York.

Holck, Per

2005   Egill Skallagrimssons gård og kirke på Island—fra utgravningene 2001–2005. *Michael Quarterly* (Norwegian Medical Society) 2: 340–48.

Jones, Gwyn

1968   *The Legendary History of Olaf Tryggvason: The Twenty-Second W. P. Ker Memorial Lecture, Delivered in the University of Glasgow, 6th March 1968.* Jackson, Glasgow.

Kaiser, Charlotte

1998   *Krankheit und Krankheitsbewältigung in den Isländersagas: Medizinhistorischer Aspekt und erzähltechnische Funktion.* Seltman & Hein Verlag, Cologne.

Kennett, Douglas J., B. Lynn Ingram, Jon M. Erlandson, and Phillip L. Walker

1997   Evidence for Temporal Fluctuations in Marine Radiocarbon Reservoir Ages in the Santa Barbara Channel, Southern California. *Journal of Archaeological Science* 24(11): 1051–59.

Martin, Sarah A., Debbie Guatelli-Steinberg, Paul W. Sciulli, and Phillip L. Walker

2008   Brief Communication: Comparison of Methods for Estimating Chronological Age at Linear Enamel Formation on Anterior Dentition. *American Journal of Physical Anthropology* 135(3): 362–65.

Miller, William I.

1990   *Blood-Taking and Peacemaking: Feud, Law and Society in Saga Iceland.* University of Chicago Press, Chicago.

Nordal, Sigurður

1933   *Egils saga Skalla-Grímsonar.* Hið íslenzka fornritafélag, Reykjavík.

Prizer, Kaethin, Jacqueline T. Eng, Per Holck, and Phillip L. Walker

2004   Stature as an Indicator of Nutritional Status in Viking Age Iceland. Paper presented at the symposium Viking Archaeology in Iceland: The Mosfell Archaeological Project at the 69th Annual Meeting of the Society for American Archaeology, Montreal.

Sarnat, B. G., and I. Schour

1941   Enamel Hypoplasia (Chronological Enamel Aplasia) in Relation to Systemic Disease: A Chronologic, Morphological and Etiological Classification. *Journal of the American Dental Association* 28: 1989–2000.

Schour, I., and M. Massler

1941   The Development of the Human Dentition. *Journal of the American Dental Association* 28: 1153–60.

Silventoinen, K.

2003   Determinants of Variation in Adult Body Height. *Journal of Biosocial Science* 35(2): 263–85.

Spitz, Werner U., and Russell S. Fisher

1993   *Spitz and Fisher's Medicolegal Investigation of Death: Guidelines for the Application of Pathology to Crime Investigation.* C. C. Thomas, Springfield, Ill.

Steffensen, Jón

1975   *Menning og Meinsemdir: Ritgerðasafn um mótunarsögu íslenskrar þjóðar og baráttu hennar við hungur og sóttir.* Sögufélagið, Reykjavík.

Thorsson, Örnólfur (editor)

2000   *The Sagas of Icelanders: A Selection.* Viking, New York.

Trotter, Mildred, and Goldine C. Gleser

1958   A Re-evaluation of Estimation of Stature Based on Measurements of Stature Taken during Life and of Long Bones after Death. *American Journal of Physical Anthropology* 16: 79.

Walker, Phillip L.

2001   A Bioarchaeological Perspective on the History of Violence. *Annual Review of Anthropology* 30: 573–96.

2005   Greater Sciatic Notch Morphology: Sex, Age, and Population Differences. *American Journal of Physical Anthropology* 127(4): 385–91.

2008   Sexing Skulls Using Discriminant Function Analysis of Visually Assessed Traits. *American Journal of Physical Anthropology* 139: 39–50.

Walker, Phillip L., and Jeffrey C. Long

1977   An Experimental Study of the Morphological Characteristics of Tool Marks. *American Antiquity* 42: 605–16.

Walker, Phillip L., Jesse Byock, Jacqueline T. Eng, Jon M. Erlandson, Per Holck, Kaethin Prizer, and Mark Tveskov

2004   Bioarchaeological Evidence for the Health Status of an Early Icelandic Population. *American Journal of Physical Anthropology* Supplement 38: 204.

Williams, Mary Wilhelmine

1920   *Social Scandinavia in the Viking Age.* Macmillan, New York.

Zori, Davide

2007   Nails, Rivets, and Clench Bolts: A Case for Typological Clarity. *Archaeologia Islandica* 6: 32–47.

4 ❖ Legendary Chamorro Strength

Skeletal Embodiment and the Boundaries
of Interpretation

*Gary M. Heathcote, Vincent P. Diego, Hajime Ishida,
and Vincent J. Sava*

Individual Profile

Site: Taga
Location: Southwest coast of Tinian, Commonwealth of the Northern Mariana Islands (CNMI)
Cultural Affiliation: Late part of Latte period (A.D. 1000–1521) or early part of Early Historic period (A.D. 1521–1700) (Moore and Hunter-Anderson 1999)
Date: Probably 16th–17th centuries, based on archaeological context
Feature: Latte 28-5-24, a 12-pillar latte structure, with shafts standing ca. 5.4 feet above the ground, and capstones measuring 5.3 feet in diameter (Spoehr 1957:89)
Location of Grave: No information other than that the burial was recovered within the boundaries of Latte 28-5-24
Burial and Grave Type: Skull and body on left side, recovered at depth of 39 inches (Hornbostel 1924)
Associated Materials: Mandibles from two other individuals placed directly over knees; shell money recovered 2½ feet from skull
Preservation and Completeness: Excellent preservation, but incomplete; at the time of study (1990), the remains were curated at the Bishop Museum and included only the skull, clavicles, long bones, and tali
Age at Death and Basis of Estimate: 45–55 years, based on dental attrition, cranial suture closure, and arthritic changes
Sex and Basis of Determination: Male, based on cranial morphology and long bone size and robusticity
Conditions Observed: Healed stab wound through the frontal process of the right malar; remarkable robusticity of clavicles, arm bones, tibiae; moderate to markedly developed expression of three posterior cranial superstructures
Specialized Analysis: Study of occipital superstructure development and covariation with long bone robusticity
Excavated: 1924, by Hans Hornbostel, for the Bernice P. Bishop Museum, Honolulu
Archaeological Report: Hornbostel 1924; Thompson 1932; Spoehr 1957
Current Disposition: CNMI Museum of History and Culture, Saipan

This chapter focuses on a protohistoric Chamorro (Chamoru) man referred to as Taotao Tagga' (a man of Tagga', Tinian), situating him within his culture, society, and historical period. Chamorros are the indigenous people of the Mariana Islands, an archipelago in the western Pacific that consists of two polities today, the unincorporated U.S. territory of Guam (Guåhan) and the Commonwealth of the Northern Mariana Islands (CNMI), which includes the island of Tinian (figure 4.1). We present and evaluate evidence suggesting that Taotao Tagga' and a considerable proportion of (mostly) male compatriots possessed great musculoskeletal strength, especially of the upper body, which lends credence to claims of extraordinary strength that appear in Chamorro legends and in the chronicles of early European visitors to the Marianas. In discussion of the skeleton, we focus on two kinds of muscle use/hypertrophy indicators: posterior cranial superstructures and an index of humeral robusticity. Regarding motor behavioral and kinesiologic reconstruction, we probe the boundaries of osteobiographical interpretation (Saul and Saul 1989), attempting to infer what we can about the muscular strength and related activity patterns of Taotao Tagga' (and fellow ancestral Chamorros) without crossing over the line of cautious interpretation.

Since 2002, forensic artist Sharon Long's facial reconstruction of this man (figure 4.2) has been featured at the CNMI Museum of History and Culture in Saipan. The reconstruction was modeled on a cast of his skull and does not portray the serious facial injury he sustained as a younger man (see below). He lived into his fifth or sixth decade, probably during the sixteenth and seventeenth centuries. His remains were interred at a former village along the southwest coast of Tinian, now known as the Taga (Tagga') site, in association with a latte house (guma' latte) situated close to the House of Taga. Latte houses consisted of A-frame superstructures of wood and thatch built atop megalithic foundation columns (haligi) with capstones (tasa). The House of Taga (listed on the National Register of Historic Places) is the largest completed latte structure in the Marianas (figure 4.3). The megalithic foundation is approximately 21 × 64.3 feet across, consisting of two rows of six limestone haligi and tasa that stood 16 feet above the ground and weighed approximately 14 tons each (Morgan 1988: 133–34). Taotao Tagga''s place of burial, labeled Latte 28-5-24 by archaeologist Hans Hornbostel (1924) and later as Latte 17 (Spoehr 1957: 87), may also have been his home and his place of work. This latte house was second in size to the House of Taga (Morgan 1988: 133) and was spatially and contextually unique among the 16 other latte structures at the site, being aligned axially with only the House of Taga. Its size and location closest to the sea suggest a special significance of this guma' latte within the community of its time, and that those buried there were individuals of societal distinction.

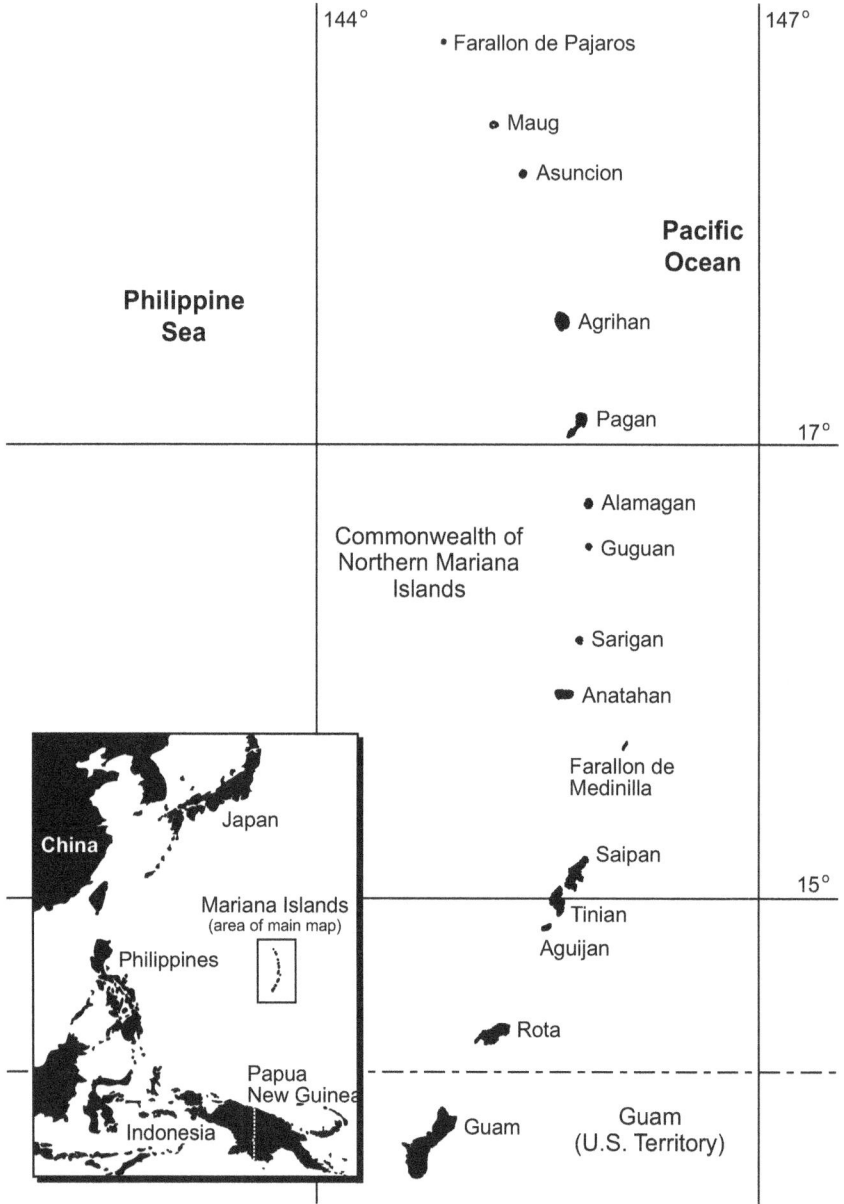

144° 147°

• Farallon de Pajaros

• Maug

• Asuncion

**Pacific
Ocean**

**Philippine
Sea**

• Agrihan

• Pagan   17°

Commonwealth of
Northern Mariana
Islands

• Alamagan

• Guguan

• Sarigan

• Anatahan

Farallon de
Medinilla

China

Japan

Mariana Islands
(area of main map)

Philippines

Papua
New Guinea

Indonesia

Saipan   15°

Tinian

Aguijan

• Rota

Guam   Guam
(U.S. Territory)

Figure 4.1. The Mariana Archipelago in the western Pacific Ocean.

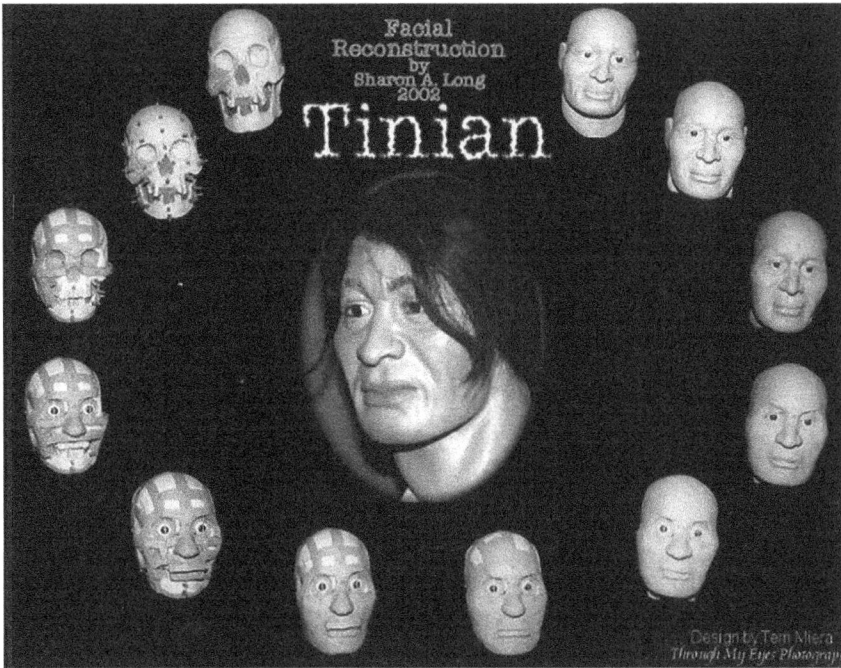

Figure 4.2. Reconstruction stages of the face and head of Taotao Tagga.' (Courtesy of Sharon Long.)

Tales of Strength: Legends to T-Shirts

A relatively common theme in Chamorro legends is that ancestors—usually *Maga'låhi siha* (chiefs)—possessed great strength and carried out astounding physical feats (Thompson 1947: 31). Folkloric themes of culture heroes with extraordinary strength are widespread throughout Oceania and elsewhere (Knapper 1995; Flood et al. 1999; Taonui 2006), but Chamorro legends are about more than the strong chiefs of old. They are about the ever-present embodied spirits of these ancestral culture heroes. Despite generations of condemnation by church officials, Chamorros maintain beliefs about the active role of ancestral spirits in their daily lives (Thompson 1946; Mitchell 1986).

A recent review of Marianas folklore, legends, and literature (Torres 2003) includes a section on the "Legends of Strength" motif, which focuses on the legendary chiefs and supernatural "before time ancestors" known as *taotaomo'na*. Frequent themes include gigantism, bravery, physical prowess, and great strength (Mitchell 1986). *Taotaomo'na* are a class of embodied ancestral spirits that are often, but not always (Cunningham 1992: 104), gigantic headless men of

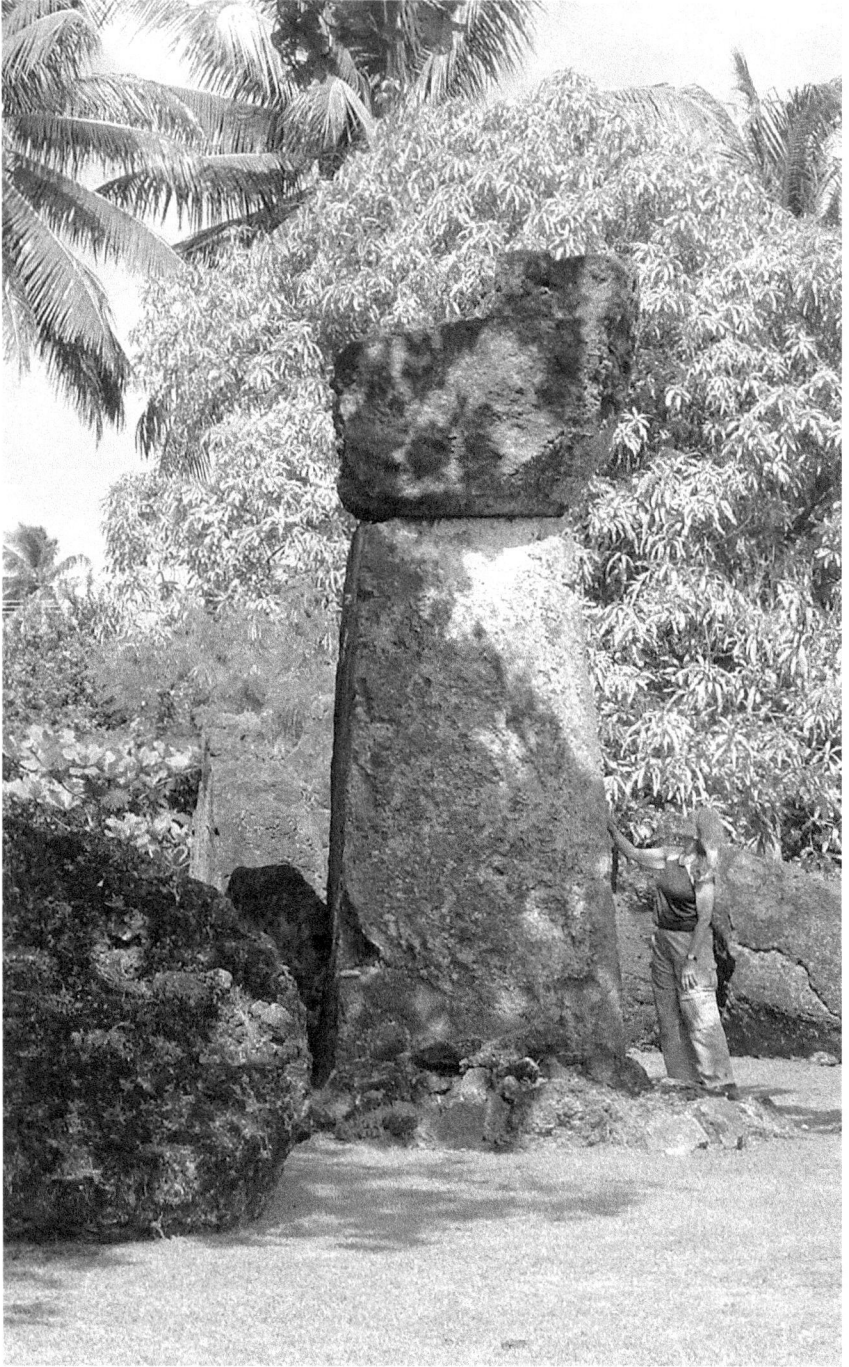

Figure 4.3. The last remaining upright *haligi* and *tasa* from the latte set foundation of the House of Taga on Tinian. (2011 photograph courtesy of Sandra Yee.)

superhuman strength who were formerly chiefs of various districts (Thompson 1945: 22; Nelson and Nelson 1992: 41). In the Guam legend of Chief Masala and the Tinian legend of Chief Taga, both are "strong and boisterous chiefs of enormous size, able to perform gargantuan feats. Each could build a huge latte house with the massive stones. Each had a precociously strong son" (Torres 2003: 11). In the story of Masala, his son's strength (uprooting a large coconut tree at age three) proved so threatening to him that he tried to kill the boy who, fearing for his life, leaped from the northernmost tip of Guam (named Puntan Patgon, or Child's Point), across more than 40 miles of ocean, to the island of Rota (Luta).

Today in the Marianas, representations of (mostly male, but sometimes female) Chamorro strength abound on T-shirts, automotive window decals, and airbrushed paintings on pickup trucks depicting iconic ancestral Chamorros. Recent projects by indigenous artists reflect a spectrum of imaginings about or connections with their ancestors through spiritual communion (Flores 1999). These include portrait series of Chamorro archetypes with faces that emanate intelligence, dignity, and fearlessness, and scenes of ancient village life in which men's physical strength is portrayed as ancillary to communal virtues including the practice and mastery of traditional skills such as stone working, house building, seafaring, and food procurement.

Early Chroniclers' Impressions: "Behold the Chamorros!"

Early European chroniclers of the people of Remote Oceania were practically unanimous in describing various Pacific Islander groups as "tall, muscular and well-proportioned" (Houghton 1996: 31). The early historical record regarding Mariana Islanders has multiple references to their stature, robust bodies, muscularity, pleasing body proportions, and great strength. One of the more interesting historical accounts is attributed to Fr. Martin Ignacio de Loyola, a Franciscan priest aboard the *Espiritu Santo* during a late-sixteenth-century Acapulco-to-Manila stopover on Guam (Lévesque 2002: 385):

> They are as tall as giants, and of such great strength that it has actually happened that one of them, while sitting on the ground, got hold of two Spaniards of good stature, seizing each of them by one foot with his hands, and lifting them thus as easily as if they were two children. (de Loyola 1581, in Lévesque 1992: Document 1581B)

Accounts of Chamorro physical appearance (e.g., Driver 1988; Lévesque 1990–96) from the early European contact period (A.D. 1521–1700) lend credibility to de Loyola's tale of Chamorro brawn, for European scribes universally described Chamorros (probably young and middle adult males) as possessing great strength. In 14 chronicles that explicitly mention strength, verdicts ranged from "they appear strong" to "among the strongest (*indios*) . . . yet discovered in either the Orient or the Occident" (York 2001: 6, 11). Regardless of the extent of exaggeration, the unanimity of multiple and independent testimonials about the great strength of Chamorros is compelling.

Chamorro Giants: Myth or Reality?

Virtually all of the historical accounts mentioning stature claim that the Chamorros were somewhat to much taller than their beholders, with descriptions ranging from "as tall as we" to "very tall" to the presumably exaggerated "gigantic" (York 2001: 4–7, 17–18). Assertions of large stature are substantiated in estimates based on long bones of prehistoric Chamorros, but those of gigantism appear to be hyperbolic. Given that these scribes encountered different regional populations in the Mariana Islands, some of the interobserver variation might reflect geographically patterned phenotypic variation, but we suggest that, when not purposefully exaggerated, most perceptions of giant Chamorros were due to eye-level differentials of the beholders relative to the observed.

Taotao Tagga"s stature is estimated at 176.6±1.57 cm (5 feet 9.5 inches) based on the length of his right femur and utilizing a regression formula for Polynesian Maori (Houghton et al. 1975). This places him near the upper range of variation for 33 prehistoric Chamorro males from nine Marianas archaeological sites whose average height is estimated at 173.1 cm (around 5 feet 8 inches) (Pietrusewsky et al. 1997). By the global standards of half a century ago, this falls within a commonly used classification range defining "tall" (170–179 cm) populations (Comas 1960: 315). Chamorro females were also tall by these standards. Pietrusewsky et al. (1997) reported a mean stature of 161.3 cm (5 feet 3.5 inches) for 33 archaeologically recovered Mariana Islanders, which falls at the low end of the "tall" range of female global variation (159–167 cm) (Comas 1960: 315).

To test the proposition that chroniclers who described early contact Chamorros as "tall" had it correct, while those who wrote of "giants" may have been diminutive themselves, appropriate comparative data were sought. The eyewitness chroniclers were mostly Spaniards from commercial sailing vessels, but the ships' crews included men of several different nationalities. These newcomers were doubtless of differing statures, but it is likely that most of them did not "measure up" to most of the Chamorros they encountered. Anthropometric data on Spaniards and other Europeans from the early contact era are limited. A study of Spanish Catalonian males from a ninth- to sixteenth-century burial ground reported the mean stature (based on femur length) as 166.2 cm (around 5 feet 5 inches) (Vives in Hernández et al. 1998: 549). The best comparative data are from records of European soldiers from Hungary, France, Bohemia, and Saxony who were born between 1735 and 1739 (Komlos and Cinnirella 2005). These studies report mean heights ranging from 164.6 to 167.4 cm (ca. 5 feet 5 inches to 5 feet 6 inches), indicating that the nearly contemporary European soldiers were, on average, at least two inches shorter than Chamorros (table 4.1).

Table 4.1. Estimated stature of Taotao Tagga' compared to prehistoric male Mariana islanders and eighteenth-century European soldiers

Individual or Population	Stature (cm)	Source
Taotao Tagga'	176.6 ± 1.57	
Prehistoric Mariana Islanders (N=33)	173.1	Pietrusewsky et al. 1997: 337
Hungary	167.4	Komlos and Cinnirella 2005
France	167.1	
Bohemia	166.1	
Saxony	164.6	

Posterior Cranial Superstructures: What Do They Mean?

A significant minority of Latte period and Early Historic Chamorro males exhibit cranial superstructures at certain muscle attachment sites on the back of the skull. We contend that these remarkable features are part of a suite of skeletal features related to upper body strength in Chamorros (Heathcote et al. in press; Heathcote et al. n.d.). The superstructures include: tubercles on the occipital torus (TOT); retromastoid processes (PR); and tubercles in the posterior supramastoid region (TSP) (figure 4.4). Collectively, they are referred to as occipital superstructures (OSS). Morphologically, OSS range from swellings or crests on the bone, to tubercles, to larger tuberosities and processes. They can be scored on a 5-point scale: a score of 0 indicates incipient or no expression, 1 indicates slight expression, 2 denotes moderate expression, and scores of 3 or 4 indicate markedly developed superstructures (Heathcote et al. 1996).

As shown in figure 4.4, TOT develop where the upper trapezius muscles originate, while TSP and PR are associated with insertions of the sternocleidomastoid and superior oblique muscles, respectively. We think that the development of these superstructures is triggered by strenuous repetitive muscle use, probably starting at a young age, in genetically predisposed individuals. More

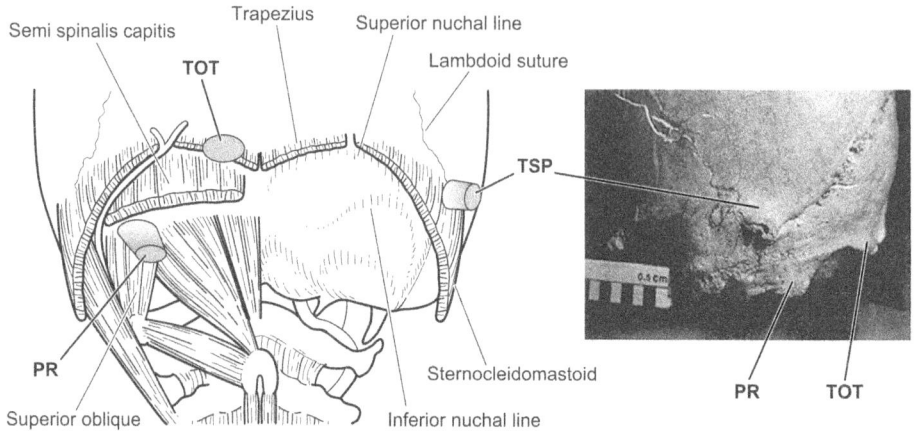

Figure 4.4. *Drawing*: posterior view of a cranium, showing locations of three occipital superstructures (PR, TOT, and TSP) in relation to associated muscle attachments. (Courtesy of Kingbernam Bansil.) *Photograph*: lateral posterior view of these three occipital superstructures on the posterior cranium of a 40- to 50-year-old male (Burial No. 123) from the Gogna-Gun Beach site, Guam.

formally, our model posits that morphogenesis and continued development of OSS are the interactive outcome of a genetically underpinned, chronic activity–induced multifactorial process, as follows: (1) predisposition for damage at enthesis sites in people with subclinical collagen abnormalities interacts with (2) chronic microtraumata from strenuous muscular overuse beginning at an early age, leading to (3) exuberant reactive or reparative processes, resulting in strong OSS developments (Heathcote et al. n.d.)

All three OSS, in all degrees of development, are far more common on crania of Pacific Islanders and aboriginal people of Australia and New Guinea than in other populations. Among Pacific Islanders, a significant minority of Chamorro males have moderate to extremely strong expressions for all three sets of superstructures. Surveys of male crania (n = 101–8) from the three largest Mariana Islands—Guam, Saipan, and Tinian—found markedly developed (and frequently co-occurring) TOT, PR, and TSP, on 29.7 percent, 39.4 percent, and 20.8 percent of the crania, respectively. Pronounced OSS are not unknown in Chamorro females, but they are rare, with markedly expressed TOT, PR, and TSP occurring, respectively, in 2.3 percent, 0 percent, and 1.2 percent of females from the largest Mariana Islands (n = 83–87) (Heathcote et al. n.d.).

In the context of fellow Chamorros, Taotao Tagga' is one of the more robustly developed individuals; his OSS vary in expression from moderate TSP to extremely marked PR and TOT (figure 4.5). While the actions of muscles associated with OSS are known, as is the case with the more commonly studied musculoskeletal stress markers (MSM) of the appendicular skeleton (e.g., Hawkey and Merbs 1995; Steen and Lane 1998), the extent to which extrapolations of specific activities can be made from markings on bone is a contentious issue (Merbs 1983; Kennedy 1989; Stirland 1991; Waldron 1994; Pearson and Buikstra 2006). While recent MSM studies have advanced the praxis of behavioral interpretation by looking very carefully at specific kinds of tool use and subsistence activities (Eshed et al. 2004; Molnar 2006), as well as the effects of body size and/or age on MSM development (Zumwalt et al. 2000; Weiss 2007), interpretive difficulties are not obviated even in the best-designed studies.

In attempting any behavioral interpretation from muscle markings on bone, a first principle is that muscles do not operate in isolation, but rather as synergistic groups (Stirland 1998). But even when (more appropriately) considering muscles within functional complex units, we are mindful that different activities utilize similar muscle groups (Bridges 1995; Peterson 2000). As a result, many activities probably do not produce bony signatures that are sufficiently distinctive to relate them to specific activities. The exceptions to this may be in the skeletons of individuals who were long-term specialists at certain tasks

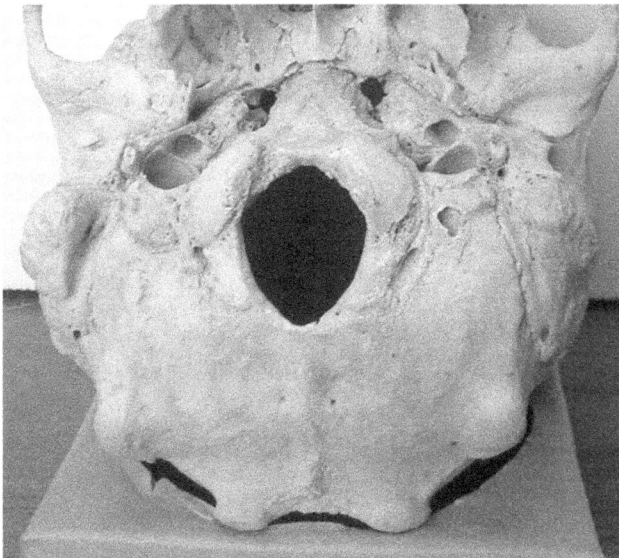

Figure 4.5. Inferior view of Taotao Tagga"s posterior cranium, showing co-occurrence of markedly developed PR and TOT occipital superstructures.

within their societies (Peterson 2000: 45, 47). We propose that activities of long duration, involved in the construction of latte house foundations, left a bony record in the OSS that developed on the posterior crania of (mostly) Chamorro men who specialized in the quarrying, dressing, transportation, and emplacement of latte stones and their capstones. The work activities outlined in table 4.2, together with attendant actions of OSS-associated muscles, render our occupational proposal a feasible hypothesis.

Table 4.2. Muscles associated with occipital superstructures (OSS) and possibly related latte construction activities

OSS Associated Muscles and Their Actions	Activities in Latte Construction (megalith transport and placement)
Occipital torus tubercles (TOT): Upper trapezius (1) Pulls head up, (2) bends the neck from side to side, (3) draws the collarbone and shoulder blade backward, (4) elevates and rotates the shoulder to raise the arms above the head, and elevates the tip of the shoulder, (5) supports the collar bone and shoulder blade when holding heavy weights with the arms down at the side.	Use of carrying poles in yoke position forces the head down, which is resisted by trapezius, associated with TOT development. Pulling ropes to move sleds or operate hoists extends the back and draws clavicles and scapulae backward, flexes the arm muscles, and flexes, rotates, and extends the neck. These exercise muscle groups associated with TOT, PR, and TSP.
Retromastoid processes (PR): Superior oblique (1) Involved in bending the neck backward and (2) rotating the neck to the side.	Carrying litters at waist level with arms at the sides stresses muscles at the TOT and possibly PR and TSP sites.
Posterior supramastoid tubercles (TSP): Sternocleidomastoid (1) Draws the neck forward, (2) raises the neck while supine, (3) raises the chest in forced breathing, (4) tilts the neck toward the shoulder, (5) rotates the neck.	Hefting objects on the shoulder involves stabilizing the load by bracing the head against the object, using PR- and TSP-associated muscles.

Infracranial Skeletal Changes

If marked developments of OSS represent part of a more widespread muscle overuse syndrome related to megalithic stone work, then we also expect other changes to the skeletons of Taotao Tagga' and his peers, such as activity-related infracranial MSM changes (bone overgrowth and remodeling at tendon and ligament attachment sites), geometric changes to long bones, degenerative arthritis, and spinal injuries (Larsen 1997; Knüsel 2000). Taotao Tagga''s vertebrae were not included in the museum collection, but physical stress-related injuries like Schmorl's nodes, vertebral compression fractures, and spondylolysis have indeed been found in individuals from Tonga with strongly expressed OSS (Sava 1996). Arriaza (1997) did not examine vertebral injury–OSS covariation, but has presented evidence of high frequencies of spondylolysis in late prehistoric Guam Chamorros, and—like us—suggested an etiological relationship to megalithic construction activities. Arthritic and remodeling changes to Taotao Tagga''s long bones are dramatic and are consistent with an upper body muscle overuse and heavy weight-bearing syndrome (Heathcote et al. in press). Strongly reactive MSM changes are found on his clavicles (origin site of pectoralis major and the insertion site of the costoclavicular ligament), humeri (deltoideus insertion site), ulnae (triceps brachii insertion site), and radii (biceps brachii insertion site) (Heathcote 2006).

Taotao Tagga''s lower limbs are generally robust and bear MSM changes, but they were not as markedly remodeled as his upper limbs. Changes in his hip joint include buildup of new bone at the fovea capitis on both femoral heads, which may be related to heavy weight bearing (Heathcote 2006). Both of his knees show evidence of the essentially traumatic activity–related changes of Osgood-Schlatter's disease: jagged spurs on the proximal tibial tuberosities where the patellar ligaments insert (Heathcote 2006). This condition likely reflects partial separation of the ligaments when Taotao Tagga' was a youth, and is common today among young athletes who strain this ligament in sudden bursts of exercise (Aufderheide and Rodríguez-Martin 1998: 85).

Skeletal Robusticity

The adaptive response of bone to biomechanical strain induced during exercise and activity is well documented (Lanyon 1992; Ruff et al. 2006). Simply put, mechanical loading, including muscular pull and torsion forces, causes long bones to become thicker during life (Martin and Burr 1989). Exercise and activity levels are important determinants of bone quality, geometry, and strength (Jones et al. 1977; Ruff 2003; Tobias et al. 2007). There is a close, but imperfect, equation of bone strength with muscle strength, given that muscle size has been shown to be positively correlated with bone strength (Ruff 2005), muscle force (Folland and Williams 2007), and amount and intensity of strength-building activities (Wernbom et al. 2007).

While bone strength is measured with ever more sophisticated imaging techniques, there is a reasonable degree of correspondence between traditionally measured external long bone shaft diameters and torsional strengths, that is, ability to resist bending (Grine et al. 1995). As such, indices derived from external measurements of long bones approximately reflect bone cross-sectional areas and cortical thickness, and thus bone strength (Wescott 2006). Traditional indices of skeletal robusticity, which express the thickness of long bone shafts relative to their lengths, are the simplest approach to approximating activity-related geometric changes to long bones (Pearson 2000: 570). These indices can be used as indirect indicators of muscularity and, by extension, provide information on lifestyle and muscle activity levels throughout life.

We focus here on Taotao Tagga''s humeral shaft index, HSRI-2, calculated from the sum of the shaft's minimum and maximum diaphyseal diameters at midshaft, and expressing these additive breadths as a proportion of maximum length. Comparative data for other populations (table 4.3) document the exceptional magnitude of Taotao Tagga''s HSRI-2 index of 15.8 (figure 4.6), which appears virtually outside the range of variation for all non-Chamorro populations that have been so measured. Taotao Tagga''s index is more than one standard deviation greater than the mean for 32 of his fellow male Chamorros (14.6±1.1). Other high-index outliers in this Mariana Island sample include two individuals from Taga, Tinian (Bernice P. Bishop Museum 892 and 912), with humeral robusticity indices of 17.8 and 15.9. Only 3 of 27 Chamorro males from Guam had humeri with larger HSRI-2 indices than Taotao Tagga', whereas two of three male compatriots from Taga had humeri exceeding his index value (Ishida n.d.); Taga may have been an epicenter of Chamorro humeral hyperrobusticity.

The relative stoutness of Chamorro humeri is perhaps even more remarkable when compared to more ancient human ancestors. The HSRI-2 index of Taotao Tagga' and the mean index for Chamorro males far exceed the means for the two most robust of the fossil groups, European and Middle Eastern Neandertals (13.7±1.3) and the Epigravettian-associated Early Modern *Homo sapiens* from Italy (13.7±0.8). As Neandertals are characterized as having massive limb bones and being more heavily muscled than anatomically modern humans (Pearson 2000), a provisional conclusion—awaiting confirmation from further

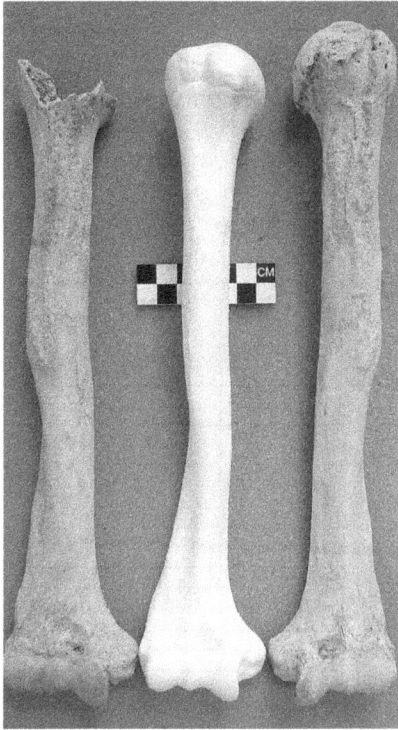

Figure 4.6. Anterior views of Taotao Tagga"s humeri with a plastic model right humerus (PS-1) in the center for reference. The HSRI-2 humeral robusticity index for the model is 13.2, which is near the median of the comparative index data in table 4.3.

comparative studies—is that in terms of upper body strength, Taotao Tagga' and company were among the strongest archaic or modern *Homo sapiens* who ever lived.

Covariation of Robusticity Indices with OSS

To seek corroboration for our hypothesis that OSS development and upper arm robusticity (and strength) are skeletal responses to the same suite of activities, we examined the bivariate relationship between indices of long bone robusticity and degree of development of posterior cranial superstructures in 16 Chamorro individuals with sufficiently complete skeletons. Pearson's correlation and linear regression analyses (SAS for Windows, Version 8.2) were used to express the strength and patterning of relationship between each individual's OSS summary score (Sum3OSS) and long bone robusticity indices, including two humeral (HSRI-1 and HSRI-2), one femoral (FSRI), and one tibia (TSRI) index (Heathcote et al. in press).

Strength of correlation between Sum3OSS and indices of upper and lower

Table 4.3. Humeral shaft robusticity index (HSRI-2) in males

Population/Individual Sampled (number measured), Source	Maximum Length Mean (SD)	Maximum Shaft Diameter Mean (SD)	Minimum Shaft Diameter Mean (SD)	Shaft Robusticity Index Mean (SD)
Taotao Tagga´, Ishida: n.d.	**322.0**	**29.0**	**22.0**	**15.8**
Chamorro excluding Taotao Tagga' (N=32), Ishida n.d.	320.8 (9.7)	26.2 (2.1)	20.7 (1.6)	14.6 (1.1)
Neolithic Tsukumo, Japan (N=15), Baba and Endo 1982	291.5 (12.4)	23.9 (1.8)	17.5 (1.4)	13.9 (-)
Mesolithic, Europe (N=4)				13.8 (1.3)
Sami, Lapland (N=34)				13.7 (0.9)
Neandertals Europe, Middle East (N=6)				13.7 (1.3)
Epigravettian (Upper Paleolithic), Italy (N=6)				13.7 (0.8)
Inuit (N=25)				13.6 (1.1)
Recent Japanese, Kinai (N=30), Baba and Endo 1982	294.2 (15.6)	22.3 (1.5)	17.4 (1.5)	13.5 (-)
Aboriginal Australians (N=17)				13.2 (0.8)
U.S. "whites" (N=25)				13.1 (0.9)
Zulu (N=31)				13.0 (0.9)
African Americans (N=41)				12.8 (0.9)
Hawaiians, Mokapu, Oahu (N=72), Ishida 1993	319.2 (13.0)	23.2 (1.5)	17.4 (1.1)	12.7 (-)
Chinese (N=27)				12.6 (1.0)
Recent Formosans (N=102), Baba and Endo 1982	313.4 (14.4)	22.4 (1.5)	17.1 (1.2)	12.6 (-)
Upper Pleistocene, Minatogawa I, Okinawa (N=1), Baba and Endo 1982	287.0	20.5	15.5	12.5
Neolithic Yang Shao Tsun, China (N=2), Baba and Endo 1982	332.6 (-)	23.5 (-)	17.7 (-)	12.4 (-)
Early modern Homo sapiens Skhūl/ Qafzeh, Israel (N=2)				11.6 (-)
Upper Paleolithic, Jebel Sahaba, Sudan (N=1)				11.4
Khoisan, SW Africa (N=21)				11.1 (0.9)
Aurignacian (Upper Paleolithic), Paviland 1 (N=1), Trinkaus and Holliday (2000)	337.0	19.4	15.7	10.4

Source: Data from Pearson 2000 except where noted. Measurements are Martin's H1 (maximum length), H5 (maximum shaft diameter), and H6 (minimum shaft diameter) (Bräuer 1988). Index = 100 × [(Max diameter + Min diameter)/(Max length)]. Sides measured: Baba and Endo: right; Ishida: right; Pearson: side not indicated; Trinkaus and Holliday: left.

limb robusticity is strikingly different. Sum3OSS does not correlate significantly with lower limb robusticity indices for the femur and tibia (FSRI: Pearson's r = 0.31, p < .261; TSRI: r = 0.24, p < .440), but correlations with the two indices of upper arm robusticity are highly significant (HSRI-1: r = 0.66, p < .006, HSRI-2: r = 0.70, p < .003). This adds support to our contention that OSS are meaningful markers of upper body strength. The physiological connectedness of these changes is also supported by regression analysis of Sum3OSS and HSRI-2, which shows a strong, positive linear relationship (R^2 = 0.48, p < .004) between additive OSS expression and upper arm robusticity (figure 4.7).

Discussion

Herein we have presented evidence in support of our contention that Taotao Tagga' and other hyperrobust Chamorro males manifested extraordinary upper body strength, and that such a paleophysiological profile can be inferred from posterior cranial superstructures and humeral robusticity. We have also presented support (albeit more problematic) for the hypothesis that well-developed OSS and accompanying infracranial changes in Taotao Tagga' and other (mostly male) Chamorros are related to the quarrying, masonry work, transport, and emplacement of pillars and capstones that were the infrastructure for *guma' latte* construction. Early eyewitness descriptions of Marianas stone working are lacking, but accounts of Tongan stone working (Beaglehole 1967;

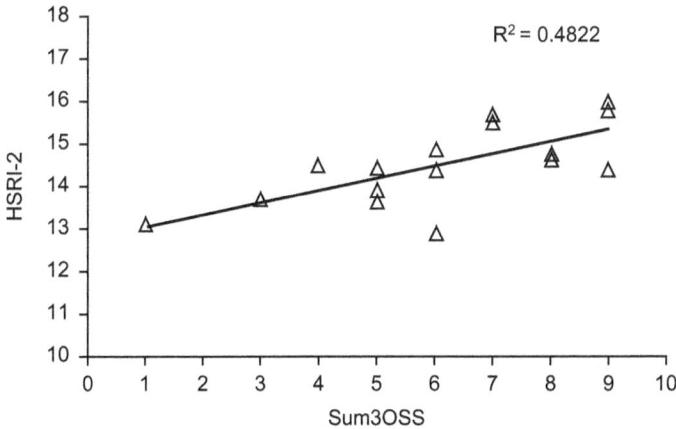

Figure 4.7. Scatterplot showing linear regression of the additive superstructure score (Sum3OSS) and HSRI-2 index of humeral robusticity in a small sample of Late Latte and Early Historic period Chamorros from Guam and Tinian.

Ferdon 1987; Spennemann 1989; Sava 1996) provide proxies for the activities (summarized in table 4.2) and technologies employed in the Marianas (Cunningham 1992; Heathcote et al. in press). Pre-European Tongans are the only other people known to have had high frequencies of OSS that were both well developed and co-occurring (Heathcote et al. 1996; Sava 1996; Heathcote et al. n.d.), suggesting that the commonalities of OSS patterning in Mariana Islanders and Tongans are due in (extragenetic) part to common occupational stressors related to coral-limestone quarrying and monument building.

The existence of a significant minority of individuals like Taotao Tagga' with codevelopment and strong expressions of OSS has important implications for social and population structure in the Marianas. Such an uneven intrapopulation distribution is consistent with the proposition that a group of specialists in Chamorro society, engaged in strenuous activities including stone quarrying and megalithic construction, were furthermore genetically predisposed to develop such superstructures.

The suggestion that there were economic specialists in protohistoric Chamorro society does not fit with the orthodox view that protohistoric Chamorro villages were essentially independent social units without much vertical stratification, and that local chiefs lacked larger regional level jurisdiction (Cordy 1986; Craib 1986; Knudson n.d.). However, a greater degree of social stratification has been suggested for Taotao Tagga''s village. The imposing House of Taga was positioned between two clusters of smaller latte sets at the Taga site, and was centrally located between two other latte settlements in Tinian. This intra- and intercommunity house patterning may reflect late protohistoric emergence of a system with a paramount chief and local chiefs, the former situated at the House of Taga (Graves 1986).

Was Taotao Tagga' primarily a builder of *guma' latte*, and secondarily a warrior, farmer, and fisherman? The discernment of such specific patterns of activity from related skeletal changes is outside the realm of bioarchaeological capability at present (Robb 1998). We can say with some confidence, however, that his location at Taga as opposed to other settlements increases the likelihood that Taotao Tagga' was a semispecialist involved in a restricted range of economic behaviors throughout much of his lifetime. While full-time specialists are absent in societies of foragers with informal political leadership, they are encountered in some semisedentary horticultural societies (Ember et al. 2007: 286), and the presence of people with a narrowed range of economic activities might reasonably be expected in communities with incipient political hierarchy. Elsewhere in Micronesia, in the northern islands of Kiribati, each residential kin group traditionally included at least one specialist builder of dwelling houses, and giant meetinghouses with their stone pillars were constructed by a specialist clan of builders within each district (Hockings 1989). This suggests that specialists (or semispecialists) could also have existed in the Marianas, especially in places like Taotao Tagga"s home district.

Fine-grained reconstruction of the relative contributions of the range of activities that shaped Taotao Tagga"s body will probably always remain beyond the boundary of empirically grounded osteobiographic interpretation, but the evidence of his extraordinary upper arm robusticity and concordant OSS development bear convincing testimony that Taotao Tagga' and a significant minority of other male Chamorros of his time and culture were possessed of upper body strength that proved to be the stuff of legend.

References

Arriaza, Bernardo T.
1997   Spondylolysis in Prehistoric Human Remains from Guam and Its Possible Etiology. *American Journal of Physical Anthropology* 104: 393–97.
Aufderheide, Arthur C. and Conrado Rodríguez-Martin
1998   *The Cambridge Encyclopedia of Human Paleopathology*. Cambridge University Press, Cambridge.
Baba, Hisao, and Banri Endo
1982   Postcranial Skeleton of the Minatogawa Man. In *The Minatogawa Man: The Upper Pleistocene Man from the Island of Okinawa*, edited by H. Suzuki and K. Hanihara, pp. 61–195. University of Tokyo Press, Tokyo.
Beaglehole, John Cawte (editor)
1967   *The Journals of Captain James Cook on His Voyages of Discovery*. Cambridge University Press, Cambridge.
Bräuer, G.
1988   Osteometrie. In *Anthropologie: Handbuch der Vergleichenden Biologie des Menschen*, Vol. 1, part 2, edited by R. Knussmann and Harold R. Barlett, pp. 160–232. Gustav Fischer, Stuttgart.
Bridges, Patricia S.
1995   Skeletal Biology and Behavior in Ancient Humans. *Evolutionary Anthropology* 4: 112–20.
Comas, Juan
1960   *Manual of Physical Anthropology*. Revised and enlarged English edition. Charles C. Thomas, Springfield, Ill.
Cordy, Ross
1986   Relationships Between the Extent of Stratification and Population in Micronesian Politics at European Contact. *American Anthropologist* 88: 136–42.

Craib, J. L.

1986   Casas de Los Antiguos: Social Differentiation in Protohistoric Chamorro Society, Mariana Islands. Ph.D. dissertation, University of Sydney.

Cunningham, Lawrence J.

1992   *Ancient Chamorro Society*. Bess Press, Honolulu.

Driver, Marjorie G.

1988   Fray Juan Pobre de Zamora: Hitherto Unpublished Accounts of His Residence in the Mariana Islands. *Journal of Pacific History* 23: 86–94.

Ember, Carol R., Melvin Ember, and Peter N. Peregrine

2007   *Anthropology*. 12th ed. Pearson Prentice Hall, Upper Saddle River, N.J.

Eshed, Vered, Avi Gopher, Timothy B. Gage, and Israel Hershkovitz

2004   Has the Transition to Agriculture Reshaped the Demographic Structure of Prehistoric Populations? New Evidence from the Levant. *American Journal of Physical Anthropology* 123: 303–15.

Ferdon, Edwin N.

1987   *Early Tonga as the Explorers Saw It, 1616–1810*. University of Arizona Press, Tucson.

Flood, Bo, Beret E. Strong, and William Flood

1999   *Pacific Island Legends: Tales from Micronesia, Melanesia, Polynesia, and Australia*. Bess Press, Honolulu.

Flores, Judy

1999   Art and Identity in the Mariana Islands: Issues in Reconstructing an Ancient Past. Ph.D. dissertation, Sainsbury Research Unit for the Arts of Africa, Oceania & the Americas, University of East Anglia.

Folland, Jonathan, and Alun G. Williams

2007   The Adaptations to Strength Training: Morphological and Neurological Contributions to Increased Strength. *Sports Medicine* 37: 145–68.

Graves, Michael W.

1986   Organization and Differentiation within Late Prehistoric Ranked Social Units, Mariana Islands, Western Pacific. *Journal of Field Archaeology* 13: 139–54.

Grine, F. E., W. L. Jungers, P. V. Tobias, and O. M. Pearson

1995   Fossil *Homo* Femur from Berg Aukas, Northern Namibia. *American Journal of Physical Anthropology* 97: 151–85.

Hawkey, Diane E.

1998   Disability, Compassion and the Skeletal Record: Using Musculoskeletal Stress Markers (MSM) to Construct an Osteobiography from Early New Mexico. *International Journal of Osteoarchaeology* 8: 326–40.

Hawkey, Diane E., and Charles F. Merbs

1995   Activity-Induced Musculoskeletal Stress Markers (MSM) and Subsistence Strategy Changes among Ancient Hudson Bay Eskimos. *International Journal of Osteoarchaeology* 5: 324–38.

Heathcote, Gary M.

2006   Taotao Tagga': Glimpses of His Life History, Recorded in His Skeleton. Non-Technical Report Series, Anthropology Resource & Research Center, University of Guam, Paper No. 3. Anthropology Resource & Research Center, Mangilao, Guam.

Heathcote, Gary M., Kingbernam L. Bansil, and Vincent J. Sava
1996   A Protocol for Scoring Three Posterior Cranial Superstructures Which Reach Remarkable Size in Ancient Mariana Islanders. *Micronesica* 29: 281–98.
Heathcote, Gary M., Timothy G. Bromage, Vincent J. Sava, Bruce E. Anderson, Douglas B. Hanson, Jean-Jacques Hublin
N.d.   Occipital Superstructures in Late Pre-Contact and Early Historic Chamorro Remains from the Marianas Islands. Ms. in senior author's possession.
Heathcote, Gary M., Vincent P. Diego, Hajime Ishida, and Vincent J. Sava
In press   An Osteobiography of a Remarkable 16th–17th Century Chamorro Man from Taga, Tinian. *Micronesica.*
Heathcote, Gary M., Ann L. W. Stodder, Hallie R. Buckley, Douglas B. Hanson, Michele T. Douglas, Jane H. Underwood, Thomas T. Taisipic, and Vincent P. Diego
1998   On Treponemal Disease in the Western Pacific: Corrections and Critique. *Current Anthropology* 39: 359–68.
Hernández, Miquel, Clara García-Moro, and Carles Lalueza-Fox
1998   Stature Estimation in Extinct Aónikenk and the Myth of Patagonian Gigantism. *American Journal of Physical Anthropology* 105: 545–51.
Hockings, John
1989   *Traditional Architecture in the Gilbert Islands: A Cultural Perspective.* University of Queensland Press, St. Lucia.
Hornbostel, Hans
1924   The Latte of Tinian; June: Notes, Sketches and Photos, 1st Installment. In *Field Notes on Guam, Saipan, Rota and Tinian*, Section 3.1. Bernice P. Bishop Museum Library, Honolulu. Copies on file at Guam Museum, Hagåtña.
Houghton, Philip
1996   *People of the Great Ocean: Aspects of Human Biology of the Early Pacific.* Cambridge University Press, Cambridge.
Houghton Philip, B. Foss Leach, and Doug G. Sutton
1975   The Estimation of Stature of Prehistoric Polynesians in New Zealand. *Journal of the Polynesian Society* 84: 325–36.
Ishida, Hajime
1993   Limb Bone Characteristics in the Hawaiian and Chamorro Peoples. *Japan Review* 4: 45–57.
N.d.   Unpublished metrical data on Chamorro long bones from the Hornbostel Collection. Bernice P. Bishop Museum, Honolulu.
Jones, H. H., J. D. Priest, W. C. Hayes, C. C. Tichenor, and D. A. Nagel
1977   Humeral Hypertrophy in Response to Exercise. *Journal of Bone & Joint Surgery (American)* 59: 204–8.
Kennedy, Kenneth A. R.
1989   Skeletal Markers of Occupational Stress. In *Reconstruction of Life from the Skeleton*, edited by M. Y. Iscan and K. A. R. Kennedy, pp. 129–60. Wiley-Liss, New York.
Knappert, Jan
1995   *Pacific Mythology: An Encyclopedia of Myth and Legend.* Diamond Books, London.

Knudson, K. E.

N.d. The Mariana Islands. In The Micronesian Region: Peoples, Places, Cultures, Pre-history and History, edited by K. E. Knudson and L. Dupertuis, pp. 171–80. Un-published ms., on file at the University of Guam Title III Program in Micronesian Studies, Mangilao.

Knüsel, Christopher

2000 Bone Adaptation and Its Relationship to Physical Activity in the Past. In *Human Osteology in Archaeology and Forensic Science*, edited by M. Cox and S. Mays, pp. 381–401. Greenwich Medical Media, London.

Komlos, John, and Francesco Cinnirella

2005 European Heights in the Early 18th Century. Munich Economics Discussion Paper 2005-05: 17. University of Munich, Munich.

Lanyon, Lance E.

1992 Control of Bone Architecture by Functional Load Bearing. *Journal of Bone and Mineral Research* 7:S2: S369–S375.

Larsen, Clark Spencer

1997 *Bioarchaeology: Interpreting Behavior from the Human Skeleton*. Cambridge University Press, Cambridge.

Lévesque, Rodrigue (compiler and editor)

1990–96 *History of Micronesia: A Collection of Source Documents*. Vols. 1–8 (of 20), edited and translated by R. Lévesque. Lévesque Publications, Gatineau, Québec.

1992 *History of Micronesia: A Collection of Source Documents*, Vol. 2, *Prelude to Conquest (1561–1595)*, edited and translated by R. Lévesque. Lévesque Publications, Gatineau, Québec.

1995 *History of Micronesia: A Collection of Source Documents*, Vol. 5, *Focus on Marianas 1670–1673*. Lévesque Publications, Gatineau, Québec.

1996 *History of Micronesia: A Collection of Source Documents*, Vol. 7, *More Turmoil in the Marianas (1679–1683)*, edited and translated by R. Lévesque. Lévesque Publications, Gatineau, Québec.

1997 *History of Micronesia: A Collection of Source Documents*, Vol. 9, *Conquest of the Gani Islands, 1687–1696*. Lévesque Publications, Gatineau, Québec.

2002 *History of Micronesia: A Collection of Source Documents*, Vol. 20, *Bibliography of Micronesia, Ships through Micronesia, Cumulative Index*, edited and translated by R. Lévesque. Lévesque Publications, Gatineau, Québec.

Martin, R. Bruce, and David B. Burr

1989 *Structure, Function, and Adaptation of Compact Bone*. Raven Press, New York.

Merbs, Charles F.

1983 Patterns of Activity-Induced Pathology in a Canadian Inuit Population. Archaeological Survey of Canada Paper No. 119. Mercury Series, National Museum of Man, Ottawa.

Mitchell, Roger. E.

1986 Patron Saints and Pagan Ghosts: The Pairing of Opposites. *Asian Folklore Studies* 45: 101–23.

Molnar, Petra

2006 Tracing Prehistoric Activities: Musculoskeletal Stress Marker Analysis of a Stone-

Age Population on the Island of Gotland in the Baltic Sea. *American Journal of Physical Anthropology* 129: 12–23.

Moore, Darlene R., and Rosalind L. Hunter-Anderson

1999   Pots and Pans in the Intermediate Pre-Latte (2500–1600 BP), Mariana Islands, Micronesia. In *The Pacific from 5000–2000 BP, Colonisation and Transformations*, edited by J. C. Gallipaud and I. Lilley, pp. 487–503. IRD Editions, Paris.

Morgan, William N.

1988   *Prehistoric Architecture in Micronesia.* University of Texas Press, Austin.

Nelson, Evelyn Gibson, and Frederick Jens Nelson

1992   *The Island of Guam: Description and History from a 1934 Perspective.* Edited by M. S. McCutcheon. Ana Publications, Washington, D.C.

Pearson, Osbjorn M.

2000   Activity, Climate and Postcranial Robusticity: Implications for Modern Human Origins and Scenarios of Adaptive Change. *Current Anthropology* 41: 569–607.

Pearson, Osbjorn M., and Jane E. Buikstra

2006   Behavior and the Bones. In *Bioarchaeology: The Contextual Analysis of Human Remains*, edited by J. E. Buikstra and L. A. Beck, pp. 207–25. Academic Press, New York.

Peterson, Jane Darden

2000   Labor Patterns in the Southern Levant in the Early Bronze Age. In *Reading the Body: Representations and Remains in the Archaeological Record*, edited by A. E. Rautman, pp. 38–54. University of Pennsylvania Press. Philadelphia.

Pietrusewsky, Michael, Michele T. Douglas, and Rona M. Ikehara-Quebral

1997   An Assessment of Health and Disease in the Prehistoric Inhabitants of the Mariana Islands. *American Journal of Physical Anthropology* 104: 315–42.

Robb, John E.

1998   The Interpretation of Skeletal Muscle Sites: A Statistical Approach. *International Journal of Osteoarchaeology* 8: 363–77.

Ruff, Christopher B.

2003   Growth in Bone Strength, Body Size, and Muscle Size in a Juvenile Longitudinal Sample. *Bone* 33: 317–29.

2005   Mechanical Determinants of Bone Form: Insights from Skeletal Remains. *Journal of Musculoskeletal Neuronal Interaction* 5: 202–12.

Ruff, Christopher B., Brigitte Holt, and Erik Trinkaus

2006   Who's Afraid of the Big Bad Wolff? "Wolff's Law" and Bone Functional Adaptation. *American Journal of Physical Anthropology* 129: 484–98.

Saul, Frank P., and Julie M. Saul

1989   Osteobiography: A Maya Example. In *Reconstruction of Life from the Skeleton*, edited by M. Y. Iscan and K. A. R. Kennedy, pp. 287–302. Wiley-Liss, New York.

Sava, Vincent J.

1996   Occipital Superstructures in Human Skeletal Remains from Tonga: Comparisons with Other Populations and Proposed Etiologies. Unpublished ms., Department of Anthropology, University of Hawai'i.

Shackelford, Laura L.

2007   Regional Variation in the Postcranial Robusticity of Late Upper Paleolithic Humans. *American Journal of Physical Anthropology* 133: 655–68.

Skerry, Tim M.

2006 One Mechanostat or Many? Modifications of the Site-Specific Response of Bone to Mechanical Loading by Nature and Nurture. *Journal of Musculoskeletal and Neuronal Interaction* 6: 122–27.

Spennemann, Dirk H. R.

1989 'Ata 'A Tonga Mo 'Ata 'O Tonga: Early and Later Prehistory of the Tongan Islands. Ph.D. dissertation, Australian National University, Canberra.

Spoehr, Alexander

1957 Marianas Prehistory: Archaeological Survey and Excavations on Saipan, Tinian and Rota. *Fieldiana: Anthropology* 48. Chicago Natural History Museum, Chicago.

Steen, Susan L., and Robert W. Lane

1998 Evaluation of Habitual Activities among Two Alaskan Eskimo Populations Based on Musculoskeletal Stress Markers. *International Journal of Osteoarchaeology* 8: 341–53.

Stirland, Ann J.

1991 Diagnosis of Occupationally Related Paleopathology: Can It Be Done? In *Human Paleopathology: Current Syntheses and Future Options*, edited by D. J. Ortner and A. C. Aufderheide, pp. 40–47. Smithsonian Institution Press, Washington, D.C.

1998 Musculoskeletal Evidence for Activity: Problems of Evaluation. *International Journal of Osteoarchaeology* 8: 354–62.

Taonui, Rawiri

2006 Polynesian Oral Traditions. In *Vaka Moana: Voyages of the Ancestors. The Discovery and Settlement of the Pacific*, edited by K. R. Howe, pp. 22–53. University of Hawai'i Press, Honolulu.

Thompson, Laura M.

1932 Archaeology of the Marianas Islands. Bernice P. Bishop Museum Bulletin No. 100. Bernice P. Bishop Museum, Honolulu.

1945 The Native Culture of the Marianas Islands. Bernice P. Bishop Museum Bulletin No. 185. Bernice P. Bishop Museum, Honolulu.

1947 *Guam and Its People*. Princeton University Press, Princeton, N.J.

Thompson, Stith

2006 *The Folktale*. Holt, Rinehart and Winston, New York.

Tobias, J. H., C. D. Steer, C. G. Mattocks, C. Riddoch, and A. R. Ness

2007 Habitual Levels of Physical Activity Influence Bone Mass in 11-Year-Old Children from the United Kingdom: Findings from a Large Population-Based Cohort. *Journal of Bone and Mineral Research* 22: 101–9.

Torres, Robert Ternorio

2003 Pre-Contact Marianas Folklore, Legends, and Literature: A Critical Commentary. *Micronesian Journal of the Humanities and Social Sciences* 2: 3–15.

Trinkaus, Erik, and Trenton W. Holliday

2000 The Human Remains from Paviland Cave. In *Paviland Cave and the "Red Lady": A Definitive Report*, edited by S. Aldhouse-Green, pp. 141–204. Western Academic & Specialist Press, Bristol, U.K.

Waldron, Tony

1994 *Counting the Dead: The Epidemiology of Skeletal Populations*. John Wiley & Sons, Chichester, U.K.

Weiss, Elizabeth

2007   Muscle Markers Revisited: Activity Pattern Reconstruction with Controls in a Central California Amerind Population. *American Journal of Physical Anthropology* 133: 931–40.

Wernbom, Mathias, Jesper Augustsson, and Roland Thomeé

2007   The Influence of Frequency, Intensity, Volume and Mode of Strength Training on Whole Muscle Cross-Sectional Area in Humans. *Sports Medicine* 37: 225–64.

Wescott, Daniel J.

2006   Effect of Mobility on Femur Midshaft External Shape and Robusticity. *American Journal of Physical Anthropology* 130: 201–13.

York, Robert (compiler and editor)

2001   Chamorro Physical Appearance & Dress—European Contact Period Accounts (A.D. 1521–1700). CNMI Museum Saipan Reference Document 2001-1. CNMI Museum, Saipan.

Zumwalt, Ann C., Christopher B. Ruff, and Cynthia A. Wilczak

2000   Primate Muscle Insertions: What Does Size Tell You? *American Journal of Physical Anthropology* Supplement 30: 331.

5 ◆ Mortuary Evidence for Maya Political Resistance and Religious Syncretism in Colonial Belize

Gabriel D. Wrobel

Individual Profile

Site: Chau Hiix

Location: Western Lagoon, northern Belize

Cultural Affiliation: Maya, Colonial era

Date: A.D. 1520–1660, based on Accelerator Mass Spectrometry (AMS) of long bone fragments.

Features: CHE70-3-80-99 (Burial 137) and CHE70-3-125-99 (Burial 149)

Location of Graves: Structure 2, southeast corner of Plaza A

Burial and Grave Type: Single primary inhumations, on back and extended, hands on hips

Associated Materials: Partial ceramic vessel covering face and unidentified copper item with B137; jade bead, metate fragment, and unidentified copper item with B149

Preservation and Completeness: Very good preservation; crania and some long bones reconstructed

Age at Death and Basis of Estimate: Young adults, based on dental attrition and tooth eruption

Sex and Basis of Determination: Males, based on pelvic and cranial morphology and long bone robusticity

Conditions Observed: Skeletal lesions indicative of anemia and nonspecific infection

Specialized Analysis: AMS dating and stable carbon isotope analysis of long bone fragments for dietary reconstruction

Excavated: 1999, directed by K. Anne Pyburn, Indiana University, Bloomington

Archaeological Report: Wrobel 2000, Andres and Pyburn 2003

Current Disposition: At Indiana University, Bloomington, on loan from the Belize Institute of Archaeology

Excavations at the Classic period Maya site of Chau Hiix, located in northern Belize, uncovered two Historic (ca. A.D. 1520–1660) burials within a palace structure. Both individuals were young males, and an analysis of their dental morphology shows them to be Maya. At the time of the interments, Chau Hiix had been abandoned for approximately 400 years, and Spaniards had firmly established themselves in Central America. The treatment and context of the burials show a form of syncretism in which the mortuary treatment reflects both Maya and Christian conventions. Selective use of elements of both cultural traditions is also evident at the nearby settlements of Lamanai and Tipu, where *visita* missions were established by Franciscans in the sixteenth century and churches continued to be used for burial even after the Spanish were no longer in control.

In his discussion of the Colonial Maya of Belize, Jones (1989: 16) states, "the Mayas used the frontier to hide both people and ideas and to maintain an underground of spirited resistance, even while transforming their own society to incorporate aspects of Spanish government and religion." Graham (1991) also stresses that the relationship of the Maya communities in Belize to the Spanish was characterized by fluctuation between cooperation and resistance, and that the form of Christianity taken by the Maya similarly reflected assimilation—on the Maya's own terms. The two Historic period burials from Chau Hiix reflect this dual relationship. The burial position and grave goods situate these mortuary features within the Colonial system, while their placement in an abandoned building that had also been used for burial by the Prehispanic Maya denotes resistance through the maintenance of selected Maya traditions. The skeletal biology of these individuals is consistent with the biological patterns of Prehispanic Colonial Lowland Maya, and when considered with the associated archaeological data, the osteobiographies reveal the impacts of biological and cultural disruptions typical of this period.

Chau Hiix

Chau Hiix is located in northern Belize approximately equidistant from the larger sites of Lamanai and Altun Ha (figure 5.1). Most archaeological research at Chau Hiix addresses the ancient community's role in the political economy of the region. Perhaps because of its location next to fertile swampy agricultural land and relatively easy access to an important riverine trade route, Chau Hiix maintained a vibrant population through the Early Postclassic period from A.D. 900 to 1200 (table 5.1), in contrast to other nearby communities that succumbed to the collapse and were abandoned at some point in the ninth century A.D.

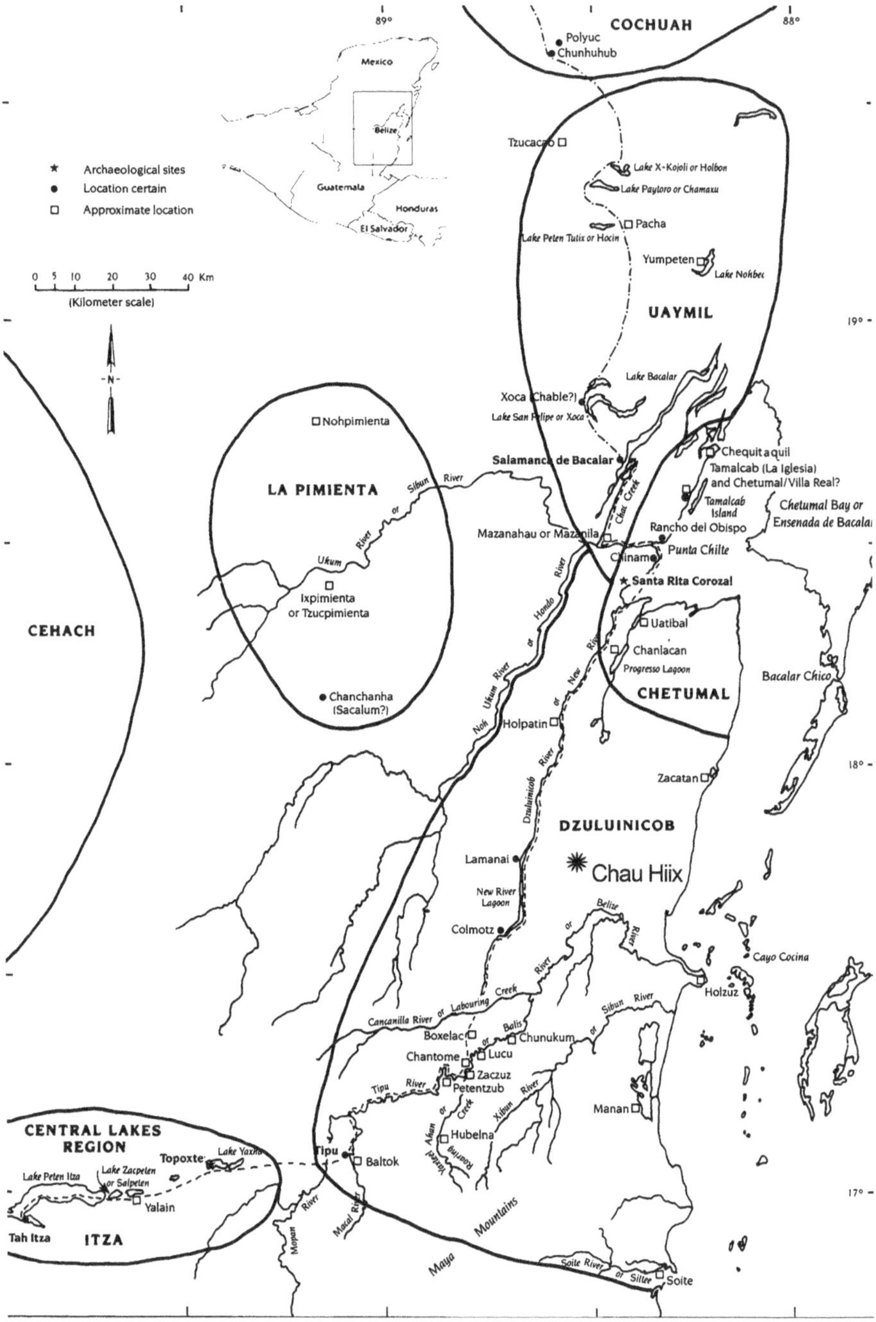

Figure 5.1. The southeastern frontier of Colonial Yucatan showing the location of Chau Hiix and other Colonial Maya sites. (Modified from Jones 1989, map 2, xvi–xvii. Inset of the Maya region courtesy of *The Electronic Atlas of Ancient Maya Sites* ©2008 Clifford T. Brown and Walter R. T. Witschey, http://mayagis.smv.org/.)

Table 5.1. Chronology of Maya in northern Belize as seen from Lamanai

Time period		
Present–1981	Independence	Economic and cultural orientation changes to greater involvement with North and Spanish America; greater participation in global economy
1964	Self-governing	Long-distance trade continues to be characterized by relationships with Britain
	British colonial	Sugar mill built at Lamanai mid-19th century; widespread use of imported British ceramics
1700	Yglesias Spanish colonial	Terminal Postclassic to Early Historic: distinctive ceramics; widespread use of the bow and arrow; appearance of European pottery and metals after 1540
1450	Cib	Late Postclassic: concentration of activity along the lagoon; continuity in forms and ceramic motifs from the Early Postclassic; a probable period of ceramic stylistic change between Cib and Yglesias
1250	Buk	Early Postclassic: distinctive elite subcomplex of pottery seems to replace Classic polychromes; no hiatus from Terminal Classic apparent in stratigraphy; continuity in organization of ceramic production; residential buildings largely of wood; apparent increase in lagoon orientation
1000	Terclerp	Terminal Classic: extensive masonry platform construction, superstructures largely perishable; distinctive pottery with some forms that herald Postclassic styles
800	Tzunun	Late Classic: very little known about this period at Lamanai; ceramic change to Terminal Classic is gradual
600	Shel	Provisional Middle Classic represented ceramically by Tzakol 3 polychromes, slab-footed cylinder vessels, stela iconographic elements
450–250	Sac	Early Classic
0–100 B.C.	Zotz	Terminal Preclassic
400 B.C.	Lag	Late Preclassic
900 B.C.	Mesh	Middle Preclassic
1500 B.C.	?	Provisional

Source: Adapted from Graham 2004.

Chau Hiix's continued viability through the tumultuous Early Postclassic is attributed to its location: the surrounding swamps make the site highly defensible, difficult to access, and relatively invisible (Andres and Pyburn 2003). Evidence for occupation and settlement at Chau Hiix ceases in the Postclassic period, most likely during the thirteenth century. However, evidence of reuse of certain features in the ceremonial center suggests that the settlement was not forgotten and was visited periodically.

This study is focused on two burials found in Structure 2, which is part of a residential *plazuela* group next to the main temple in the ceremonial core of Chau Hiix. Following the pan-Maya sociopolitical transformations in the ninth century, Structure 2 became a focus of mortuary activity for the community, and more than 70 individuals were buried there. Variations in burial treatments, with some graves being richly furnished and some not furnished at all, may represent use by different socioeconomic groups or the changing fortunes of a single family using the plot. Regardless, the last two people buried there are temporally distinct from the others. Burials 137 and 149 were placed in deep pits in the center of the structure (figure 5.2). Several pieces of human bone were found carefully placed next to both burials, and these pieces have been matched with broken (but in situ) elements of nearby earlier burials, which were disturbed when the Historic graves were dug. This practice of reburying disturbed elements of earlier Christian burials is still seen today in the modern Maya town of Succotz (Elizabeth Graham, personal communication 2008), and is not uncommon in any Christian cemetery where bones are disturbed. The relatively deeper pits used for the two final interments indicate that sufficient time had elapsed since the last burials were placed in Structure 2 to allow substantial erosion of buildings in the long-abandoned site center. This also explains the extreme shallowness of the majority of the other burials, which were originally placed in deeper pits or beneath plastered floors.

The bodies of the two young men were placed on their backs and extended, with their hands crossed on their pelves, their heads pointing east. A crypt formed by three pieces of cut limestone (two on either side of the head supporting a capstone) was constructed to protect the head of B149. The head of B137 was protected by a large piece of a broken ceramic vessel, which was placed over his face.

Both men had green copper stains on their hands and pelves, and an eroded and nondiagnostic piece of metal about the size of a grain of rice was recovered from around B137. No other grave goods were found with B149, but B137's grave also included a metate fragment and a small jade bead, which was found on his chest.

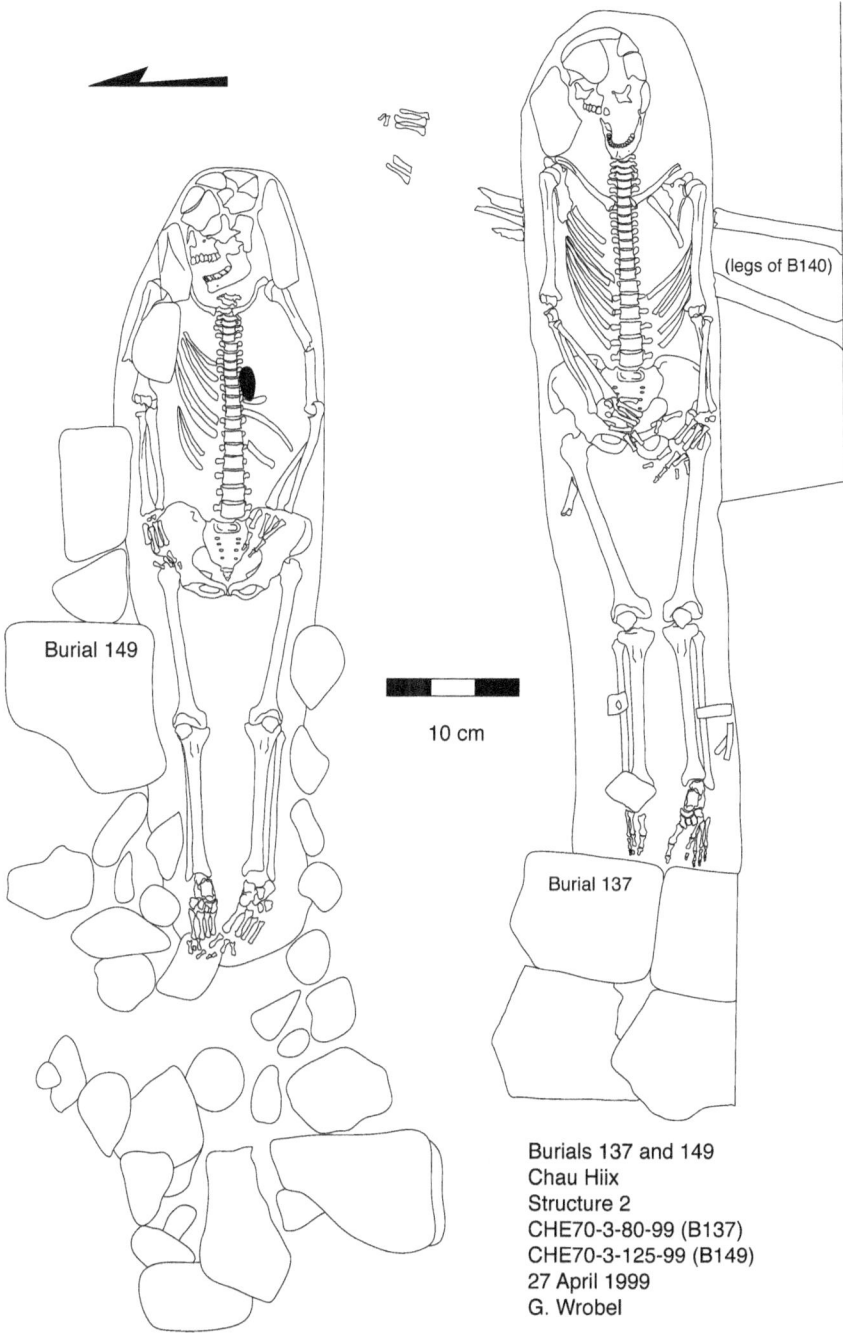

Burial 149

10 cm

(legs of B140)

Burial 137

Burials 137 and 149
Chau Hiix
Structure 2
CHE70-3-80-99 (B137)
CHE70-3-125-99 (B149)
27 April 1999
G. Wrobel

Figure 5.2. Burials 137 and 149.

Osteobiography

The morphological sex indicators on the pelvis (greater sciatic notch) and cranium (nuchal lines, mandible, and mastoid process) of B137 are all masculine. In the case of B149, sex indicators of the pelvis (pubis) and the cranium (mastoid process, nuchal lines) are also clearly male, although his brow ridges are relatively gracile. The excellent preservation of both individuals also allowed the collection of metric data for use in discriminant functions created using a contemporaneous skeletal population from the nearby Historic period site of Tipu (Wrobel et al. 2002). These data also indicated that the individuals were relatively robust males (table 5.2). It should be noted that measurements on the leg bones affected by the areas of infection (discussed below) were not included in these calculations.

Table 5.2. Long bone measurements, Chau Hiix burials and Tipu males and females

Bone	B137	B149	Tipu male mean (mm)	Tipu female mean (mm)
Femur				
Midshaft a-p* diameter	29	29	27.55	23.90
Midshaft circumference	86	89	82.78	75.05
Subtrochanteric a-p diameter	24	26	23.48	21.22
Maximum a-p diameter of shaft	29	30	28.78	25.46
Tibia				
Midshaft a-p diameter	31	30	29.34	25.25
Midshaft circumference	84	80	77.85	67.07
Minimum circumference of shaft	77	72	72.20	62.55
a-p diameter at nutrient foramen	33	34	32.78	27.85
Humerus				
Minimum circumference of shaft	61	61	60.53	51.93
Diameter at deltoid tuberosity	21	23	22.59	19.5
Radius				
Minimum circumference	43	43	41.54	36.69
Diameter at radial tuberosity	17.5	16.5	16.12	13.97
Ulna				
Minimum circumference	36	36	34.84	29.81

*a-p denotes anterior-posterior.

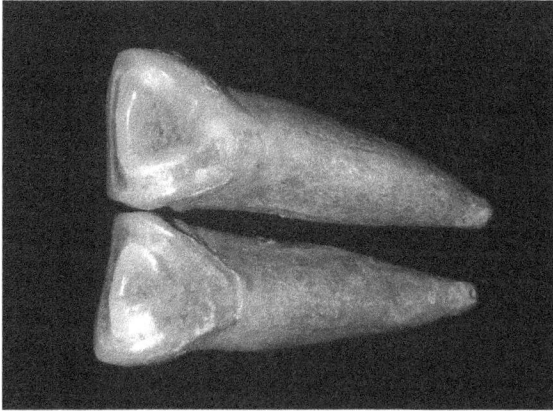

Figure 5.3. Shovel-shaped incisors, Burial 149. (Photograph by Robert Taylor.)

In an effort to confirm the individuals' Maya ancestry, morphological features of the teeth were compared to standards from the Arizona State University Dental Anthropology System (ASUDAS). Both individuals displayed specific dental traits that are found in very high frequency in Native American groups, and in low frequency in European and African groups. Examples of such diagnostic traits include the presence of raised ridges, or "shoveling," on the labial and lingual surfaces of the anterior maxillary teeth (figure 5.3), and "L"-shaped wrinkles in the distal side of the mesiolingual cusp, known as deflecting wrinkles, on the lower first molars. These observations confirm that these individuals are of Maya rather than European descent (Wrobel 2004), as was shown in a similar study by Jacoby (2000) of the contemporaneous population from Tipu.

Burial 137 was an adult, with slight to moderate dental attrition, suggesting a young individual with a coarse diet, typical of Maya populations. No other distinct age indicators, such as arthritis, are visible, and the age indicators of the pelvis are not preserved. No evidence of pathology is evident on the postcranial skeleton of B137, although his cranial vault does show some signs of healed porotic hyperostosis, a condition indicating anemia in which the usually smooth surfaces of the cranial bones become porous. The teeth of B137 are extremely small when compared to other prehispanic Maya teeth from Chau Hiix and other sites. Jacobi's (2000) Historic Tipu population had smaller average dentitions than Classic period Maya populations (Wrobel 2004). This trend parallels similar reductions over time found in agricultural populations with high carbohydrate consumption and seems to result from selection for smaller, more caries-resistant teeth (Brace et al. 1991). Some calculus buildup is present, especially on his anterior teeth, and this, too, is typical of Maya populations with a heavy reliance on starchy maize diets. As a result of this high carbohydrate diet, he had numerous interproximal and cervical caries on his premolars and molars.

Burial 149 was clearly an adult, since his third molars were completely erupted. Arthritic changes of the skeleton are minimal, suggesting that he died at a relatively young age. His teeth had no pathology other than moderate calculus buildup and very slight occlusal attrition. The tibiae and fibulae of B149 exhibit signs of infection in the legs that seems to be focused on the vasculature (figures 5.4a, 5.4b). The bone around the nutrient foramina on both legs (tibiae and fibulae) shows remodeling and general periostitis. The femora show some evidence of healed infection, resulting in a smooth but uneven surface, and there is active periostitis on the central metacarpals and phalanges of his left hand.

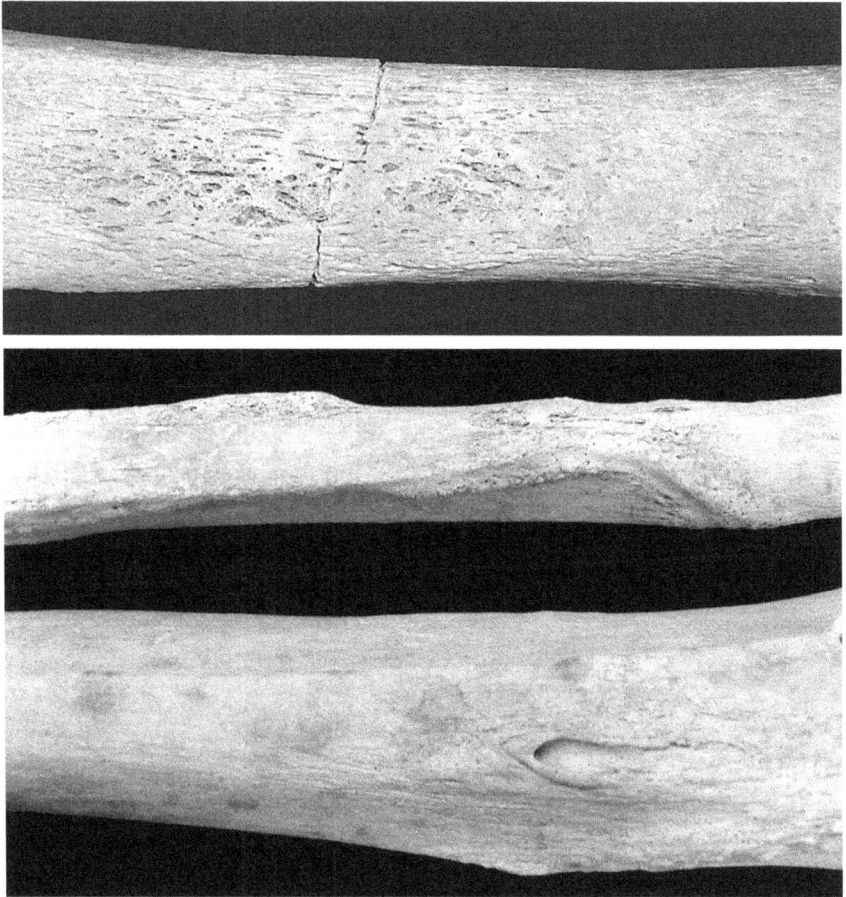

Figures 5.4a–b. Infection on legs of Burial 149. 5.4a (*above*): distal third of the right tibia; 5.4b (*below*): proximal third of the left tibia and fibula shafts.

Like B137, B149 also shows evidence of some porosity on the cranial vault, likely healing porotic hyperostosis. No arthritis was visible on his vertebrae or on the rest of the skeleton, with the possible exception of the left wrist; the surface of the distal ulnar head shows a slight pinprick texture, which might indicate mild arthritis, or might be related to the infection seen on the left hand bones.

Interpretation

These two burials at Chau Hiix clearly date to the Historic period, based on preservation, stratigraphy, and burial treatment. This is confirmed with Accelerator Mass Spectrometry (AMS) radiocarbon dates from the bones of both individuals. The ranges with 2-sigma calibration are A.D. 1470–1660 for B137 and A.D. 1520–1670 for B149. Since these individuals appear cotemporaneous, we can consider their overlapping dates as most viable (i.e., A.D. 1520–1660). While there is no convincing evidence that people lived at Chau Hiix during the Historic period, the nearby population of Lamanai, approximately 20 km west of Chau Hiix, would appear to be an excellent candidate for the source of these two individuals. So why were these men buried at Chau Hiix instead of at Lamanai?

The date of the burials corresponds to a point in time representing the initial Christianization of Maya in Belize. The first church at Lamanai was constructed as early as 1544, and missions at Tipu and Lamanai were established then (Graham 2011, 1998; Jones 1989). A second, larger church was built at Lamanai, probably in the 1560s, but possibly as late as the early seventeenth century (Graham 2011). Though the Spanish were dominant in the northern Yucatan, Belize was still something of a colonial outpost. Lamanai and Tipu were *visita* missions, which were visited only sporadically by Spanish Franciscan friars.

During the Colonial period, Lamanai and the surrounding area, including Chau Hiix, may have been part of a region known as Dzuluinicob, of which Tipu was the capital (Jones 1989). The Dzuluinicob province was made up of a series of indigenous villages and *visita* missions that were governed by the small outpost town of Bacalar, which was charged with the difficult task of exerting colonial control over this province by maintaining forced Indian service and collecting taxes and tribute. Dzuluinicob was economically significant for its production of cacao, and strategically important as a staging ground for military and missionary expeditions to the neighboring Itza Maya of the central Peten, who remained independent of Spanish rule until 1707.

Graham et al. (1989: 1256) note that "because it was closer to the administrative seat of Salamanca de Bacalar, Lamanai was more vulnerable than Tipu to Spanish economic controls, and Spanish *encomenderos* had difficulty keeping inhabitants from running away." The lack of a consistent Spanish presence in these communities, as well as the excessive tribute demanded of them, led to several revolts. These were often led by Maya elites trained in Franciscan monasteries, who "brought to their followers newly syncretized, holistic amalgamations of Maya and Christian religious ritual and belief" (Jones 1989: 51). By 1638, the Belize Maya were in full revolt; the churches at Lamanai were burned down. The Spanish military intervened sporadically during this period, causing the dispersal of many Maya fleeing Spanish retaliation. Spanish authorities eventually reestablished communication and contact with the frontier outposts in Belize in 1695, but not administrative control.

Chau Hiix would have offered an excellent sanctuary for these refugees. Local people were obviously aware of its location, and there is ample evidence that the Maya continued to visit the site for ritual purposes after it was abandoned in the Postclassic. Visitors built a small shrine on the main plaza and left offerings in the form of smashed pottery, *incensarios*, and other objects (Andres and Pyburn 2003). Since this use seems to have been related to traditional Maya religious (that is, "pagan") pilgrimages rather than Catholic-based ritual, the Spanish were probably unaware of the continued use of Chau Hiix.

Contextual evidence from the burials shows the amalgamation of Christian and traditional Maya religion and ritual. For instance, Christian influence can be seen in the burial position. The position of the bodies, on their backs, extended, with hands crossed over the pelves, is consistent with other Maya burials from Christianized communities (Jacobi 2000). However, Christians of this era in the Yucatan and in Belize were almost always buried with their heads toward the west, whereas the Chau Hiix burials were placed with their heads toward the east. This discrepancy may be a local variant, and several other Historic period cases are known from northern Yucatan (Vera Tiesler, personal communication 2008). These other east-heading burials have been variously interpreted as church personnel and also as unsanctified individuals. Another possible explanation is that Spanish custom dictated that the deceased be positioned so that their feet pointed toward the church, or toward the altar if they were buried within the church (Jacobi 2000: 32). The feet of the Chau Hiix burials pointed west, toward Lamanai.

Other aspects of mortuary treatment seem to indicate the role of these individuals within their communities. In addition to the jade bead from B137, grave goods in both burials included the evidence of copper, which was present very late in the prehistoric era in Belize. These could also be the remnants of copper-alloyed artifacts imported from Europe. Prehistoric copper at Lamanai appears to be limited to the grave goods of a few richly furnished individuals from the Early Postclassic Buk phase (A.D. 1000–1200) (Pendergast 1981; Graham 2004). But later components at Lamanai have yielded more copper and copper-alloyed artifacts from controlled archaeological excavations than any other Southern Lowland Maya site (Simmons 2005: 237). These are mostly status display objects: bells, tweezers, rings, buttons, and other ornaments. Simmons's (2005) study of metallurgy at Lamanai shows evidence that the elites were producing their own copper artifacts beginning in the Late to Terminal Postclassic (fourteenth to fifteenth centuries) and continuing through the Historic period. Copper was relatively rare at Historic Lamanai, and still probably was a status indicator. Most of the copper comes from the area surrounding Structure N11-18, which is thought to have been the home of the principal Maya administrator during the Contact period (Simmons 2005: 234).

While the corroded copper artifact found with B137 at Chau Hiix was unidentifiable, the stains on the phalanges of both individuals suggest that they wore copper rings. The stains around the pelves may be from needles used to hold shrouds, similar to the practice found in burials at Tipu (Graham 1991), or perhaps small bells worn around the waist, as found at Lamanai (Pendergast 1981). In any case, the very presence of these objects hints at relatively high status for these individuals.

The biological data from the two skeletons are comparable to the extensively studied Colonial Tipu population (Cohen et al. 1993, 1997; Danforth et al. 1997; Jacobi 2000; Hartnett 2002; Wrobel et al. 2002). Unfortunately, no such data exist for the Historic population of Lamanai. Neither individual at Chau Hiix displayed cranial or dental modification, both of which were very rare in Historic populations, though fairly common among the Postclassic Maya in the area (White 1998; Williams and White 2006). Both individuals have shovel-shaped incisors, a trait characteristic of Native American, rather than European, heritage. No European burials have been discovered at Tipu or Lamanai, either. The relatively small dentition of B137 and the congenitally absent lower third molars of B149 are consistent with a dental reduction trend found in Mesoamerica between the Preclassic and the Historic eras, thought to result from selection against large, caries-prone teeth (Wrobel 2004).

The mild, inactive porotic hyperostosis found on both burials is also typical of the Tipu burials, among whom 55.3 percent of the adults had at least some porosity on the skull interpreted as evidence of anemia (Cohen et al. 1997: 84). As in the Tipu population (Cohen et al. 1997), there is systemic infection (B149) but no suggestion of treponemal infection. Neither individual displayed linear enamel hypoplasias, which are shallow depressions on the teeth indicating a general disturbance to an individual's development at the time the affected tooth was forming. The absence of linear enamel hypoplasias in the two young men buried at Chau Hiix is also in keeping with data from Tipu where hypoplasias were rare, especially compared to earlier, Preclassic Maya populations (Danforth 1997).

None of the pathologies noted were severe, and no evidence of trauma exists on either individual; thus cause of death is unknown.

The skeletal robusticity data in table 5.2 show that the long bone dimensions of the two individuals generally exceed the averages for Tipu males, which may be related to diet. Analysis of stable carbon isotopes in the Chau Hiix skeletons shows that, like Postclassic and Historic era people at Lamanai, the diets of B137 and B149 show a decrease in terrestrial animal protein and an increase in reliance on marine or reef resources compared to the Classic period (Metcalf et al. 2009). Faunal studies by Emery (1999: 77) show that animal taxonomic diversity was lower at Lamanai than at Tipu. Animal-related dietary breadth was lower, and more riverine species and birds were exploited, as were more species from agricultural (rather than forested) habitats. The transitions seen at Lamanai from Postclassic to Colonial are continuing trends from the Mid– Late Postclassic transition. However, they are more dramatic than they are at Tipu. It is hard to know whether this indicates a change in hunting practices or expanded agricultural land. What we may be seeing is significant disruptions of Precolonial patterns in towns—such as Lamanai and Bacalar—which were closer to Spanish centers of control and hence received more monitoring than remote communities such as Tipu.

Conclusion

The burials of these two young men at Chau Hiix show an interesting combination of cultural elements from both Western Christian and Maya traditions. Biologically and culturally, they were typical members of the Colonial era Maya population. Their burial at this abandoned ceremonial center tells part of the story of the sociopolitical climate of northern Belize at that time.

Most of what we know about this period comes from ethnohistoric accounts, which give a Westernized view of Maya reactions to Spanish rule, and the documentary evidence diminishes markedly after the Spanish were expelled from Belize in 1638. Archaeological studies supplement the ethnohistory of this area and help to answer questions about the social, political, and economic adaptation of these frontier communities. Graham et al. (1989: 1259) elucidate the postcontact cultural processes of the Maya in this period, in which we see the simultaneous rejection of Spanish rule and the selective integration of Christian belief systems. The burials at Chau Hiix indicate assimilation and syncretism, but they also represent acts of resistance and traditionalism on the part of these two men and their survivors.

Acknowledgments

Thanks to Elizabeth Graham, Anne Pyburn, Della Cook, and Krista Jordan. This research was made possible by funding from the Indiana University Anthropology Department and the Foundation for the Advancement of Mesoamerican Studies (FAMSI). As always, many thanks to the Belize Institute of Archaeology and the Village of Crooked Tree.

References Cited

Andres, Christopher, and K. Anne Pyburn
2003   Out of Sight: The Postclassic and Early Colonial Periods at Chau Hiix. In *The Terminal Classic in the Maya Lowlands*, edited by A. Demarest, D. Rice, and P. Rice, pp. 402–23. Westview Press, Boulder, Colo.
Brace, C. Loring, Shelley L. Smith, and Kevin D. Hunt
1991   What Big Teeth You Had Grandma! Human Tooth Size, Past and Present. In *Advances in Dental Anthropology*, edited by M. A. Kelley and C. S. Larsen, pp. 33–57. Wiley-Liss, New York.
Cohen, Mark N., Kathleen O'Conner, Marie E. Danforth, Keith P. Jacobi, and Carl Armstrong
1993   Health and Death at Tipu. In *In the Wake of Contact: Biological Responses to Conquest*, edited by C. S. Larsen and G. R. Milner, pp. 121–33. Wiley-Liss, New York.
1997   The Archaeology and Osteology of Tipu. In *Bones of the Ancestors*, edited by S. L. Whittington and D. M. Reed, pp. 78–89. Smithsonian Institution Press, Washington, D.C.
Danforth, Marie E.
1997   Childhood Health Patterns in the Late Classic Maya: Analysis of Enamel Microdefects. In *Bones of the Maya*, edited by S. L. Whittington and D. M. Reed, pp. 127–38. Smithsonian Institution Press, Washington, D.C.
Danforth, Marie E., Keith P. Jacobi, and Mark N. Cohen
1997   Gender and Health among the Colonial Maya of Tipu. *Ancient Mesoamerica* 8: 13–22.
Emery, Kitty F.
1999   Temporal Trends in Ancient Maya Animal Use. In *Reconstructing Ancient Maya Diet*, edited by C. D. White, pp. 61–81. University of Utah Press, Salt Lake City.
Graham, Elizabeth
1991   Archaeological Insights into Colonial Period Maya Life at Tipu, Belize. In *Colum-*

bian Consequences, Vol. 3, *The Spanish Borderlands in Pan-American Perspective*, edited by D. H. Thomas, pp. 319–35. Smithsonian Institution Press, Washington, D.C.

1998 Mission Archaeology. *Annual Review of Anthropology* 27: 25–62.

2004 Lamanai Reloaded: Alive and Well in the Early Postclassic. *Research Reports in Belizean Archaeology* 1: 23–41.

2011 *Maya Christians and Their Churches in Sixteenth-Century Belize.* University Press of Florida, Gainesville.

Graham, Elizabeth, David M. Pendergast, and Grant D. Jones

1989 On the Fringes of Conquest: Maya-Spanish Contact in Colonial Belize. *Science* 246: 1254–59.

Hartnett, Kristen Marie

2002 Habitual Activity Patterns at the Historic Period Maya Site of Tipu, Belize. Master's thesis, Department of Anthropology, Arizona State University.

Jacobi, Keith P.

2000 *Last Rites for the Tipu Maya.* University of Alabama Press, Tuscaloosa.

Jones, Grant D.

1989 *Maya Resistance to Spanish Rule.* University of New Mexico Press, Albuquerque.

Metcalfe, Jessica Z., Christine D. White, Fred J. Longstaffe, Gabriel Wrobel, and Della Collins Cook

2009 Hierarchies and Heterarchies of Food Consumption: Stable Isotope Evidence from Chau Hiix and the Northern Belize Region. *Latin American Antiquity* 20(1): 15–36.

Pendergast, David M.

1981 Lamanai, Belize: Summary of Excavation Results, 1974–1980. *Journal of Field Archaeology* 8: 29–53.

Simmons, Scott

2005 Investigations in the Church Zone: Maya Archaeometallurgy at Spanish Colonial Lamanai, Belize. *Research Reports in Belizean Archaeology* 2: 231–39.

White, Christine D.

1998 Sutural Effects of Fronto-Occipital Cranial Modification. *American Journal of Physical Anthropology* 100: 397–410.

Williams, Jocelyn, and Christine D. White

2006 Dental Modification in the Postclassic Population from Lamanai, Belize. *Ancient Mesoamerica* 17: 139–51.

Wrobel, Gabriel

2000 Mortuary Patterning in Structure 2 Burials: The 1999 Excavations. In The Chau Hiix Archaeological Project 1999 Interim Report, edited by C.R. Andres, pp. 7–20. Unpublished report submitted to the Belize Institute of Archaeology, Belmopan.

2004 Metric and Nonmetric Dental Variation among the Ancient Maya of Northern Belize. Ph.D. dissertation, Department of Anthropology, Indiana University.

Wrobel, Gabriel, Marie Danforth, and Carl Armstrong

2002 Estimating Sex of Maya Skeletons by Discriminant Function Analysis of Long Bone Measurements from the Protohistoric Maya Site of Tipu, Belize. *Ancient Mesoamerica* 13: 255–63.

TWO ◈ Ancient Travelers and "Others"

6 ◆ Social Marginalization among the Chiribaya

THE *CURANDERO* OF YARAL, SOUTHERN PERU

María Cecilia Lozada, Kelly J. Knudson,
Rex C. Haydon, and Jane E. Buikstra

Individual Profile

Site: El Yaral

Location: Osmore drainage of southern Peru

Cultural Affiliation: Unknown

Date: Four radiocarbon dates suggest that this site was occupied around A.D. 1000

Feature: Burial 213

Location of Grave: Cemetery 2, Trench 4

Burial and Grave Type: A single primary burial in an irregular and unlined shallow pit; placed on his left side and facing north, knees and right arm flexed, left arm internally rotated and slightly extended, hips extended, neck and head rotated over 90°

Associated Materials: Ceramic vessel, wooden tablet, yarn of wool, wooden spoon, 2 textile bags, and wooden "comb"

Preservation and Completeness: Excellent skeletal preservation; some soft tissue present

Age at Death and Basis of Estimate: 35–40 years, based on pubic symphysis and auricular surface

Sex and Basis of Determination: Male, based on pelvic morphology and femur dimensions

Conditions Observed: Multiple fractures in the skull and mandible

Specialized Analysis: Radiography, strontium isotopes from tooth enamel

Excavated: 1990, Chiribaya Bioarchaeological Project, directed by Jane E. Buikstra, Arizona State University

Archaeological Report: Lozada and Torres 1991

Current Disposition: Mallqui Center of Bioarchaeological Research, Ilo, Peru

Curanderos in the Andes

Curanderos, or healers, represent essential components of Andean communities, both today as well as in the past. Guaman Poma de Ayala, a native Peruvian who documented many aspects of the preconquest Inka world, acknowledged their importance in his *Nueva Corónica y Buen Gobierno* [1613] (1987). Guaman Poma de Ayala classifies this specialized group, depicted as healers, according to their powers and/or curing techniques (Millones and Platt 1989). Other colonial accounts found in the Huarochiri manuscript, originally written in Quechua immediately after the conquest, portray the *curandero* as a charismatic and powerful male figure. The healer was an outsider whose main role was to restore health to individuals or even communities (Urioste 1981).

Ethnographic studies of *curanderos* in contemporary Peru indicate that these Andean healers are community leaders who serve as mediators between perceived reality and the supernatural (Millones 1987). Furthermore, *curanderos* are charismatic and highly respected members of the community because of their healing powers as well as their role as spiritual guides. They are extremely knowledgeable about the environment, often traveling and collecting herbs and special items from diverse areas such as the jungle, highlands, and coast (Millones 1997). Although highly respected by the communities, *curanderos* are also characterized as loners whose social acceptance depended on the success of their powers. As such, their status in society is often variable and extremely fluid.

Burials of *curanderos* are rarely encountered in archaeological sites. In his seminal work, Henry Wassén (1972) suggests that the Niño Korin excavated in northeastern Bolivia at an altitude of 3,500 m is one of the earliest archaeologically documented burials of a young *curandero*. The individual was buried with his working tools, including snuff trays, bamboo tubes, spoons, spatulas, baskets, and fur/skin pouches. Based on a stylistic examination of these artifacts, the burial dates to the Middle Horizon between A.D. 800 and 1,000 (Wassén 1972).

Along the coast of northern Peru, Elera (1994) documented the presence of an itinerant *curandero*. This burial was found in Morro de Eten, dating to the Middle Formative period around 500–200 B.C. Similar to the Niño Korin, this coastal *curandero* was buried with his belongings such as stone mirrors, shells, and spatulas. Interestingly, he was buried with a rattle that had been implanted into his right leg and may have been used as part of rituals.

Although these archaeological findings attest to the antiquity and widespread existence of "*curanderismo*" in the ancient Andes, many questions remain unanswered. For example, there is basic agreement in the ethnohistorical and ethnographic literature regarding the pivotal role of these specialists; however, their treatment at death may have depended on how they were perceived by the community in which they lived. *Curanderos* have often been broadly divided into those who used their powers to help individuals and communities through healing and divining and those who used their powers to harm (Giese 1989). The sickness and eventual death of a *curandero* would have been an extraordinary event in the community, and the perception of the *curanderos* by the local community can perhaps be interpreted through how they were treated after death. In this chapter, we present the case of an archaeologically documented *curandero* from southern Peru. This burial was excavated from the Chiribaya site known as El Yaral in 1991.

El Yaral, Chiribaya, and the Late Intermediate Period of Southern Peru

The Chiribaya people flourished in southern Peru between A.D. 700 and 1350 and centralized their power in the coastal region of the Osmore Valley (figures 6.1a–b). Extensive mortuary excavations at four sites were conducted as part of the Chiribaya Project in 1991 (Lozada and Buikstra 2002). These sites are: San Geronimo, Chiribaya Alta, Chiribaya Baja, and Yaral. Using mortuary data derived from approximately 500 burials, as well as studies of biological distance, cranial modification styles, and dietary reconstruction, we know that the Chiribaya emerged from earlier coastal populations and were divided into specialized groups of *pescadores*, or fishermen, and *labradores*, or agriculturalists (Lozada and Buikstra 2002; Tomczak 2003). Yaral is located in the mid valley of the Osmore drainage approximately 50 km from the Pacific Ocean at approximately 1,000 MASL (figures 6.1a–b). Radiocarbon dates from both domestic and mortuary contexts indicate that the site was occupied around A.D. 1000. This was a community of agriculturalists within the larger Chiribaya polity.

Tombs can be viewed as highly symbolic spaces. Mortuary theorists believe that the social identity of the deceased, as perceived by his or her living counterparts, can often be gleaned from mortuary treatment (Binford 1971). It has also been proposed that burial treatment may reflect emotional responses that promote group solidarity or express feelings of anger and fear (Tarlow 2000). Among the burials excavated from the four Chiribaya sites, the majority exhibit standard practices and symbols associated with Chiribaya; however, there are a few burials that stand in stark contrast and represent individuals who either rose above or stood apart from the norms of Chiribaya society. One such individual was the *curandero* interred in Burial 213 at El Yaral.

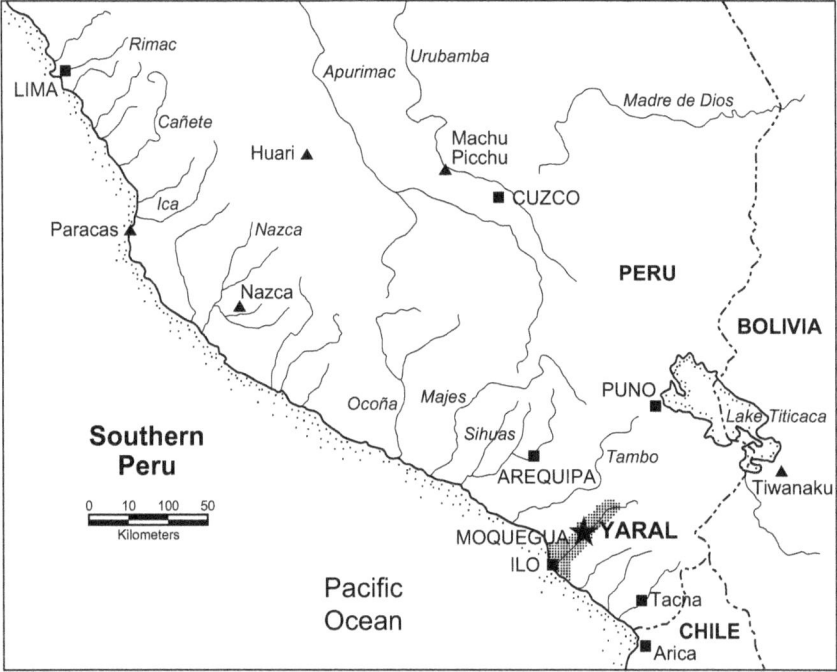

Figure 6.1a. Map of the Southern Andes with the site of El Yaral marked.

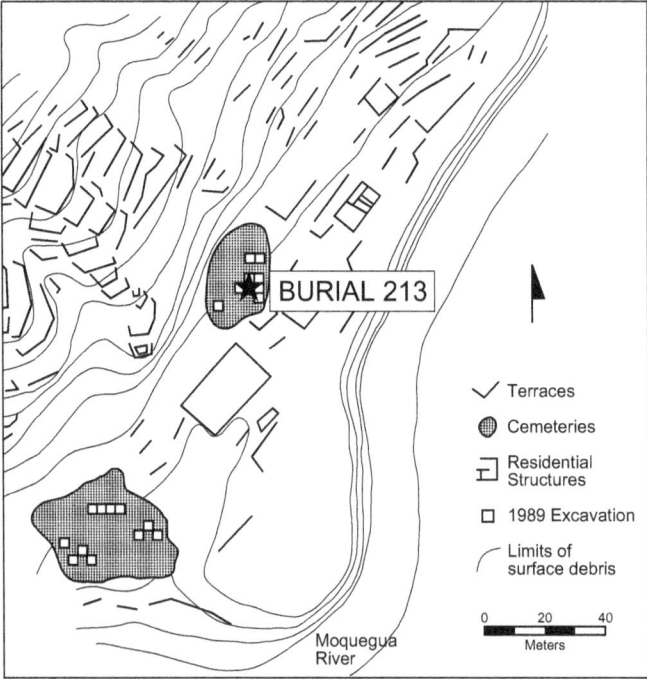

Figure 6.1b. The site of El Yaral and the location of Burial 213.

The *Curandero* of El Yaral

Burial 213 was excavated from cemetery 2 at El Yaral. The typical tombs at El Yaral are modest and constructed in a standardized manner. Tombs are circular and lined with stones. Following Chiribaya tradition, the body was buried in a flexed position, facing east with grave goods placed close to the feet. The average burial at El Yaral included two ceramic vessels, a spoon, a basket, and some botanical and animal remains—relatively few items compared to burials at other Chiribaya sites (Lozada and Buikstra 2002).

The individual from Burial 213 was an adult male between 35 and 40 years, interred in an irregular and unlined shallow pit (figures 6.2a–b). Instead of being buried in a flexed position, this individual was placed on his left side facing north. His knees and right arm were flexed, yet the left arm is internally rotated and extended, and his hips are extended. His ankles were bound together with a heavy wool material. His neck is extended over 90 degrees, and rotated. His head abuts the side of the shallow pit and is also rotated to the right, suggesting that the body was crudely placed or even thrown into the pit. Unlike any other burial uncovered among the Chiribaya, he was covered with stones and gravel, with a large stone directly over the right side of his face. Immediately beneath the stones, we could see facial fractures in the mandible, midface, and zygomatic arches that were likely caused by the stones, although it is not clear whether these were inflicted before or after the individual's death.

The individual from Burial 213 was interred with a textile bag; a wooden spoon, tablet, and spatula; and a comblike object made of marine mammal bone and cactus spines (figures 6.3 a–c). These grave goods were placed along his back. Finally, a ceramic globular vessel with a small handle and short neck was found next to the body. Compared to typical items from other burials at El Yaral or other Chiribaya sites, these items are distinct in both style and manufacture. The spoon, tablet, and spatula are made of a dense black wood known locally as chonta. Chonta wood (*Astrocarym chonta*) is an exotic wood that is only found in the tropical areas of the Andes. The ceramic vessel is of nonlocal manufacture, and it does not show any features of typical Chiribaya ceramics. Even the individual's attire was unusual. He was buried wearing an old raglike textile made from a coarse wool fiber.

Close examination of his head revealed the multiple fractures that can also be seen on radiographs (figures 6.4a–b). The absence of remodeling or associated deep hemorrhage suggests that these wounds were postmortem, and may have resulted from an attempt to damage or disfigure the corpse.

To test whether the individual from Burial 213 was of nonlocal origin, we

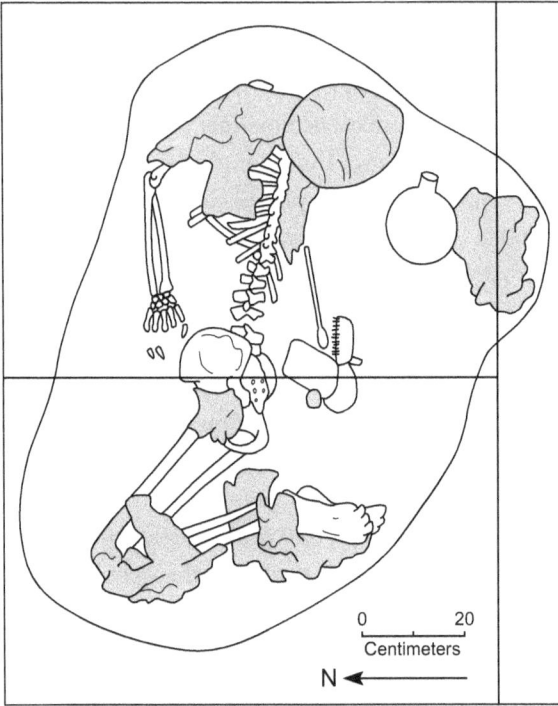

Figure 6.2a–b. Drawing (a) and photograph (b) of Burial 213, demonstrating the position of the body and important features of the burial.

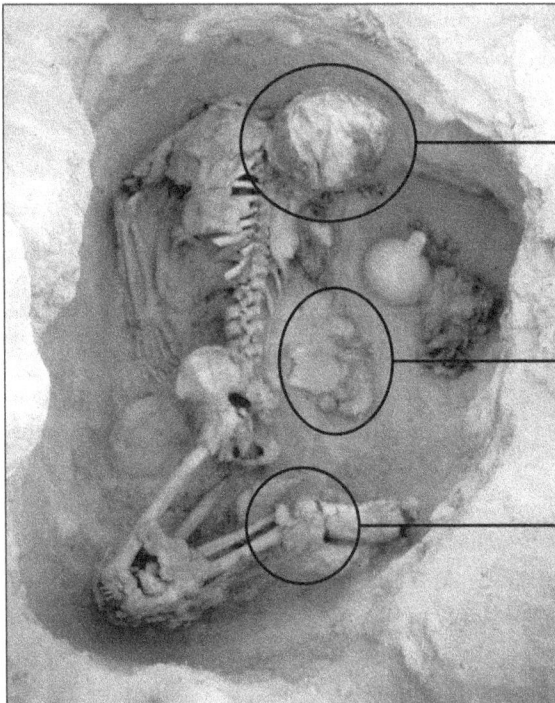

Overlying stone & facial trauma

Wooden tablet, spatula, comb & spoon

Feet bound with wool material

0   20
Centimeters

N ←

Large Comb Made of Bone and Cactus Spines

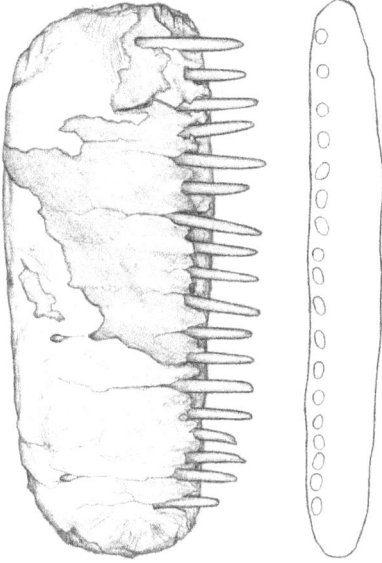

Comb Layers

Feathers

Animal Fur

Resin

Cactus Spines

Bone

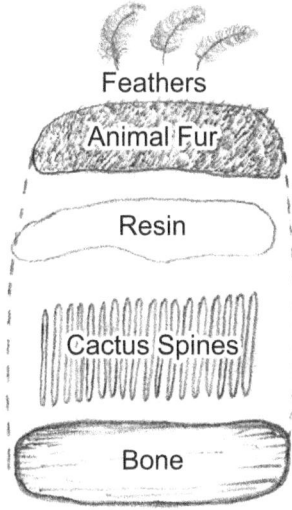

Canteen/Bottle

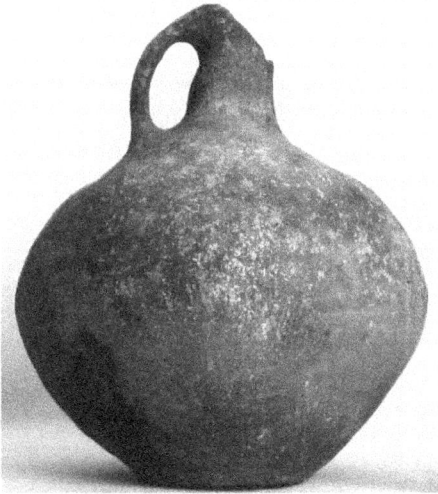

Wooden Tablet and Spatula (Burned)

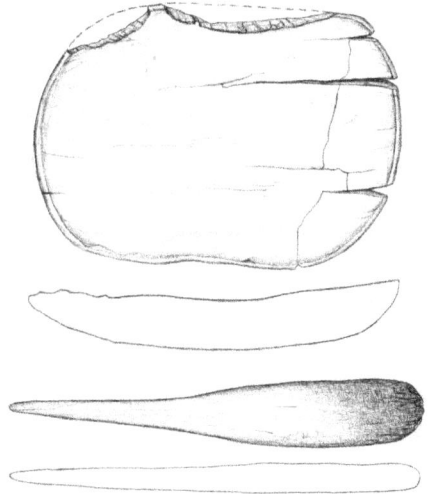

Figure 6.3a–c. Funeral offerings included with Burial 213.

compared strontium isotope signatures from the tooth enamel of this individual to other burials from El Yaral. Strontium isotope analysis represents a powerful tool to identify migrations between different geographic zones using skeletal material, instead of through proxy measures such as material culture. Briefly, strontium isotopes in an individual's tooth enamel and bone can show where that individual lived for the first and last years of his or her life, provided that local food constituted the majority of that individual's diet (Knudson and Price 2007). Based on modern guinea pigs from the Osmore Drainage, the local range is defined as $^{87}Sr/^{86}Sr = 0.7059–0.7066$. In the case of the *curandero*, the strontium isotope ratios in first molar tooth enamel, typically formed during the initial years of life, is outside of this local range (M8-10395, $^{87}Sr/^{86}Sr = 0.708087$), unlike the majority of other individuals buried at Yaral. This suggests that this individual may have spent parts of his life, including his first three to four years, in a different geologic zone.

Conclusion

The bioarchaeological study presented in this chapter suggests that the individual interred in tomb 213 was unique among the Chiribaya. In fact, he may not have been either biologically or culturally affiliated with the other members of Chiribaya society. Furthermore, evaluation of strontium isotope data from his teeth suggests that he spent parts of his life outside the area where he was buried, and may have been itinerant, carrying his belongings and tools. The globular ceramic vessel with a short and narrow neck allows the easy transportation of liquids. His funerary goods are unique and have some similarities to those artifacts buried with the Korin child, identified as a young *curandero* in the highlands of Bolivia. The fact that his wooden artifacts are made from a tropical plant suggests that this individual was in contact with communities in the jungle. The inclusion of snuff tablets and a spatula may indicate that he prepared hallucinogenic snuff, a practice that was common in the highlands and in San Pedro de Atacama (Berenguer and Dauelsberg 1989), but not among the Chiribaya. The rough manner in which he was interred indicates that he was brutally mistreated during burial, and may even have been murdered. The shallow pit in which he was interred was crude, intruding into the neighboring tomb, and appears to have been hastily made.

Interestingly, his legs were bound, and his body was covered with stones. Apart from physically binding and maiming the body, such practices may have also been meant to limit mobility in the afterlife. In this manner, the living may have used this mortuary treatment to limit his spirit or powers even after death.

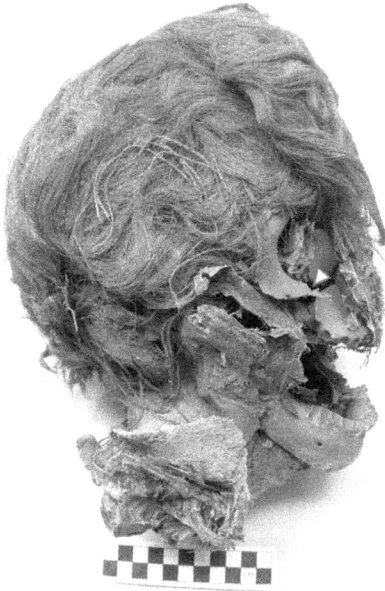

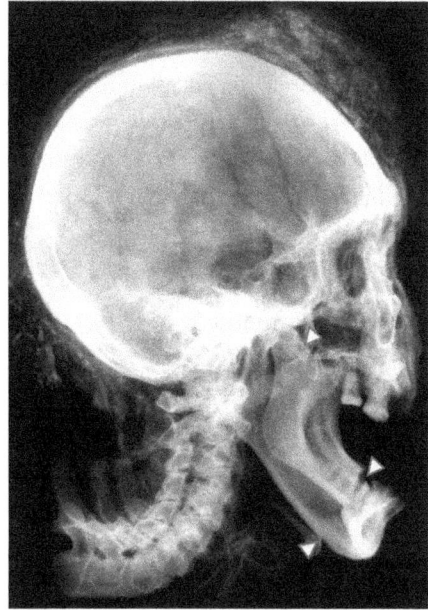

Figure 6.4a. Side view, photograph and corresponding radiograph, of the head from Burial 213. Arrows indicate fractures identified in the skull and mandible.

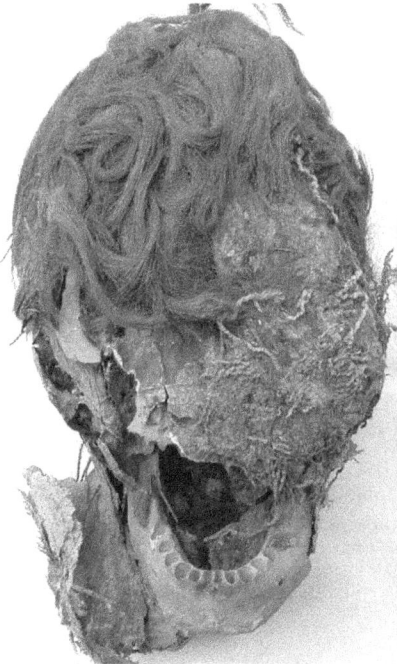

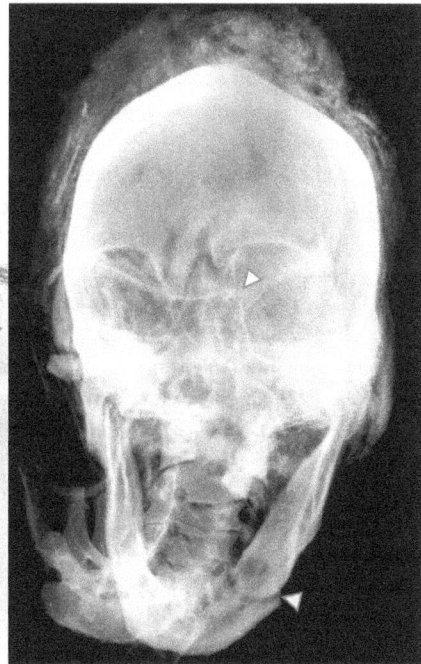

Figure 6.4b. Frontal view, photograph and corresponding radiograph, of the head from Burial 213. Arrows indicate fractures identified in the skull and mandible.

Based on the ethnographic accounts, ethnohistorical documents, and our own bioarchaeological research, we propose that this individual was a *curandero* who was either unsuccessful or was perceived by the Chiribaya as harmful. In spite of this sentiment, he was still buried within the cemetery used by the Chiribaya in southern Peru, underscoring the often conflicting emotions of dependence and fear that characterize how many *curanderos* were seen by their local communities.

Acknowledgments

The authors wish to thank Dr. Sonia Guillén, Bertha Vargas, and Elizabeh Schaeffer who graciously assisted wih this research and publication.

References Cited

Berenguer, José, and Percy Dauelsberg

1989   El Norte Grande en la Orbita de Tiwanaku. In *Culturas de Chile, Prehistoria*, edited by J. Hidalgo, V. Schiappacasse, F. H. Niemeyer, C. A. del Solar, and I. Solimano, pp. 129–90. Editorial Andrés Bello, Santiago.

Binford, Lewis

1971   Mortuary Practices: Their Study and Their Potential. In *Approaches to the Social Dimensions of Mortuary Practices*, ed. J. A. Brown, pp. 6–29. Memoirs of the Society for American Archaeology No. 25. Society for American Archaeology, Washington, D.C.

Elera, Carlos G.

1994   El Shaman del Morro de Etén: Antecedentes Arqueológicos del Shamanismo en la Costa y Sierra Norte del Perú. In *El Nombre del Señor*, edited by L. Millones and M. Lemlij, pp. 22–51. Biblioteca Peruana de Psicoanálisis, Lima.

Giese, Claudius Cristobal

1989   *Curanderos: Traditionelle Heiler in Nord-Peru, Küste und Hochland*. Münchner Beitrage zur Americanistik Bd. 20. K. Renner, Hohenschäftlarn.

Guaman Poma de Ayala, Felipe

1987 [1613]   Nueva Corónica y Buen Gobierno. In *Nueva Corónica y Buen Gobierno*, Vol. 1, edited by J. V. Murra, R. Adorno, and J. L. Urioste, pp. 272–74. Historia 16. Madrid.

Knudson, Kelly, and T. Douglas Price

2007   The Utility of Multiple Chemical Techniques in Archaeological Residential Mobility Studies. *American Journal of Physical Anthropology* 132: 25–39.

Lozada, María Cecilia, and Elva Torres

1991   Mortuary Excavations at El Yaral, Southern Peru. Manuscript in senior author's possession.

Lozada, María Cecilia, and Jane E. Buikstra

2002   *El Señorío de Chiribaya en la Costa Sur del Perú*. Instituto de Estudios Peruanos, Lima.

Millones, Luis

1987   *Historia y Poder en los Andes Centrales (Desde los Origenes al Siglo XVII)*. Alianza Editorial, Madrid.

1997   *El Rostro de la Fe: Doce Ensayos Sobre Religiosidad Andina*. Universidad Pablo de Olavide, Fundación El Monte, Sevilla.

Millones, Luis, and Mary Platt

1989   *Amor Brujo: Imagen y Cultura del Amor en los Andes*. Instituto de Estudios Peruanos, Lima.

Tarlow, Sarah

2000   Emotion in Archaeology. *Current Anthropology* 41: 713–46.

Tomczak, Paula

2003   Prehistoric Diet and Socio-economic Relationships within the Osmore Valley of Southern Peru. *Journal of Anthropological Archaeology* 22(3): 262–78.

Urioste, George L.

1981   Sickness and Death in Preconquest Andean Cosmology: The Huarochiri Oral Tradition. In *Health in the Andes*, edited by J. W. Bastien and J. M. Donahue, pp. 9–18. American Anthropological Association, Washington, D.C.

Wassén, Henry S.

1972   *A Medicine-Man's Implements and Plants in a Tiahuanacoid Tomb in Highland Bolivia*. Ethnologiska Studier Vol. 32. Ethnographic Museum, Gothenburg, Sweden.

7 ◆ A Neolithic Nomad from Dakhleh Oasis

Jennifer L. Thompson

Individual Profile

Site: Sheikh Muftah, Dakhleh Oasis, Egypt
Location: 25° 28.99′ north, 29° 06.53′ east
Cultural Affiliation: Sheikh Muftah Cultural Unit, Predynastic
Date: ca. 3200–2000 B.C., radiocarbon dates on charcoal from hearths at several Sheikh Muftah sites (McDonald et al. 2005)
Feature: 365-2
Location of Grave: Northwest corner of Spring Mound, southwest of present-day village of Ezbet Sheikh Muftah
Burial and Grave Type: Single primary inhumation with legs tightly flexed
Associated Materials: Copper pin
Preservation and Completeness: Fair preservation, some skeletal elements highly fragmentary, cranium largely complete, long bones fairly complete
Age at Death and Basis of Estimate: 40–45 years, based on dental wear and pubic symphysis morphology
Sex and Basis of Determination: Male, based on skull and pelvic morphology and overall size and robusticity
Conditions Observed: Peripheral enthesopathies, degenerative joint disease, cervical vertebral fracture, caries, antemortem tooth loss
Specialized Analysis: None
Excavated: 1998, 1999, Dakhleh Oasis Project, Anthony Mills, director, and under the auspices of the Society for the Study of Egyptian Antiquities
Archaeological Report: Thompson 2002, forthcoming; Thompson and Madden 2003, 2006
Current Disposition: Curated, Dakhleh Oasis, Egypt

When thinking about ancient Egypt, most people envision the massive pyramids and pharonic tombs of the dynastic period. But people lived in, and journeyed through, Egypt for millennia before this. Predynastic Neolithic people were not pyramid builders. Instead, they were hunter-gatherers and nomadic pastoralists. It was only fairly recently, during the mid-to-late Holocene, that dramatic climate change resulted in a massive diaspora out of the expanding desert and into the Nile Valley. This influx of people into the Nile Valley is thought to have precipitated the development of the first dynasties in Egypt and culminated in an agricultural revolution. While this scenario is largely correct, it implies that all people migrated to the Nile Valley and became settled agriculturalists and that the desert was completely abandoned. It is now clear that some people remained in the Western Desert oases, and it is likely that some trade and movement persisted between these outlying areas and the Nile region until pharonic times, when regular, frequent travel was more common.

Since 1977 archaeologists, geologists, physical anthropologists, geomorphologists, botanical and faunal experts, and a host of other scientists have been investigating prehistory and history here, from the mid-Pleistocene to Roman times, as part of the Dakhleh Oasis Project (DOP). Through the study of individuals from the cemetery at Kellis (also known as Ismant el-Kharab), a Roman period site (ca. A.D. 100–450) at Dakhleh, we know details of the people who lived here in historic times (Cook et al. 1988; Fairgrieve and Molto 2000; Molto 2000, 2002; Tocheri et al. 2005; Dupras and Tocheri 2007). And we know a great deal about the predynastic people who lived in and near the Nile Valley (Starling and Stock 2007; Zakrzewski 2007). But far less is known about the lives and health status of the earlier, predynastic people who lived at Dakhleh and the other outlying oases. How different were their lives from those in agricultural settlements of the Nile region, and how much contact was there with the Nile Valley? Were they still nomadic pastoralists, or did they grow crops? How did they cope with climate change? Seven Neolithic skeletons have been recovered from Dakhleh Oasis. One of these is the focus of this chapter, and his osteobiography allows us to address some of these questions.

People and Climate at Dakhleh Oasis

Dakhleh Oasis is in the Western Desert of Egypt, roughly 800 km south and west of Cairo and 250 km west of Luxor (figure 7.1) (Mills 1979). One of five major oases in the Western Desert, Dakhleh spans about 100 km east to west and 25 km from north to south (Cook et al. 1988). To the north and east there is a limestone-capped escarpment, rising about 1,000 feet above the terrain and providing an impressive backdrop for the region. To appreciate the impact climate has had on this region, it is important to understand how conditions have changed over time. Today about 75,000 people live in Dakhleh Oasis—a vast, sandy sea dotted with small agricultural villages, cultivations, and palm groves, creating splashes of greenery here and there, connected by a main highway. Dakhleh has electricity, televisions, cell phones, and schools, yet ancient traditions and habits still survive here. It is not uncommon to see farmers traveling with their crops in carts pulled by donkeys, and many buildings are still made of mud bricks. While the term "oasis" conjures up images of sparkling blue ponds of water, Dakhleh's water is pumped from aquifers located deep underground, and that is what allows crops like wheat and dates to be grown here.

Humans and their predecessors (*Homo erectus*) have passed through or lived in Dakhleh from ca. 400,000 B.C. onward as evinced by the stone tools they left

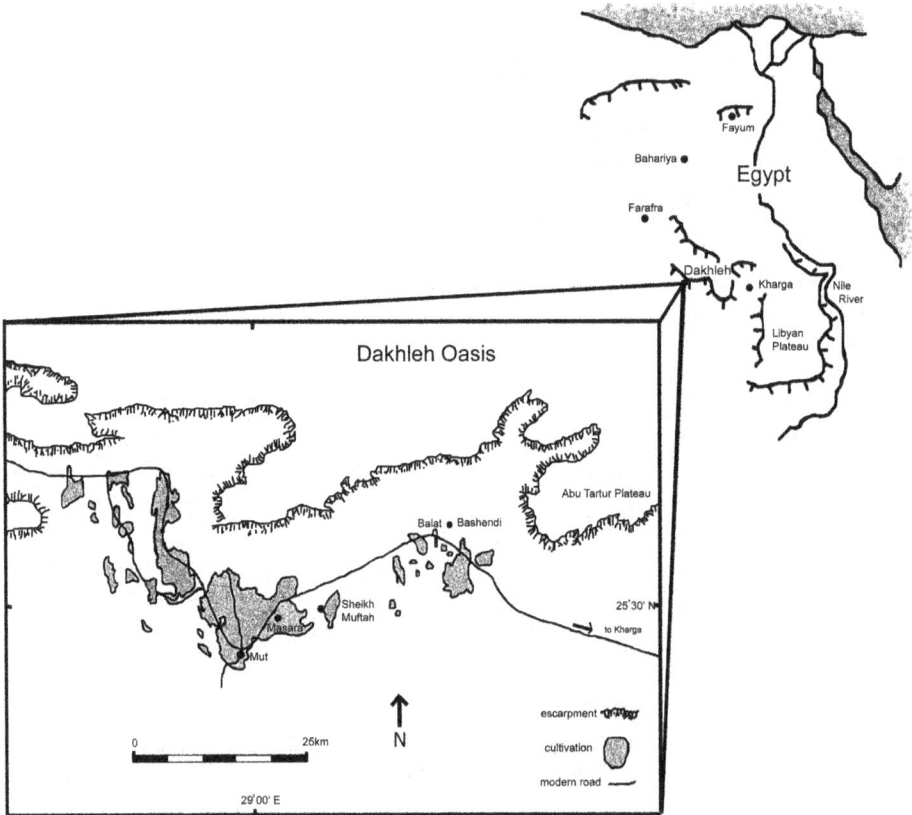

Figure 7.1. Map of Dakhleh Oasis and Egypt. (Courtesy of Colin Hope.)

behind (Kleindienst 2003). At that time shallow lakes covered much of the oases, providing freshwater environments capable of supporting a savanna fauna (Kleindienst et al. 1999; Kleindienst 2003; Kieniewicz and Smith 2009). The ancient lakeshore is described as "bounded with reed thickets, with sandstone ridges separating the shoreline into bays, to which animals from a hinterland of grassy areas interspersed with woodland came to water" (Churcher et al. 1999: 308–9). This would have provided rich floral and faunal resources for the small bands of hunter-gatherer people in the region.

The climate history of the oasis reveals several humid and dry phases that affected its inhabitants' choice of subsistence strategy, particularly in the Holocene period—from about 10,000 B.C. onward. Prior to 5000 B.C. the Western Desert of Egypt experienced a humid phase, but with a couple of dry episodes that each lasted 100–200 years (McDonald 1998). After 5000 B.C. it became increasingly drier, and by 3000 B.C. the climate was similar to what it is today, making the Western Desert largely uninhabitable. By 4300 B.C. (McDonald 2002) the lack of archaeological sites beyond the oasis indicates the region was being depopulated, the refugees moving south and east to resettle in more hospitable environments in the Nile Valley (McDonald 1998). Despite aridification of the region, the inhabitants of Dakhleh, the largest oasis in the Western Desert (McDonald 2002), were somewhat buffered by the continued presence of water. The archaeological record provides evidence of shifts in the economic adaptations of people in Dakhleh in response to that climate change.

As summarized in table 7.1, the Masara people were hunter-gatherers who spent part of their year in the oasis during the Early and Middle Holocene, from around 8300 to 6500 B.C. (McDonald 1990, 1993, 1998, 2001, 2009; Warfe 2003). Hut circles and storage areas dating toward the end of this time span provide evidence of increased sedentism, but grinding stones, stone tools, and faunal remains indicate that wild grain and wild animals (hartebeest, gazelle, hare, birds) were consumed (McDonald 1990, 1998, 2009). As the Middle Holocene desert became less habitable, archaeological evidence from the Bashendi cultural unit (Bashendi A, 6400–5650 B.C., and the later Bashendi B, 5400–3800 B.C.) again indicates increased, perhaps seasonal, use of the oasis. One site dated to late Bashendi A had at least 200 small huts, which suggests a fairly large population of several hundred people. Larger stone structures may have served as pens for herd animals (McDonald 2009).

While the Western Desert was being depopulated after 5000 B.C., Dakhleh Oasis was the exception to this trend, becoming a refugium for the local mobile herder-foragers. The Bashendi B people were mobile herders of cattle and goats (McDonald 2009), but there are no structures suggesting animal pens like

Table 7.1. Dakhleh cultural periods cited in chapter 7

Periods and Dates	Culture	Subsistence
Early–Middle Holocene		
8300–6500 B.C.	Masara	Hunter-gatherers
Middle Holocene		
6400–5650 B.C.	Bashendi A	Mobile herder-foragers
5400–3800 B.C.	Bashendi B	Mobile herder-foragers
Late Holocene		
3200–2000 B.C.	Sheikh Muftah	Mobile herder-foragers (incipient agriculture?)
2200 B.C.	Old Kingdom	Agriculturalists
A. D. 100–450	Roman	Agriculturalists

Sources: Roman Kellis dates from Molto 2002. Other dates modified to B.C. from dates in McDonald 2009, McDonald et al. 2001, and McDonald et al. 2005.

those at older sites. As the drying of the surrounding region required Bashendi B people to rely more heavily on the resources in the oasis, it is *possible* that a shift from nomadic pastoralism to incipient agriculture occurred. However, archaeological evidence is mixed. They herded goats and cattle, but grinding stones and sickle blades indicate plant use (possibly wild sorghum and/or millet), while projectile points and faunal remains again point to hunting. The shift to a primarily agricultural economy did not take place until much later in Old Kingdom times (after 2200 B.C.), but some shift in subsistence strategy is likely during the increasing aridity of the region (MacDonald 2002, 2009).

By Sheikh Muftah times, the late Holocene oasis dwellers were more restricted in mobility, and climatic change would have affected available food resources. The majority of the Sheikh Muftah sites (named after Ezbet Sheikh Muftah, a small village in the area) were located near the center of the oasis, where some water remained available (Churcher 1982; McDonald et al. 2001). At this time Dakhleh was a well-watered, low-lying area with marshes and lakes surrounded by woodland and savanna (Churcher 1981: 210). There is no evidence of the shelters or storage units seen in earlier sites, only what appear to be temporary campsites close to wetlands and artesian springs. Pottery is common on the Sheikh Muftah sites, with some coarse wares showing signs that they were involved in preparing food, dry cooking, and indirect boiling, while finer pottery wares were perhaps used for serving, storage, or transportation (McDonald et al. 2001). Grinding stones, hoes, and sickles are rare, and the sparse paleobotanical evidence does not include any cultigens, although variation in the artifact assemblage suggests increased sedentism.

Faunal remains from Sheikh Muftah sites include cattle, goat, gazelle and hartebeest, wild pig (or warthog), and ostrich eggs. Cattle were herded but were likely not used for their meat; instead, their milk and blood would have been collected (McDonald et al. 2001). Meat came from wild game like gazelle and hartebeest, the remains of which are highly fragmented, suggesting that bones were broken open to obtain marrow, perhaps as a means of maximizing food resources in a time of scarcity (Churcher 1983: 183; Churcher 1999; McDonald 1999: 124). According to Fagan, desert populations "responded to drier conditions by settling closer to permanent water, where they faced the same problem as the people of the Nile—seasonal food shortages and the constant threat of starvation" (1995: 284).

By about 2200 B.C. regular ties with the Nile Valley were reestablished, and the region became controlled by outsiders for political reasons—first by the pharaohs and their representatives, and later by the Romans as part of their political expansion. Thus the archaeological record provides a detailed outline of the occupation of the oases from the mid-Pleistocene to present day. However, what is lacking are the physical remains of the people themselves.

The Neolithic Nomad

During the initial phases of the DOP, the oasis was surveyed to discover the extent and nature of the archaeological remains, from lithic scatters to Roman aqueducts depending upon the time period. Several skeletons were observed (but not excavated) eroding out of sediments beneath (or from) a cultural surface associated with the Sheikh Muftah unit. In 1996 three of these burials (in an extremely fragmentary state of preservation) were formally recorded south and west of the village of Ezbet Sheikh Muftah. In subsequent field seasons, the remains of two additional (nearly complete) individuals were recovered, although any indications of burial walls had long been obliterated. The adult male, the "Neolithic Nomad" discussed here, reflects some of the biological and cultural responses of the people of his time to an increasingly arid and inhospitable environment.

The Neolithic Nomad (figure 7.2) was discovered at the end of the 1998 field season at locality 365, a low mound about 1 m at its highest, with a north–south axis located southwest of Ezbet Sheikh Muftah village and its cultivated fields (Thompson 2002). The most prominent part of the mound is about 3 m long and 1 m wide, with the sides sloping away in all directions to cover a 10 × 7 m area. The burial area was once capped by fist-size sandstone fragments, which had to be carried from at least several hundred meters away. Several ancient eroded-down artesian spring mounds are in the vicinity of the burials (M. Kleindienst, personal communication 1997). This was not a place people lived permanently; it was a place of lakes, streams, and spring mounds, where people brought their herds and where some of their dead were interred.

The Neolithic Nomad has the catalog number 365-2, reflecting the fact that he was the second of three individuals discovered at that locality. Sex was determined on the basis of skull and pelvic morphology and overall size and robusticity following the methods outlined in Buikstra and Ubelaker (1994). His skull was excavated at the time of discovery, but his postcranial skeleton was left in situ to be excavated the following year. The soil of the mound had become hardened mud over the millennia and was reluctant to "give up its dead." The careful excavation of the bones took almost a week. At some point while I was digging with dental picks and brushes alone in the desert, catalog number 365-2 became "George." Despite its European, not Egyptian, roots, the name just came to me. Looking back, perhaps I thought that somehow it was wrong to call him after an Egyptian god. Lying on my side, ignoring the blowing sand and occasional visiting fly, paying no attention to the donkey's braying and prayer calls drifting across the desert from Sheikh Muftah, I breathed in his bone dust, and he became real to me, and I felt compelled to name him as a person, not a god.

The mound was some distance from the modern village and outside the cultivation area, and because the ancient bones were of little interest to the local residents, no guards were posted at the site. But one night during the excavation vandals ripped George's femur out of the ground and hacked into the mound in search of treasure. The leg bone was left in fragments on the ground next to the disturbed area, but luckily they did no more damage to George's skeleton.

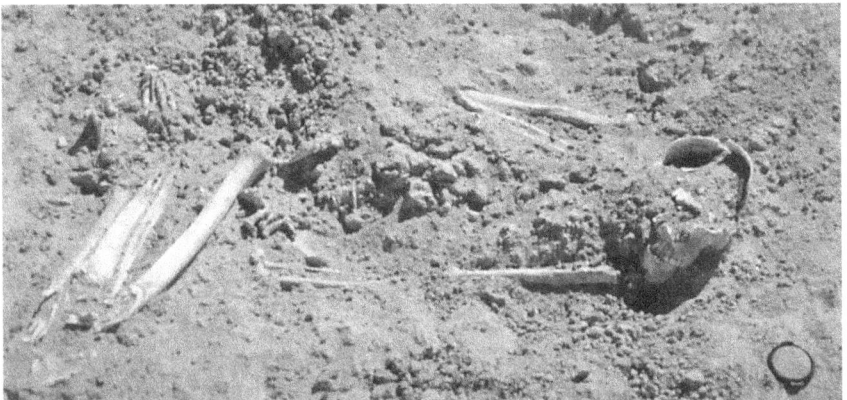

Figure 7.2. Skeleton of the "Neolithic Nomad" in situ.

The local police were sent for, but all they could see were traces of footprints heading away from the site toward the village. After that two guards kept vigil at night until all of George's bones had been excavated.

He had been buried with his legs in a flexed position, his head at the west end of the grave, his right arm across his chest, and his left arm parallel to the body (Thompson 2002). A young male (about 20 years of age) and a female (about 20–25 years of age) were buried in the same mound. Four additional individuals from the same time period have also been discovered and analyzed. Their relationship to George is not known, but it is clear that the dead were buried with some ceremony at this time. Although George was the only individual found with any grave goods, four of the other burials were also buried in a similar manner, with legs in a flexed position.

Osteobiography

George was about 40–45 years of age (based on the degree of dental wear on his teeth and morphology of the pubic symphysis) when he died, and as a result his skeleton reveals a great deal about the lifestyle of this time period. George was about 168.1 cm (5 feet 6 inches) in height, which was about average for predynastic Egyptian males. His skull has widely flaring zygomatic arches; his face is long and relatively narrow, with a deep mandible. His teeth are of interest as he had a maloccluded premolar tooth in his upper jaw. His lower jaw shows definite evidence of periodontal disease in the form of vertical bone loss on the buccal side of several mandibular teeth. He lost several teeth during life, likely the result of caries and periodontal disease.

The occlusal (chewing) surface of George's molars exhibit cupped wear (figure 7.3). Studies of dental wear show that foragers tend to wear their teeth flat, while agriculturalists present with cupped wear. This cupped wear likely results from the use of grinding stones to process grain, thus introducing fine particles into the mouth that cause more rapid wear (Smith 1984). Grinding stones were used to process wild plant food at Dakhleh since at least Masara times, so cupped wear does not, by itself, tell us that George and his people were processing domesticated plants, only that they were processing some type of plant remains (for example, wild millet or sorghum as at Nabta Playa—see below) or ingesting some grit along with the food they were eating.

Burials from Nabta Playa, a desert site south of Dakhleh, also show cupped wear on their teeth (Irish 2001). These people are from late Masara and Bashendi times, predating George. Like the previous inhabitants at Dakhleh, the Nabta Playa people were not agriculturalists, but instead they gathered wild

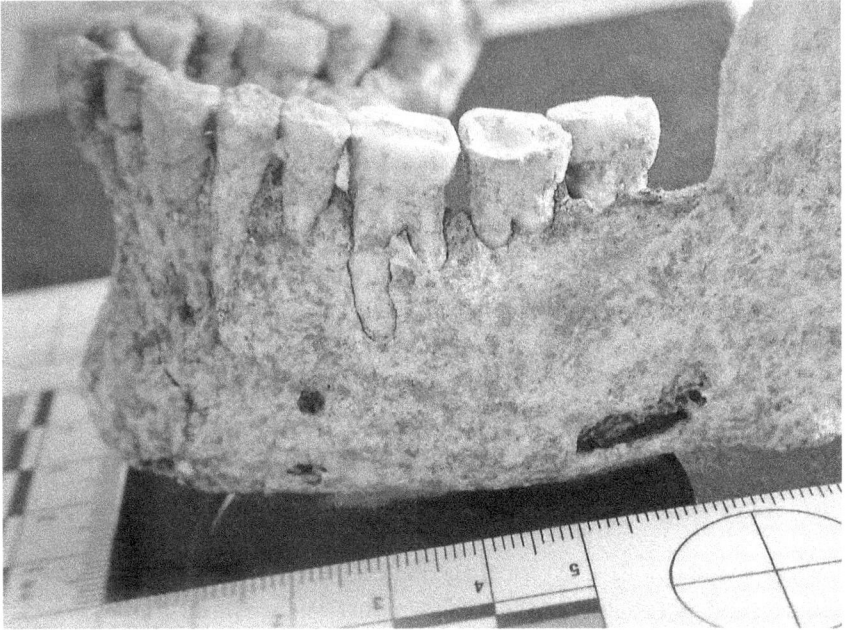

Figure 7.3. George's mandible showing the molar wear pattern.

seeds like sorghum and millet, and processed and stored them in pots. Unlike true agriculturalists, they do not exhibit the extensive caries lesions or calculus deposits that result from eating plant foods high in carbohydrates (Irish 2001: 523). With the increase of starch in the diet, linked to the introduction of cereal agriculture, root caries are more common, especially in adults, and root caries are also linked to periodontal disease (Hillson 1996).

George also suffered from root caries (on two upper left molars) and had lost two upper right molars (only roots remain). He had periodontal disease and had some calculus deposits on his teeth (as did some of the other Sheikh Muftah burials). Together, these data are suggestive of increased carbohydrate consumption during Sheikh Muftah times.

Turning to the postcranial skeleton, George presented with a compression fracture in one of his cervical vertebrae at stage 2–3 in terms of its severity (Rah and Errico 1998). This was possibly the result of the microtrauma (small tears or breaks in the tissue) experienced during repetitive mechanical stress associated with daily tasks (Thompson and Madden 2006) and may suggest that George may have regularly carried heavy objects on his head—heavily laden baskets or pots, for example (Bridges 1991, 1994; Lovell 1994). An alternative explanation is that this incidence of osteoarthritis is age related. The large deltoid muscle attachment areas on his humeri indicate that George made repetitive use of his arms to undertake strenuous activities. George also presented with degenerative joint disease, or arthritis, on all vertebrae. In addition, George showed arthritic changes in his shoulders and elbows: lipping at the glenoid fossa of the scapula, the distal humerus, the proximal radius and ulna, and the clavicle. All these arthritic changes point to everyday wear and tear. In George's case, these skeletal changes point to an active lifestyle and accumulating evidence of physical stress over his relatively long life.

George had calcaneal (heel) spurs on both feet (figure 7.4). These are seen as a small buildup of bone on the bottom of the heel at the attachment area of the *abductor hallucis* muscle (Larsen 1997; Capasso et al. 1999; Cox and Mays 2000). These are markers of strenuous activity and may result from high levels of walking and running. Sometimes called medial process spurs, they have been seen in modern-day athletes and in Neolithic long-distance travelers from Nigeria (Dutour 1986; Capasso et al. 1999). People with heel spurs suffer continuing pain, and the etiology of the spur may be related not only to increased activity but also to increased weight bearing (Smith et al. 2007). While in living people these spurs are more commonly associated with increased body weight, given George's compressed neck vertebrae his heel spurs seem likely to be the result of carrying heavy objects as well as traveling over long distances.

Another measure of activity level in ancient people is the pilasteric index, which reflects robusticity of the femur. The index is based on measurements of

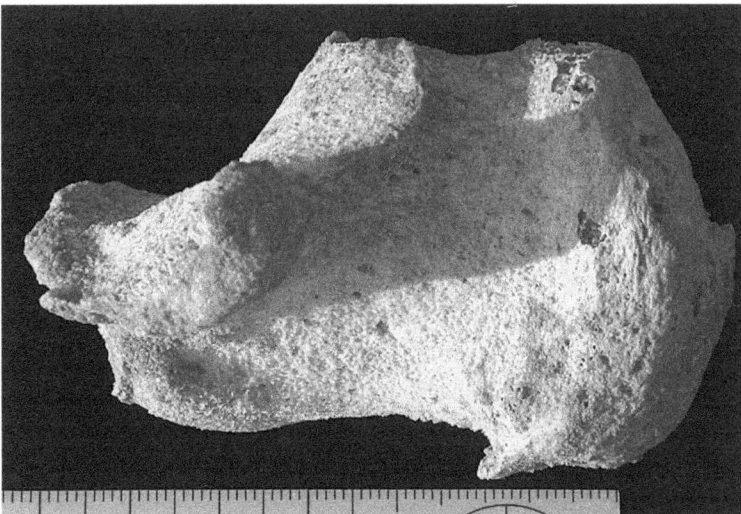

Figure 7.4. Spur (at bottom right) on George's calcaneus.

the femur at midshaft and relates the width to the length of the bone. People with a more active lifestyle typically have narrower femora at midshaft than those who are more sedentary, whose femora tend to be rounder. A ratio of close to 100 is most common in sedentary, agricultural populations, suggesting a decrease in running or long-distance travel (Bridges 1995). George's pilasteric index is 111, and while this is not as high as in some hunter-gatherer populations from North America (as high as >115 in some males, according to Bridges et al. 2000), it is comparable to the pilasteric index in male Badarians, nomadic pastoralists who lived, before George's time, near and in the Nile Valley (Thompson forthcoming). All these skeletal features support the idea that George's lifestyle was an active, nomadic one.

Clues to Social and Economic Organization in the Neolithic

A small copper pin, about two inches long and an eighth of an inch wide (figure 7.5), was found under George's pelvis. Males from the Nile Valley are known to have carried copper pins (of unknown function) in leather pouches at their waists (Friedman 1998), and so it is likely that George did also. This common practice reinforces the notion of contact between the Nile Valley and Dakhleh. Additional evidence comes from ceramics from Sheikh Muftah contexts, which include Badarian and Naqadan pottery from the Nile Valley (McDonald 1996; Hope 2002; Warfe 2003). In addition, pottery recently discovered in Kharga Oasis, located between Dakhleh and the Nile Valley, resembles pottery found at Bashendi and Sheikh Muftah sites, suggesting "the existence of an over-arching pottery tradition linking the two oases" (McDonald et al. 2005: 6). The two oases are over 100 km apart, but they are linked by the edge of the Libyan plateau, which bounds them both, with evidence of a number of Holocene localities along the foot of the escarpment between them (McDonald 2009: 10).

Archaeologist Mary McDonald (2008, 2009: 27, 37) notes that owning livestock can often lead to the accumulation of wealth and increases in status differences between people in a group, and she argues indications of "competitive prestige technologies" appear late in Bashendi A times (labrets; marine shell pendants; larger, carefully made arrowheads; some pottery) and become more varied by Bashendi B, to include small polished axes, arm rings, and beads made of semiprecious stone. She suggests that the emergence of elite groups in the predynastic Nile Valley might owe its origins to mobile pastoralists like the Bashendi people, many of whom migrated to the Nile Valley to escape the expanding desert.

Returning to our individual, does the possession of a copper pin mean that

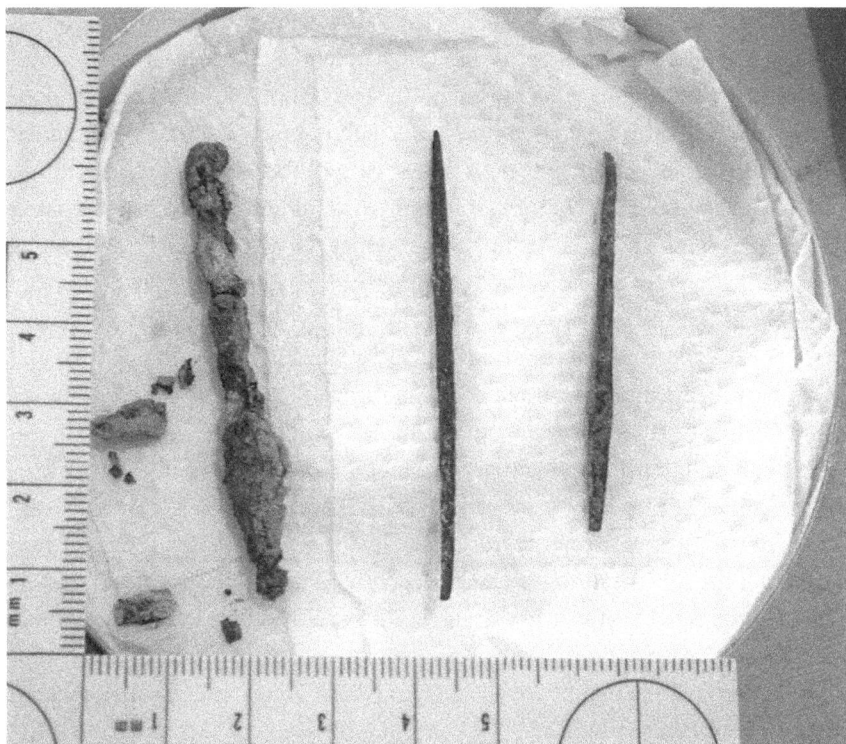

Figure 7.5. The highly corroded copper pin found with George (on left), next to two better preserved pins from another feature.

George was wealthy? Not necessarily. The Nile Valley males who were found with similar pins came from a cemetery of Hierakonpolis's working-class inhabitants (Friedman 1998). Other than this pin, no archaeological materials are directly associated with any of the seven burials excavated. Among the Sheikh Muftah people, the "lack of noticeable burial monuments or of elaborate grave goods . . . reinforces the picture of small, egalitarian groups" (McDonald et al. 2001: 9).

Conclusion

During the Sheikh Muftah cultural period, the region surrounding Dakhleh Oasis was increasingly inhospitable (McDonald et al. 2001), and diminishing water sources led to the restriction of people to the more central part of the oasis. George gives us special insight into the lifeways of the Neolithic pastoral people of Dakhleh Oasis at this particular time. George lived to about 40 years, long enough to develop age-related arthritis throughout his body. In addition to evidence of arthritis linked to repetitive activities, the massive deltoid attachment areas, his pilasteric index, and the presence of mechanically induced enthesopathic lesions on his heels suggest a highly active lifestyle. His particular dental pathologies and form of dental wear suggest that the response to climate change included the cultivation of plants here, or at least an increased reliance on wild plants high in carbohydrates. The copper pin buried with George, along with ceramic evidence, indicates that the Dakhleh people maintained contact with other areas in Egypt, including the Nile Valley. This pin is the only suggestion of grave goods in the small assemblage of burials from George's time and place. Future research may provide a clearer understanding of what this means about George as an individual in an egalitarian culture.

Skeletal remains in Dakhleh become much more plentiful in the later Holocene, in Roman times, when burial in cemeteries was more common. Those populations of primarily agricultural people provide rich sources of information about the diet, health, and social structure of late Holocene people in this oasis. Comparatively little is known about the earlier people living in Dakhleh, but the study of individuals like George, interpreted as part of the rich archaeological record (McDonald 2009), is helping us to better understand the Neolithic, nomadic oasis dwellers of Dakhleh and the Western Desert.

Acknowledgments

In addition to the Society for the Study of Egyptian Antiquities, the Dakhleh Oasis Project is supported by a number of universities and organizations, including the Dakhleh Trust. Funding for the 1999 season was provided by the Department of Anthropology, University of Nevada, Las Vegas. Thanks to Maxine Kleindienst, Rufus Churcher, Mary McDonald, and Anthony Mills for inviting me to join the Dakhleh Oasis Project. Special thanks to Mary McDonald for identification of associated lithic artifacts and assistance in the field, and to Colin Hope for his assessment of the pottery and copper artifacts associated with these finds. I thank the editors for their invitation to be part of this volume. Finally, thanks to the staff on the project for facilitating the excavations in the Dakhleh Oasis.

References Cited

Bridges, Patricia S.

1991   Degenerative Joint Disease in Hunter-Gatherers and Agriculturalists from the Southeastern United States. *American Journal of Physical Anthropology* 85: 379–91.

1994   Vertebral Arthritis and Physical Activities in the Prehistoric Southeastern United States. *American Journal of Physical Anthropology* 93: 83–93.

1995   Skeletal Biology and Behavior in Ancient Humans. *Evolutionary Anthropology* 4: 112–20.

Bridges, Patricia S., with J. H. Blitz and M. C. Solano

2000   Changes in Long Bone Diaphyseal Strength with Horticultural Intensification in West-Central Illinois. *American Journal of Physical Anthropology* 112: 217–38.

Buikstra, Jane E., and Douglas H. Ubelaker (editors)

1994   *Standards for Data Collection from Human Skeletal Remains.* Arkansas Archeological Survey Research Series No. 44. Arkansas Archeological Survey, Fayetteville.

Capasso, Luigi, Kenneth A. R. Kennedy, and Cynthia A. Wilczak

1999   *Atlas of Occupational Markers on Human Remains.* Journal of Paleopathology Monographic Publication 3. Edigrafital S.p.A., Termano, Italy.

Churcher, Charles S.

1981   Geology and Paleontology: Interim Report on the 1980 field Season. *Journal of the Society for the Study of Egyptian Antiquities* 11: 193–212.

1982   Geology and Paleontology: Interim Report on the 1981 Field Season. *Journal of the Society for the Study of Egyptian Antiquities* 12: 103–14.

1983   Dakhleh Oasis Project—Palaeontology: Interim Report on the 1982 Field Season. *Journal Society for the Study of Egyptian Antiquities* 13: 178–87.

1999   Holocene Faunas of the Dakhleh Oasis. In *Reports from the Survey of the Dakhleh Oasis, Western Desert of Egypt, 1977–1987,* edited by C. S. Churcher and A. J. Mills, pp. 133–51. Oxbow Books, Oxford.

Churcher, Charles S., Maxine R. Kleindienst, and Henry P. Schwartz

1999   Faunal Remains from a Middle Pleistocene Lacustrine Marl in Dakhleh Oasis, Egypt: Palaeoenvironmental Reconstructions. *Palaeogeography, Palaeoclimatology, Palaeoecology* 154: 301–12.

Cook, Megan, J. Eldon Molto, and Colin Anderson

1988   Possible Case of Hyperparathyroidism in a Roman Period Skeleton from the Dakhleh Oasis, Egypt, Diagnosed Using Bone Histomorphometry. *American Journal of Physical Anthropology* 75: 23–30.

Cox, Margaret, and Simon Mays

2000   *Human Osteology in Archaeology and Forensic Science.* Greenwich Medical Media, London.

Dupras, Tosha L., and Matthew W. Tocheri

2007   Reconstructing Infant Weaning Histories at Roman Period Kellis, Egypt, Using Stable Isotope Analysis of Dentition. *American Journal of Physical Anthropology* 134: 63–74.

Dutour, Olivier

1986   Enthesopathies (Lesions of Muscular Insertions) as Indicators of the Activities of Neolithic Saharan Populations. *American Journal of Physical Anthropology* 71: 221–24.

Fagan, Brian
1995   *People of the Earth*. Harper Collins, New York.

Fairgrieve, Scott I., and J. Eldon Molto
2000   Cribra Orbitalia in Two Temporally Disjunct Population Samples from the Dakhleh Oasis, Egypt. *American Journal of Physical Anthropology* 111: 319–31.

Friedman, Renée
1998   More Mummies: The 1998 Season at HK 43. *Nekhen News* 10: 4–6.

Hillson, Simon
1996   *Dental Anthropology*. Cambridge University Press, Cambridge.

Hope, Colin A.
2002   Early and Mid-Holocene Ceramics from the Dakhleh Oasis: Traditions and Influences. In *Egypt and Nubia Gifts of the Desert*, edited by R. Friedman, pp. 39–61. British Museum Press, London.

Irish, Joel
2001   Human Skeletal Remains from Three Nabta Playa Sites. In *Holocene Settlement of the Egyptian Sahara*, Vol. 1, *The Archaeology of Nabta Playa*, edited by F. Wendorf and R. Schild, pp. 521–28. Kluwer Academic/Plenum, New York.

Kieniewicz, Johanna M., and Jennifer R. Smith
2009   Paleoenvironmental Reconstruction and Water Balance of a Mid-Pleistocene Pluvial Lake, Dakhleh Oasis, Egypt. *Geological Society of America Bulletin* 121: 1154–71.

Kleindienst, Maxine R.
2003   Strategies for Studying Pleistocene Archaeology Based upon Surface Evidence: First Characterization of an Older Middle Stone Age Unit, Dakhleh Oasis, Western Desert, Egypt. In *The Oasis Papers III: Proceedings of the Third International Conference of the Dakhleh Oasis Project*, edited by C. A. Hope, pp. 1–42. Oxbow Books, Oxford.

Kleindienst, Maxine R., Charles S. Churcher, Mary M. A. McDonald, and Henry P. Schwarcz
1999   Geography, Geology, Geochronology, and Geoarchaeology of the Dakhleh Oasis Region: An Interim Report. In *Reports from the Survey of Dakhleh Oasis, 1977–1987*, edited by C. S. Churcher and A. J. Mills, pp. 1–54. Oxbow Books, Oxford.

Larsen, Clark S.
1997   *Bioarchaeology: Interpreting Behavior from the Human Skeleton*. Cambridge University Press, Cambridge.

Lovell, Nancy C.
1994   Spinal Arthritis and Physical Stress at Bronze Age Harappa. *American Journal of Physical Anthropology* 93: 149–64.

McDonald, Mary M. A.
1990   New Evidence from the Early to Mid-Holocene in Dakhleh Oasis, South-Central Egypt, Bearing on the Evolution of Cattle Pastoralism. *Nyame Akuma* 33: 3–9.
1993   Cultural Adaptations in Dakhleh Oasis, Egypt, in the Early to Mid-Holocene. In *Environmental Change and Human Culture in the Nile Basin and Northern Africa until the Second Millennium B.C.*, edited by L. Krzyżaniak, M. Kobusiewicz, and J. Alexander, pp. 199–209. Poznań Archaeological Museum, Poznań.
1996   Relations Between Dakhleh Oasis and the Nile Valley in the Mid-Holocene: A Dis-

cussion. In *Interregional Contacts in the Later Prehistory of Northeastern Africa*, edited by L. Krzyżaniak, K. Kroeper, and M. Kobusiewicz, pp. 93–99. Poznań Archaeological Museum, Poznań.

1998   Early African Pastoralism: View from Dakhleh Oasis (South Central Egypt). *Journal of Anthropological Archaeology* 17: 124–42.

1999   Neolithic Cultural Units and Adaptations in Dakhleh Oasis, Egypt. In *Dakhleh Oasis Project*, edited by A. J. Mills and C. S. Churcher, pp. 117–32. Oxbow Press, Oxford.

2001   The Late Prehistoric Radiocarbon Chronology for Dakhleh Oasis within the Wider Environmental and Cultural Setting of the Egyptian Western Desert. In *The Oasis Papers I: The Proceedings of the First Conference of the Dakhleh Oasis Project*, edited by C. A. Marlow and A. J. Mills, pp. 26–42. Oxbow Press, Oxford.

2002   Dakhleh Oasis in Predynastic and Early Dynastic Times: Bashendi B and the Sheikh Muftah Cultural Units. *Archéo-Nil* 12: 109–20.

2008   Emerging Social Complexity in the Mid-Holocene Egyptian Western Desert: Site 270 and Its Neighbours in Southeastern Dakhleh Oasis. In *The Oasis Papers 2, Proceedings of the Second International Conference of the Dakhleh Oasis Project*, edited by M. F. Wiseman, pp. 83–106. Oxbow Books, Oxford.

2009   Increased Sedentism in the Central Oases of the Egyptian Western Desert in the Early to Mid-Holocene: Evidence from the Peripheries. *African Archaeology Review* 26: 3–43.

McDonald, Mary M. A., Charles S. Churcher, Ursula Thanheiser, Jennifer L. Thompson, Ines Teubner, and Ashton Warfe

2001   The Mid-Holocene Sheikh Muftah Cultural Unit of Dakhleh Oasis, South Central Egypt: A Preliminary Report on Recent Fieldwork. *Nyame Akuma* 56: 4–10.

McDonald, Mary M. A., Jennifer R. Smith, Ashten R. Warfe, Johanna M. Kieniewicz, and Katherine A. Adelsberger

2005   Report on the 2005 Field Activities of the Kharga Oasis Prehistoric Project (KOPP). *Nyame Akuma* 64: 2–9.

Mills, Anthony J.

1979   Dakhleh Oasis Project: Report on the First Season of Survey, October–December, 1978. *Journal of the Society for the Study of Egyptian Antiquities* 9: 163–85.

Molto, J. Eldon

2000   The Comparative Skeletal Biology and Palaeoepidemiology of the People from Ein Tirghi and Kellis, Dakhleh Oasis, Egypt. In *The Oasis Papers I: The Proceedings of the First Conference of the Dakhleh Oasis Project*, edited by C. A. Marlow and A. J. Mills, pp. 81–100. Oxbow Books, Oxford.

2002   Bio-archaeological Research of Kellis 2: An Overview. In *Dakhleh Oasis Project: Preliminary Reports on the 1994–1995 to 1998–1999 Field Seasons*, edited by C. A. Hope and G. E. Bowen, pp. 239–55. Oxbow Books, Oxford.

Rah, Andrew D., and Thomas J. Errico

1998   Classification of Lower Cervical Fractures and Dislocations. In *The Cervical Spine*, edited by C. Clark, pp. 499–556. Lippincott-Raven, Philadelphia.

Smith, B. Holly

1984   Patterns of Molar Wear in Hunter-Gatherers and Agriculturalists. *American Journal of Physical Anthropology* 63: 39–56.

Smith, Simon, Paul Tinley, Mark Gilheany, Brian Grills, and Andrew Kingsford

2007   The Inferior Calcaneal Spur—Anatomical and Histological Considerations. *Foot* 17: 25–31.

Starling Anne P., and Jay T. Stock

2007   Dental Indicators of Health and Stress in Early Egyptian and Nubian Agriculturalists: A Difficult Transition and Gradual Recovery. *American Journal of Physical Anthropology* 134: 520–28.

Thompson, Jennifer L.

2002   Neolithic Burials at Sheikh Muftah, Dakhleh Oasis, Egypt: A Preliminary Report. In *Dakhleh Oasis Project: Preliminary Reports on the 1994–1995 to 1998–1999 Field Seasons*, edited by C. A. Hope and G. E. Bowen, pp. 43–45. Oxbow Books, Oxford.

Forthcoming   Neolithic People from Dakhleh Oasis. In *The Oasis Papers V: Proceedings of the Fourth and Fifth International Conference of the Dakhleh Oasis Project* (volume in preparation), edited by Olaf Kaper, Fred Leemhuis, Anthony Mills, and Verena Obrecht. Oxbow Books, Oxford.

Thompson, Jennifer L., and Gwyn D. Madden

2003   Health and Disease of Neolithic Remains from Sheikh Muftah, Dakhleh Oasis. In *The Oasis Papers III: Proceedings of the Third International Conference of the Dakhleh Oasis Project*, edited by G. E. Bowen and C. A. Hope, pp. 71–76. Oxbow Books, Oxford.

2006   Skeletal Biology of Neolithic Human Remains from Dakhleh Oasis, Egypt. In *Archaeology of Early Northeastern Africa*, edited by K. Kroeper, M. Chłodnicki, and M. Kobusiewicz, pp. 527–38. Poznań Archaeological Museum, Poznań.

Tocheri, Matthew W., Tosha L. Dupras, Peter Sheldrick, and J. Eldon Molto

2005   Roman Period Fetal Skeletons from the East Cemetery (Kellis 2) of Kellis, Egypt. *International Journal of Osteoarchaeology* 15: 326–41.

Warfe, Ashton R.

2003   Cultural Origins of the Egyptian Neolithic and Predynastic: An Evaluation of the Evidence from the Dakhleh Oasis (South Central Egypt). *African Archeological Review* 20: 175–202.

Zakrzewski, Sonia R.

2007   Population Continuity or Population Change: Formation of the Ancient Egyptian State. *American Journal of Physical Anthropology* 132: 501–9.

8 ◆ Lesley

A Unique Bronze Age Individual from Southeastern Arabia

Debra L. Martin and Daniel T. Potts

Individual Profile

Site: Tell Abraq

Location: Sharjah, United Arab Emirates (on the coast about 16 km north of Dubai) N25°29.36.5, E55°33.03.0

Cultural Affiliation: Bronze Age

Date: Ca. 2100–2000 B.C.

Feature: Collective tomb

Location of Grave: Within a multiperiod settlement mound, 10 m west of a contemporary fortification tower

Burial and Grave Type: Circular Umm an-Nar–type burial built of beach rock and limestone ashlar masonry

Associated Materials: In the collective tomb—ceramics, soft-stone and alabaster vessels, bronze weaponry, jewelry including carnelian, lapis, gold, silver, agate beads

Preservation and Completeness: Complete but fragmentary with much exfoliation of bone surfaces

Age at Death and Basis of Estimate: 18–20, based on pubic symphysis, epiphyseal union, dental eruption

Sex and Basis of Determination: Female, based on pelvis morphology including sciatic notch, subpubic angle, and ventral arc

Conditions Observed: Neuromuscular disease of unknown origin

Specialized Analyses: Radiography

Excavated: 1993–1998

Archaeological Report: Potts 2000a

Current Disposition: Department of Anthropology and Ethnic Studies, University of Nevada, Las Vegas, Human Remains Storage Facility WRI C206

Tell Abraq is a multiperiod settlement on the Persian Gulf coast of the United Arab Emirates that was occupied continuously from ca. 2200 to 400 B.C., with evidence of limited reuse in the first and third centuries A.D. (Potts 2000a) (figure 8.1). The site consisted originally of a massive fortification tower, about 40 m in diameter and 8 m high, built of a combination of mudbrick and stone, around which the inhabitants lived in palm-frond houses, similar to the traditional *barasti* or *'arish* constructions that can still be found in the mountains and along the coast to the north of the site (Dostal 1983).

The people of Tell Abraq herded sheep, goats, and cattle (Stephan 1995; Uerpmann 2001); grew date palms; and intercropped domesticated wheat and barley (Willcox and Tengberg 1995), probably in the shade of the date palms. These resources were supplemented by locally available fish and shellfish, marine mammals like dugong, green turtle (*Chelonia mydas*), and wild terrestrial fauna such as oryx, gazelle, and dromedary camel (Uerpmann and Uerpmann 2002). Although rainfall in this part of Arabia is insufficient for dry-farming, a 16 m deep well in the center of the fortification tower provided a stable source of water for drinking and irrigation. While Tell Abraq today is located slightly inland from the coast, on the edge of a *sabkha*, or salt flat, local geomorphology indicates that in the third millennium B.C., when the site was founded, the fortification tower and surrounding houses were less than 100 m from the water's edge (Dalongeville 1990).

Until the late first millennium B.C., the dead in this part of Arabia were typically buried in collective rather than individual tombs. In the late third millennium B.C. (Umm an-Nar period, ca. 2500–2000 B.C.) such tombs were circular (Blau 2001; Potts 2001: 40) and were typically constructed of unworked local stone, faced with finely masoned blocks of limestone. For use at Tell Abraq, this stone had to have been transported from a distance of at least 50 km. Tombs of this sort vary from about 4 to 14 m in diameter, with a variable number of internal walls dividing the space into separate chambers.

One such tomb, about 6 m in diameter, was discovered 10 m west of the fortification tower at Tell Abraq (Potts 1990, 1991, 2000a, 2000b) (figure 8.2). The tomb was constructed of beach rock, a calcareous concretion that forms immediately offshore in the shallow waters of coastal lagoons, faced with standard cut limestone blocks. A single internal wall running south from the northern side of the tomb divided the internal space into two chambers. The wall stopped short of the southern side of the tomb, creating a passageway between the eastern and western chambers. This passageway was situated almost directly opposite a large, trapezoidal stone in the outer wall, which gave the appearance of being removable, perhaps functioning as a portholelike point of entry to the

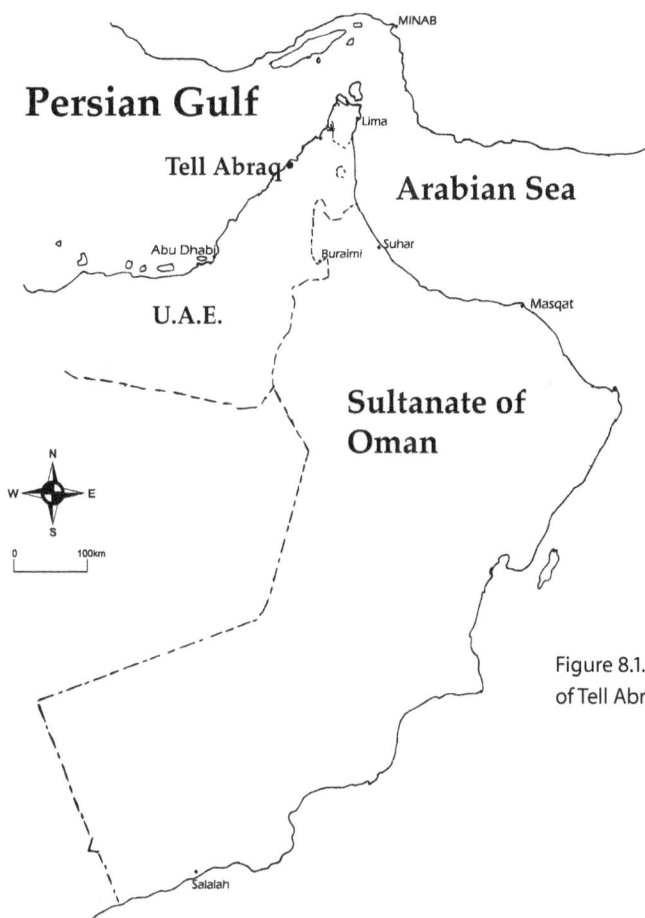

Figure 8.1. The location of Tell Abraq.

interior of the tomb. The entry would have been used for the addition of the dead over the one or possibly two centuries that the tomb was in use. Several large, flat slabs of beach rock on the eastern side of the tomb were probably some of the tomb's original roof slabs. Thus we imagine a structure that was somewhat like an igloo, albeit with a flat roof and a point of entry raised about 75 cm above the external ground surface.

This collective tomb at Tell Abraq contained well over 300 individuals. Excavations revealed a rather a dense bone bed of commingled remains. Working in small units (1 × 1 m squares, subdivided further into four 50 × 50 cm sectors), layer by layer, we mapped, photographed, and excavated jumbled bones representing individuals of every age and sex. On rare occasions several vertebrae or long bones were found in articulation, but the vast majority of the remains were commingled.

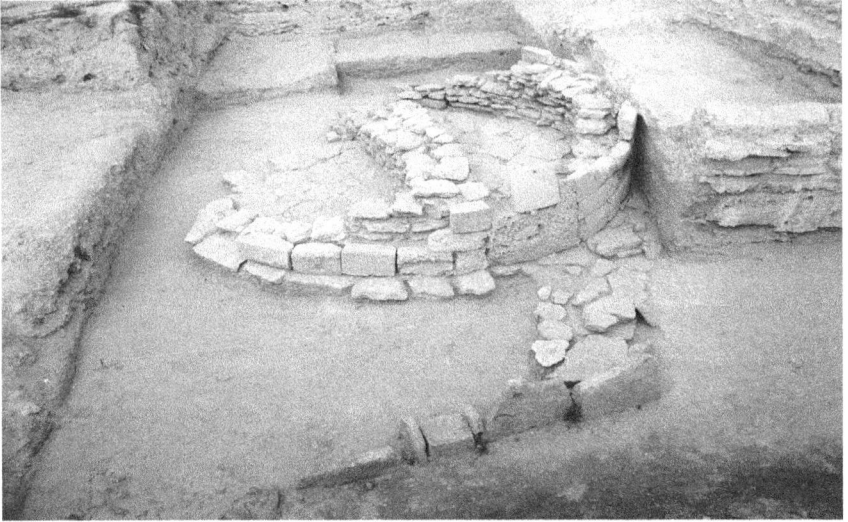

Figure 8.2. The Tell Abraq tomb fully excavated showing the flagstone floor, the central dividing wall, and the only entrance through the keyhole-style ashlar stone door. Lesley was located in the passageway space between the wall and the ending of the dividing wall.

Lesley

The only exception was Lesley. Her complete, articulated, and fairly well preserved skeleton was found in the passageway linking the eastern and western chambers, directly opposite the presumed entrance to the tomb. Her body was lying in a flexed position in the passageway, with disarticulated and jumbled bones of other adults and subadults both below her and above her (figures 8.3, 8.4).

The excavation of a commingled tomb of this magnitude was an arduous and physically demanding task in a dusty and very hot climate. Perhaps it was the exhausting conditions that made the revelation of a complete human skeleton cause for emotional celebration amid shock and surprise. The skeleton was easily aged and sexed while still in situ. The young Australian archaeologists in charge of the excavation of the tomb (Soren Blau and Jodie Benton) may have identified with this young woman from the past, and for reasons now forgotten, she was dubbed "Lesley." The name, certainly unconventional given her Arabian ancestry, stayed with us as a way to quickly refer to this remarkable and unique individual.

In use for two centuries, and containing well over 300 individuals of all ages and both sexes, this tomb was likely a repository for more individuals than those who died at this particular settlement. Lesley represents the only primary, undisturbed interment. While we do not yet know the full range of mortuary

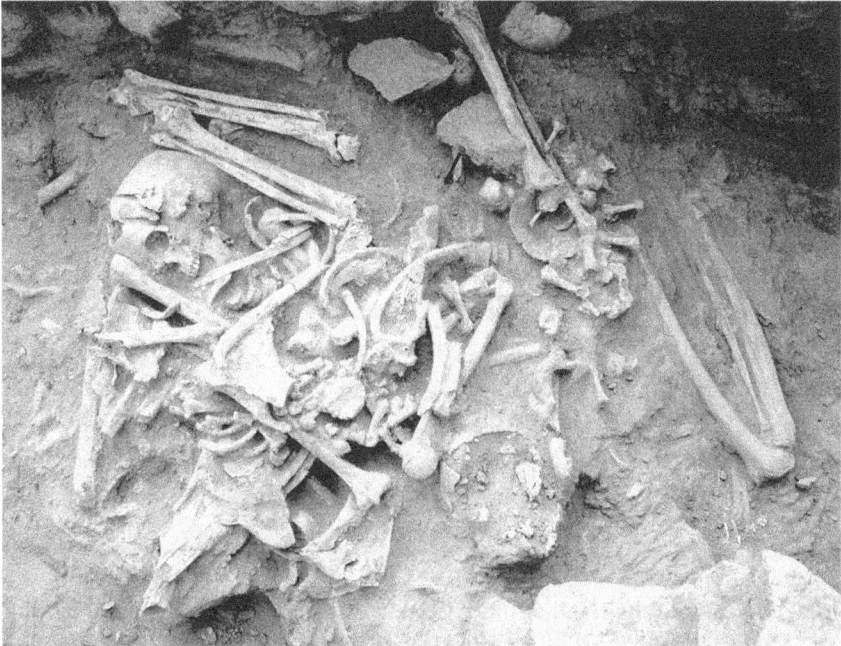

Figure 8.3. A view from on top of the inside dividing wall, looking down at the commingled remains of many individuals. Lesley is partially revealed with her cranium in the upper left and her long, thin lower legs (bent at the knees) on the far right.

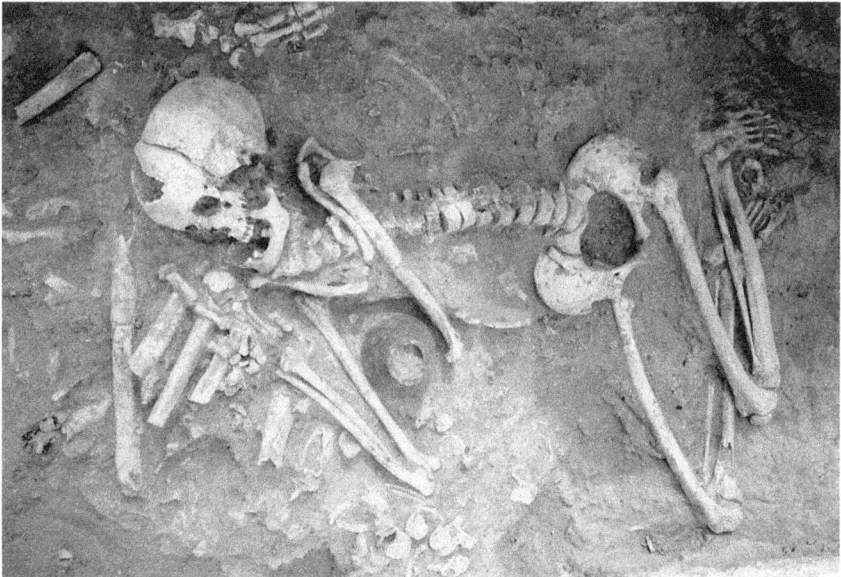

Figure 8.4. Lesley's skeleton fully exposed. View from atop the outer wall of the tomb, looking into the passageway between the outer wall and the inner dividing wall. The pottery may or may not have been associated with Lesley. Note the long, thin, and featureless femora and the extreme thinness of the right fibula.

programs employed at Tell Abraq, a predominant practice of secondary burial would account for the disarticulation of every individual except for Lesley. There are a small number of bones that have spiral fractures (indicating that they were broken around the time of death) and slight burning. But why was this one individual buried such that her skeleton remained articulated? One hypothesis is that her unusual medical condition marked her as different and perhaps dangerous, and her body was put in some very durable bag or shroud that eroded more slowly than the body did. By the time the container (perhaps a bag of leather or fiber or perhaps a wood box) eroded, the body remained in its original articulated position, which was surprising given the disarticulated nature of the bones above and below her.

We estimate that Lesley died between the ages of 18 and 20, based on her well-preserved pubic symphysis, auricular surface morphology, and stage of epiphyseal union. Diagnostic features of the pelvis indicate that she was female. A huge range of variation in robusticity, shape, and size is represented among the many adult long bones retrieved from the tomb. Even so, Lesley's extremely long, thin femora stand out as unique. With the opportunity to radiograph her long bones at the local hospital in the Emirate of Umm al Quwain, the attending radiologist pronounced that this individual had poliomyelitis. The technician offered that he had seen many cases such as this on the Arabian Peninsula, with long and thin leg bones.[1] He suggested that this was an endemic problem in the region for those living in poverty. If only diagnosis of paleopathologies were that easy. In the last 15 years, several physicians and many students have studied Lesley in order to confirm or reject the hypothesis that she was suffering from poliomyelitis at the time of death. What follows is our process of differential diagnosis.

Major skeletal observations are summarized here, moving from subclinical (less serious) to more clinically significant (and possibly debilitating) changes:

1. The long bones of the legs are markedly gracile, long, and thin (see figures 8.3 and 8.4).
2. In the pelvic girdle there is abnormal upward curvature of the sacrum-coccyx, at least 30 degrees beyond the limits of the normal range (figure 8.5), and lateral deviation of the ischial tuberosities is 15 to 20 degrees more than normal.
3. There are early osteoarthritic changes in the right patella (knee) and talo-calcaneal (ankle) joint.
4. Reconstruction of the feet using modeling clay and sand suggested a mild and recent cavovalgus deformity of the left foot. This is a type of clubfoot characterized by an overly high longitudinal arch and outwardly turned heel.

5. Periosteal reactions (in the form of raised, striated, and pitted bone) are present along all the major growth plates of the arms and legs, both proximally and distally, and are most pronounced on the anterior tuberosity and crest on both the right and left tibiae.
6. The left radius has enlarged and irregular muscle attachment areas (enthesopathies) at the proximal and distal ends.
7. There has been perimortem destruction of the nasal conchae and septum, with hyperplastic reconfiguring of the nasal aperture (figure 8.6).

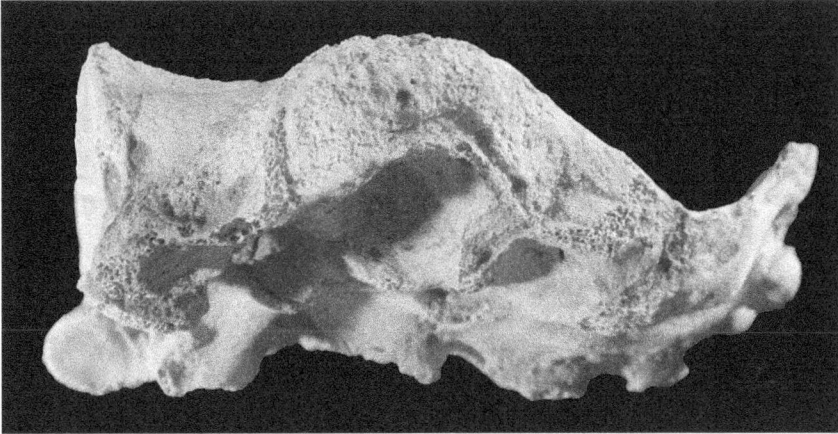

Figure 8.5. Lesley's sacrum showing abnormal upward curvature.

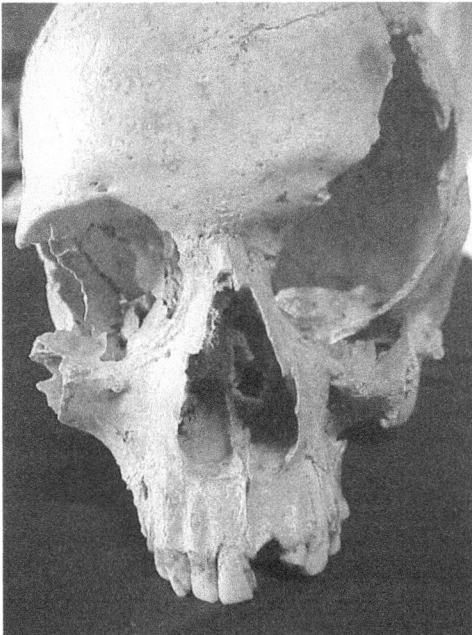

Figure 8.6. Perimortem destruction of the nasal conchae and septum with hyperplastic remodeling of the nasal aperture. In the remodeled nose, the vomer is skewed to the right with an enlarged and remodeled area near the nasospinale.

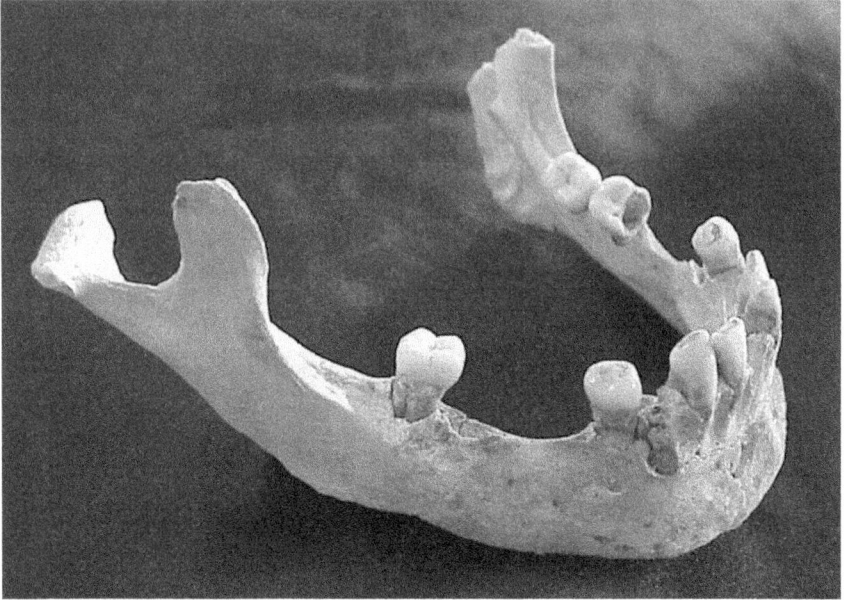

Figure 8.7. Lesley's mandible showing antemortem tooth loss of the second premolar and first molar on the left side and a large carious lesion in the second molar. On the right side there is loss of the second premolar and the first and second molars. Remodeling is evident in several of the tooth sockets.

8. Stress-related changes are present in the vertebrae of the mid and lower back, especially marked on the third lumbar, suggesting unusual stress and minor trauma to the lower back.

9. Dental caries are common in Southwest Asia (Rathbun 1984: 150; Blau 2007: 198–99), but given Lesely's young age, she had markedly poor dental health with antemortem loss of seven teeth from the mandible and five from the maxilla. The complete resorption of the root sockets indicates passage of at least several months from when the tooth was lost to Lesely's death (Peterson et al. 2002: 55) (figure 8.7).

Differential Diagnosis

Back in the United States, Dr. Donald Crisman, a physician with extensive experience in paleopathology (now deceased, formerly of Northampton, Massachusetts), examined Lesley's remains and concluded that her suite of skeletal symptoms did not conform perfectly to poliomyelitis, but that she did have some form of mild neuromuscular disease at the time of death. After Dr. Crisman's untimely death, we renewed our efforts to diagnose Lesley with the broad notion that she had a neurological disease of a few years duration. The combined observations of abnormalities on her bones suggested she had been at least partially crippled and had some physical impairment. The changes in the shape and orientation of the bones of her pelvic girdle seem to indicate chronic sitting, and the signs of early arthritis indicate overuse of the right leg and a neuromuscular imbalance of the left lower leg. This imbalance is evident in relative weakness of the muscles that invert the foot (especially the posterior tibialis muscle), which would have increased the effect of the peroneal and intrinsic muscles that evert (turn out) the foot in a relatively mild, late-onset type of clubfoot.

Poliomyelitis fits some, but not all, of the changes observed on her skeleton. Poliomyelitis is an ancient disease. Mitchell (1900) radiographically showed that the left femur of an Egyptian mummy (ca. 3700 B.C.) was more than 8 cm shorter than the right femur. Later researchers suggested that this individual had been interred with a cane that could have been used to compensate for the asymmetry in the limbs while walking (Janssens 1970). A famous stele of an Egyptian priest (ca. 1400 B.C.) shows a man with clubfoot typical of people with polio (Wyatt 2003: 260). Whitehouse (1980: 293) discusses the pharaoh Siptah from the nineteenth dynasty, whose mummified remains demonstrate the hyperextension of the foot from a leg that is shorter than the other. Roberts and Manchester (1995: 134) describe a skeleton from eighth-century England with poliomyelitis showing the extreme shortening of the right leg versus the left.

Atrophy of bones in the leg can result from poliomyelitis, but the nature of deformation depends upon the age at which polio was contracted. The case described here is relatively mild, which indicates that the infection was not contracted at an early age. Later onset of polio is common, but the muscle paralysis is characterized by a significant decrease in vascularization of the surrounding tissues (Debré and the WHO 1955). Dystonia (muscle contractions and twitching) in one foot is also an indicator of poliomyelitis, but in Lesley's case there is only a hint of cavovalgus (chronic hyperflexion), and this could be attributed to frequent use of the flexor digitorum longus muscle of the tibia used in curling the toes (excluding the big toe) of the foot under. Since she has arthritic lipping in her vertebral column (indicating biomechanical wear and tear from using the upper body) and normal-appearing muscle attachments on the arms and legs, Lesley does not appear to have been completely immobilized.

The late age of onset (late teens) of the neurological disorder affecting muscle use further suggests that the condition might not have been poliomyelitis. Poliomyelitis is a viral infection, and where endemic it generally affects young children who then become immune to it. However, if Lesley was not a native of the Gulf region and was not exposed to the virus in childhood, contracting the virus at a later age (say 15 or so) could have produced the symptoms observed.

We also considered leprosy as a possible cause of Lesley's skeletal changes. Leprosy may affect the cranium and can manifest on skeletons as periostitis and osteomyelitis, particularly on the extremities (Ortner 2003). Leprosy is also associated with destruction of the anterior maxillary and nasal bones (especially the nasal septum and anterior nasal spine), and of the digits of the hands and feet. Osteoarthritis accompanies these other patterns of bone destruction, particularly at the weight-bearing joints. Lesley does have lytic lesions around the nasal and palatine bones, as well as an enlarged nasal aperture (figure 8.6). However, the patterning of inflammation in most of her joints, the pronounced inflammation at the knee, and the severe atrophy of the fibulae near the knee again suggest poliomyelitis, which results in a decrease in vascularization in the tissues and joints.

Asymmetry in the femora can also be diagnostic of tuberculosis (Ortner 2003: 239). Symptoms of tuberculosis can include problems with walking, inflammation and lesions on various bones, and osteoarthritis. These changes are usually in association with pronounced destructive lesions in the vertebral bodies and other skeletal regions, which are not present in Lesley's remains.

Other neurological disorders such as multiple sclerosis, muscular dystrophy, myasthenia gravis, amyotrophic lateral sclerosis, and spinal muscular atrophy are possibilities, but the age of onset, patterning of the irregularities across the body, and severity of these conditions do not quite match Lesley's skeletal symptoms. And because of the later onset, congenital disorders such as clubfoot and uniform muscular disease with uniform type 1 fiber are also not a good fit with her indications.

It is clear Lesley was suffering from some type of late-onset progressive neural muscular atrophy. Given all of the symptoms and the possible diagnosis, contagious poliomyelitis is still the most likely culprit. First diagnosed by a hospital laboratory technician during the field excavation of Lesley, and later analyzed bone by bone by a physician who has diagnosed patients with it, poliomyelitis remains the leading likely cause of Lesley's problems and her early death. Aufderheide and Rodriguez-Martin (1998: 212) report that although the antiquity of poliomyelitis is not well documented, its symptomology is likely to be diffuse bone loss involving cortical and cancellous bone in the limbs and disuse atrophy. This is exactly what we do see with Lesley.

Unusual Bones, Unusual Burial Treatment, Unusual Individual

What can be said of this young woman with certainty? It appears that Lesley contracted some neuromuscular disease in her midteens. Mild inflammation (periosteal pitting) in almost all of the joint systems of the appendages suggests she may have suffered some level of discomfort. She also experienced tooth loss, caries, and abscessing at an early age. Features of Lesley's pelvis (forward molding of the sacrum and coccyx and lateral splaying of the ischia) suggest she experienced chronic sedentism. Muscle development, pelvic asymmetry, and osteoarthritis on the right side suggest she was using her body in ways that compensated for the more pronounced muscular atrophy on the left side. She has mild cavovalgus deformity of the left foot. The extreme atrophy of both fibulae suggests little use of her legs toward the end of her life. Taken together, these developments suggest restricted movement and less weight bearing than normal for a 20-year-old. In contrast, Lesley appears to have had use of her arms, perhaps undertaking work tasks from a sitting position. Or Lesley may have used her arms to move her body around since she may not have been able to coordinate and use her legs to walk.

What might Lesley's symptoms have been? How was she experiencing this health problem? Physicians typically report that the early stage of poliomyelitis is a cluster of "flulike" symptoms including malaise, headache, slight fever, and vomiting. Nonparalytic poliomyelitis would include leg pain particularly in the calves, muscle stiffness and tenderness, irritability, and excessive tiredness (Seytre and Schaffer 2005: 6–8). One of the early screening methods for poliomyelitis in schoolchildren was to assess for acute flaccid paralysis (AFP), in which there is a loss of muscle tone with generally flaccid muscles (Andrus et al. 1992).

While we cannot be sure which suite of symptoms Lesley was dealing with, she likely experienced general malaise and tiredness associated with most neuromuscular diseases.

There were many grave goods in and around the area where Lesley was located—pottery, soft-stone and alabaster vessels, bronze weaponry, and jewelry (carnelian, lapis, gold, silver, and agate beads). Some or all (or none) of these might have been Lesley's. We do know that the people who buried Lesley took the unique extra step of wrapping the body in some very durable material, keeping it intact among the scattered remains of hundreds of others. This departure from typical funerary practice suggests that Lesley was also unique during life. Was she a revered member of the community, her body kept intact at death by those who loved her? How did her increasing disability change her role in the community and her social persona? Was she buried thus because she was considered dangerous to the group because of her increasing disability and deformities? Was she cared for or ostracized? We cannot accept or reject any of these scenarios for certain, but additional studies of Lesley's bone strontium will yield further insights into her origin and her life.

Acknowledgments

Many individuals have examined and pondered Lesley's condition. We thank them all here and acknowledge their aid in helping us better understand Lesley's life and death. These include Dr. Donald Crisman (deceased), Dr. Ronald Huckstep from Australia, the Umm al Quwain Radiology Department, Dr. Richard Wright, and Hampshire College students Melanie Wilkes, Toby Stillman, and Tasha Loader. Ryan Harrod deserves special thanks for aiding us with bibliographic details and editorial assistance. Finally, Dr. Douglas M. Huber, DDS, was especially helpful in understanding Lesley's poor oral health.

Note

1. Unfortunately, we no longer have those original X-rays of the leg bones, but we hope to have an opportunity to have Lesley fully radiographed and digitized using a CT-scanner.

References Cited

Aufderheide, Arthur. C., and Conrado Rodríguez-Martin
1998   *The Cambridge Encyclopedia of Human Paleopathology*. Cambridge University Press, New York.
Andrus, Jon K., Ciro A. de Quadros, Jean-Marc Olive, and Harry F. Hull
1992   Screening of Cases of Acute Flaccid Paralysis for Poliomyelitis Eradication: Ways to Improve Specificity. *Bulletin of the World Health Organization* 70(5): 591–96.
Blau, Soren
2001   Fragmentary Endings: A Discussion of 3rd-millennium B.C. Burial Practices in the Oman Peninsula. *Antiquity* 75: 557–70.
2007   Skeletal and Dental Health and Subsistence Change in the United Arab Emirates. In *Ancient Health*, edited by M. N. Cohen and G. M. Crane-Kramer, pp. 190–206. University Press of Florida, Gainesville.
Dalongeville, Rémi
1990   L'environnement du Site de Tell Abraq. In *A Prehistoric Mound in the Emirate of Umm al-Qaiwain: Excavations at Tell Abraq in 1989*, edited by Daniel T. Potts, pp. 139–40. Munksgaard, Copenhagen.
Debré, Robert, and the World Health Organization (WHO)
1955   *Poliomyelitis*. World Health Organization, Geneva.

Dostal, Walter

1983   *The Traditional Architecture of Ras al-Khaimah (North)*. Tübinger Atlas des Vorderen Orients Beiheft Bd. 54. L. Reichert, Wiesbaden.

Janssens, Paul A.

1970   *Palaeopathology: Diseases and Injuries of Prehistoric Man*. J. Baker, London.

Mitchell, John K.

1900   Study of a Mummy Affected with Anterior Poliomyelitis. *Transactions of the Association of American Physicians* 15: 134–36.

Ortner, Donald J.

2003   *Identification of Pathological Conditions in Human Skeletal Remains*. 2nd ed. Academic Press, New York.

Peterson, Larry J., James R. Hupp, and Myron Tucker

2002   *Contemporary Oral and Maxillofacial Surgery*. 4th ed. Mosby, New York.

Potts, Daniel T.

1990   *A Prehistoric Mound in the Emirate of Umm al-Qaiwain: Excavations at Tell Abraq in 1989*. Munksgaard, Copenhagen.

1991   *Further Excavations at Tell Abraq: The 1990 Season*. Munksgaard, Copenhagen.

2000a   *Ancient Magan: The Secrets of Tell Abraq*. Trident Press, London.

2000b   Arabian Time Capsule: An Undisturbed Trove of Relics Reveals the Trading Patterns of a Bronze Age Society. *Archaeology Magazine* 53(5): 44–48.

2001   Before the Emirates: An Archaeological and Historical Account of Developments in the Region c. 5000 B.C. to 676 A.D. In *United Arab Emirates: A New Perspective*, edited by E. I. Al Abed and P. Hellyer, pp. 28–69. Trident Press, London.

Rathbun, Ted Allan

1984   Skeletal Pathology from the Paleolithic through the Metal Ages in Iran and Iraq. In *Paleopathology at the Origins of Agriculture*, edited by M. N. Cohen and G. J. Armelagos, pp. 137–67. Academic Press, New York.

Roberts, Charlotte A., and Keith Manchester

1995   *The Archaeology of Disease*. 2nd ed. Cornell University Press, Ithaca, N.Y.

Seytre, Bernard, and Mary Schaffer

2005   *The Death of a Disease: History of the Eradication of Poliomyelitis*. Rutgers University Press, New Brunswick, N.J.

Stephan, E.

1995   Preliminary Report on the Faunal Remains of the First Two Seasons of Tell Abraq/Umm al-Qaiwain/United Arab Emirates. In *Archaeozoology of the Near East*, Vol. 2., edited by H. Buitenhuis and H. P. Uerpmann, pp. 53–63. Backhuys, Leiden.

Uerpmann, Hans-Peter, and Margarethe Uerpmann

2002   The Appearance of the Domestic Camel in South-east Arabia. *Journal of Oman Studies* 12: 235–60.

Uerpmann, Margarethe

2001   Remarks on the Animal Economy of Tell Abraq (Emirates of Sharjah and Umm al-Qaywayn, UAE). *Proceedings of the Seminar for Arabian Studies* 31: 227–33.

Whitehouse, Walter M.

1980   Radiological Findings in the Royal Mummies. In *An X-Ray Atlas of the Royal Mum-*

mies, edited by J. A. Harris and E. F. Wente, pp. 286–327. University of Chicago Press, Chicago.

Willcox, George, and Margareta Tengberg

1995   Preliminary Report on the Archaeobotanical Investigations at Tell Abraq with Special Attention to Chaff Impressions in Mud Brick. *Arabian Archaeology & Epigraphy* 6: 129–38.

Wyatt, Harold V.

2003   Poliomyelitis. In *The Cambridge Historical Dictionary of Disease*, edited by K. F. Kiple, pp. 258–61. Cambridge University Press, New York.

9 ◆ The "African Queen"

A Portuguese Mystery

Mary Lucas Powell, Della Collins Cook, Maia M. Langley,
Susan Dale Spencer, Jennifer Raff, and Frederika Kaestle

Individual Profile

Site: Torre de Palma
Location: 5 km northwest of the town of Monforte, Alto Alentejo, Portugal; geographic coordinates: Lisbon datum 07° 24′ 50″.070, 38° 57′ 43″.441
Cultural Affiliation: Medieval Portugal
Date: A.D. 1469–1648 (radiocarbon date calibrated for eastern Portugal)
Feature: Unknown; Museu Nacional de Arqueologia catalog number 4769 v.2
Location of Grave: Exact location unknown, but the word "Capela," written on the right parietal, indicates that the individual was buried inside the church precinct
Burial and Grave Type: Unknown
Associated Materials: None reported
Preservation and Completeness: This individual is represented only by the cranium and mandible, first and second cervical vertebrae, and two hand phalanges
Age at Death and Basis of Estimate: 30–40 years, based on dental eruption and wear and ectocranial suture closure
Sex and Basis of Determination: Female, based on cranial morphology
Conditions Observed: Marked maxillary and mandibular prognathism; long, low cranial vault (cranial index 70.4); guttering at nasal inferior margin; missing right and left maxillary incisors suggesting deliberate avulsion; no skeletal pathology observed
Specialized Analysis: Radiocarbon dating, aDNA analysis, stable carbon isotope analysis
Excavated: 1950s–1960s, excavations directed by Manuel Heleno, Museu Etnológico, Lisbon
Archaeological Report: Heleno 1962; Maloney and Hale 1996
Current Disposition: Curated at the Museu Nacional de Arqueologia (series #0241), Lisbon

In the spring of 1947 a young farmer named Joaquim Inocêncio Militão began plowing a field on a large agricultural estate, the Herdade de Torre de Palma, located 5 km northwest of the town of Monforte in the Alto Alentejo, eastern Portugal. His plow struck the granite base of a column in an open area south of the Monte, the venerable estate farmhouse whose central fortified tower dates from the medieval era (figure 9.1). This happy accident led to the discovery of the largest Roman villa identified so far in Portugal, the center of a large agricultural estate devoted, in part, to the breeding of horses for the Roman racing circuit. One of the mosaic floors in the villa features full-length portraits of five horses, each one identified by name with a palm tree branch attached to his bridle, such as were awarded to victorious athletes. The name of "Palma," associated with this estate since ancient times, may preserve the memory of this tradition.

Some 150 m northwest of the villa and 750 m south of the Monte lay the remains of one of the earliest Christian churches in the Iberian Peninsula (Langley et al. 2007), distinguished by its unusual pair of double-apsed basilicas placed end to end. The eastern basilica was constructed in the mid-fifth century A.D., with the adjacent western basilica added during the following century. The site was evidently abandoned during the late eighth century, probably as part of the movement of rural populations into nearby fortified towns such as Monforte, 5 km to the east, during the first period of Moorish occupation of the southern

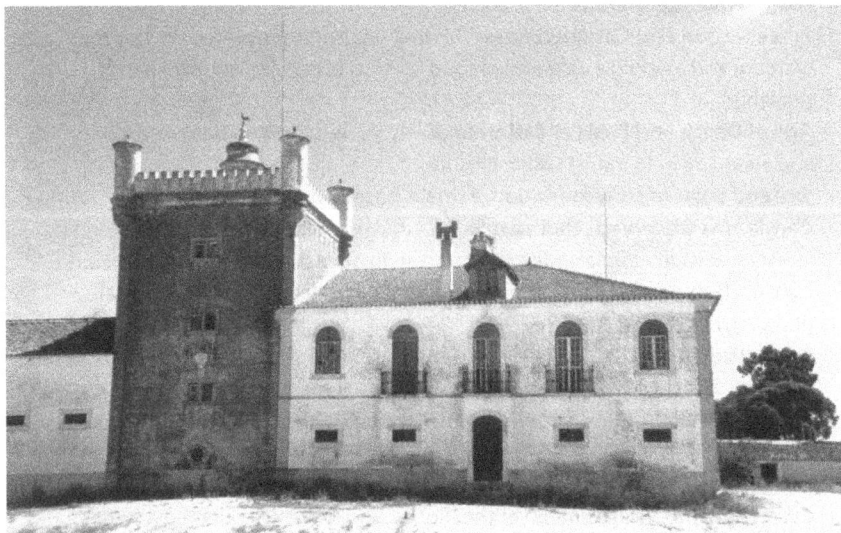

Figure 9.1. The Monte. Note the medieval-era fortified central tower. (Photograph by Mary Lucas Powell.)

half of the Iberian Peninsula. Some time during the eleventh or twelfth century, the eastern apse of the western basilica was rebuilt, and over the following three centuries numerous burials of young children were placed underneath its elevated floor. The lower part of the stone apse wall remained visible above ground long after the rest of the structure had collapsed and was still known locally as the Ermidas de São Domingos (Hermitage of Saint Dominic) in 1947 (Maloney and Hale 1996).

The initial excavations at Torre de Palma were conducted from 1947 until 1964 under the direction of Manuel Heleno and again by Fernando de Almeida in 1971—both former directors/archaeologists of the Museu Nacional de Ethnológico (now called the Museu Nacional de Arqueologia, or MNA), Lisbon. In 1984 Stephanie Maloney (project director) and John R. Hale (field director) of the University of Louisville, Kentucky, initiated a second series of excavations focusing initially on the church (called the "Capela" by the original Portuguese excavators but renamed the "Basilica" by the Maloney-Hale project) and then moving on to refine the construction sequences and chronologies of the villa and Basilica. The human skeletal remains recovered during both excavation campaigns from tombs in and around this church, its two associated small cemeteries, and other site areas comprise one of the largest Late Classical/medieval population samples from Portugal, although many of the 255 identified individuals are represented only by fragmentary remains. The site is located midslope in a northwest–southeast-oriented range of hills, below an extensive deposit of limestone; soils developed from this deposit gradually covered the underlying bedrock (schist and granite). These soils enhanced the preservation of both animal and human bone.

Discovery of 4769 v.2

In 1985 Maloney and Hale spent part of the summer at the MNA studying previously excavated materials from Torre de Palma. Hale was photographing a set of complete skulls from the site displayed in a large *vitrine* (glass display case) in the MNA laboratory when he noticed that the last skull in the top row had a distinctly different appearance from the others in the series: a long, low cranial vault (instead of the high, rounded vault typical of other Portuguese archaeological crania that he had seen), marked maxillary and mandibular prognathism, and bilateral absence of the lateral maxillary incisors. This unusual appearance recalled to his mind certain descriptions of craniofacial morphological variations between individuals of European and West African ancestry, and Hale immediately wondered if this particular individual might be African. Although the skull had not yet been cleaned of the adhering soil matrix, the words "Torre de Palma—Capela" were clearly visible written on the right parietal.

When the senior author (MLP) joined the University of Louisville Torre de Palma Archaeological Project in 1996 as project bioarchaeologist, Hale directed her attention to this very interesting individual (whom he had dubbed the "African Queen"). Because the MNA had originally contained both ethnological and archaeological collections from Portugal and its overseas colonies (including sub-Saharan Africa), Hale was worried that this skull might actually have entered the MNA as part of an ethnological collection from Africa and subsequently been mislabeled. However, a check of the relevant accession records by one of the authors (MML) indicated that all materials belonging to the ethnological collections from Africa had been transferred when a new Museu Etnológico was built during the 1980s.

The MNA catalog card for this individual (Museu Nacional de Arqueologia series 243, contentor 4769, Vol. 2) lists the specimen as "avulso" (that is, "isolated") with no associated tomb number or intrasite location. The word "Capela" on the skull provides the sole contextual information. Within the MNA series, only a very few sets of human remains are listed as "avulso," most of them being assigned to one of the tombs ("sepulturas") in the church ("Capela") or its two adjacent cemeteries that appear on the maps drawn during the MNA excavations.

Skeletal Individual 4769 v.2 is represented by a well-preserved, complete cranium and mandible (figure 9.2). When Powell and her assistant, Nathalie Antunes-Ferreira, began to clean the skull in 1999, they discovered two cervical vertebrae (C1 and C2) and two small carpal phalanges embedded in the soil around the base of the cranium. This discovery strongly suggests that the specimen had been interred with flesh still covering the bones, possibly with one hand resting on or near the face. No skeletal pathology was evident.

The determination of female sex for Individual 4769 v.2 was based on features of cranial morphology considered to be reliable indicators of sex in adult crania and mandibles (Krogman 1962): gracile supraorbital torus, thin superior orbital margins, relatively gracile mastoid processes, occipital condyles, temporal lines, and nuchal region of the occipital, and a rounded (not squared) chin. Not only is skull 4769 v.2 more gracile morphologically in appearance than the adult male crania from the Torre de Palma sample (who are generally fairly robust), but it is also generally more gracile and pedomorphic (childlike) than the other female crania and mandibles from that site. Table 9.1 presents cranial metric data for the eight most complete adult female crania from Torre de Palma; the sex estimates for these individuals were based on both cranial

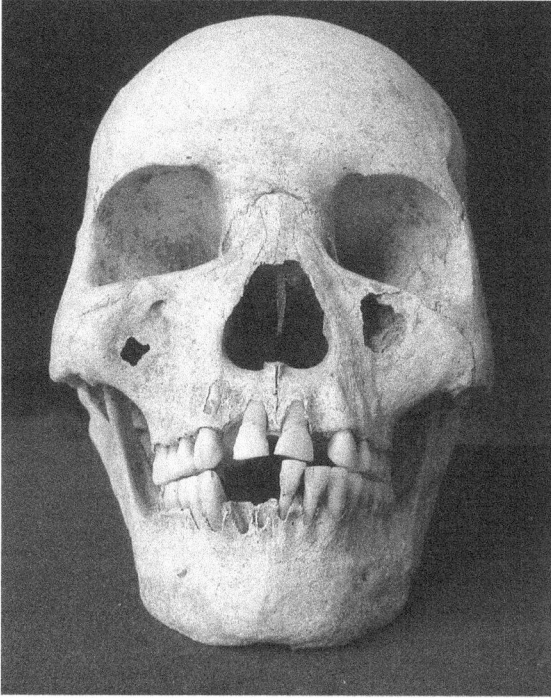

Figure 9.2. Frontal view of skull 4769 v.2. (Photograph by Maia M. Langley.)

and postcranial metric data and morphology. The last line of the table summarizes comparable cranial metric data (mean values) for 11 adult males from the sample whose sex estimates were derived by the same methods employed for the females (both cranial and postcranial metric data and morphology). Over the past 25 years (1985–2010), the sex estimates for the skull labeled MNA 4769 v.2, recorded independently by at least six experienced skeletal analysts (John R. Hale, Mary Lucas Powell, Nathalie Antunes, Cristina Pombal, Della Collins Cook, and Cristina Cruz), have unanimously been female.

All four of the third molars had fully erupted, and one was lost near the time of death. Her teeth display light to moderate wear on the occlusal (chewing) surfaces, with very small islands of exposed dentine, suggesting an age at death of 30–40 years. No cranial suture fusion is evident ectocranially; the sutures could not be examined endocranially because the cranial cavity was filled with soil. Since the excavation the soil inside the skull had hardened into a very dense ball; the most practical way to remove this material would have been to immerse the skull in water to soften the soil, but the MNA was reluctant to give permission for this procedure because of the risk that this very complete, well-preserved cranium would fall to pieces once the supporting soil had been removed.

Table 9.1. Cranial metrics, Torre de Palma females

Females	Ba-Pr Ht	G-O Ln	Max W	Ba-Br Ht	Ba-Na Ht	BZ Dia
4769 v.2 African Queen	105.0	187.5	132.0	130.5	100.0	131.0
4818 v.1 Capela sep 1A	84.6	182.5	137.5	130.5	100.0	*
4779 v.2 Capela sep 7A	92.5	186.0	146.0	136.5	104.5	132.0
4817 v.2 Capela sep 6A	81.0	175.0	139.0	134.0	98.0	125.0
4723 v.2 Capela sep D	91.0	177.0	142.0	125.0	98.0	*
4767 v.1 Capela sep E	*	171.0	128.5	*	*	125.0
4400 v.2 Cem PdE sep 1	*	167.0	125.0	*	*	125.5
4511 v.3 Cem PdE sep 7	*	183.0	134.0	131.0	97.5	126.0
4381 v.1 Sep 25	85.3	181.0	144.5	128.0	96.0	*
Female Means (w/o AQ)	86.89	177.81	137.06	130.83	99.00	126.70
Male Means	91.75	191.68	142.68	135.50	101.36	135.75

Exploring the Ancestry of Individual 4769 v.2

Assessment of biological ancestry from a skeletonized cranium is not an easy task, even with well-preserved remains: the physical anthropologists Eugene Giles and Orville Elliott note that "race determination from the cranium is more difficult than sex determination" (1962: 147), and the eminent forensic anthropologist W. M. Krogman commented, "This is a difficult, and indeed, a controversial area" (1962: 189). In the following sections, we consider six different categories of biological evidence relevant to the determination of geographical ancestry: craniofacial morphology, anthropometric craniofacial data, dental morphology, culture-specific artificial modifications of the dentition, developmental disorders that affect the shape and size of the cranium, and the analysis of ancient DNA.

Craniofacial Morphology

Individual 4769 v.2 displays several specific features of craniofacial morphology that are widely accepted by forensic anthropologists as characteristic of sub-Saharan ancestry: marked prognathism (Brooks et al. 1990); guttered nasal border (Byers 2002); broad, flared nasal aperture (Byers 2002); a broadly arched "Quonset hut" configuration of the nasal bones (Brues 1990); and inverted posterior/

Pr-Na Ht	N Br	DF S	CI
65.6	27.3	13.06	70.4
59.2	21.7	6.73	75.3
66.7	25.2	7.43	78.5
*	*	5.64	79.4
62.2	23.1	7.50	80.2
61.0	22.0	6.94	75.1
62.5	23.4	7.19	74.8
*	22.5	8.37	73.2
*	25.3	7.73	79.8
62.32	23.31	7.19	77.04
66.0	23.62	——	74.43

Note: Key to measurements (defined in Bass 1987: 66–69, except DF S, defined in Giles and Elliot 1962: 152).

Ba-Pr Ht = basion-prosthion height.

G-O Ln = glabello-opisthocranion length.

Max W = maximum width.

Ba-Br Ht = basion-bregma height.

Ba-Na Ht = basion-nasion height.

BZ Dia = maximum bizygomatic diameter.

Pr-Na Ht = prosthion-nasion height.

N Br = maximum nasal breadth.

DF S = discriminant function score derived from "White-Negro" formula for females constructed by Giles and Elliott 1962: 152.

CI = cranial index (maximum width × 100/maximum length).

*Sample mean inserted for calculation of DF S.

inferior mandible ramus border (Angel and Kelley 1990). In this regard, she differs markedly from *all* of the other adults from Torre de Palma (eight females and 11 males) in which these features can be observed. Her marked maxillary and mandibular prognathism are perhaps her most distinctive features (figures 9.3a–b), but her broad "nasal gutter" is also quite distinctive: it stands in sharp contrast to the bony "sill" that characterizes the lower margin of the nasal opening in the other observed Torre de Palma adult crania. The breadth of her nasal aperture, 27.3 mm, measured from the anatomical landmarks alare (right) to alare (left), is greater than in the other measurable adult female crania from the site (mean = 23.31 mm), as listed in table 9.1. The shape of her nose is more flared, and the smoothly rounded arch of her nasal bones matches the "Quonset hut" shape described by Brues (1990) (figure 9.2), in contrast to the more sharply peaked nasal bones displayed by the other Torre de Palma adults observed for these features. Finally, the posterior/inferior borders of both of her mandibular rami show a slight inward curvature, comparable to that illustrated by Angel and Kelley (1990: 37).

Anthropometric Analysis

In 1962 Giles and Elliott pioneered a method for objective "race identification" (1962: 147) based on a series of eight craniofacial skeletal measurements (listed

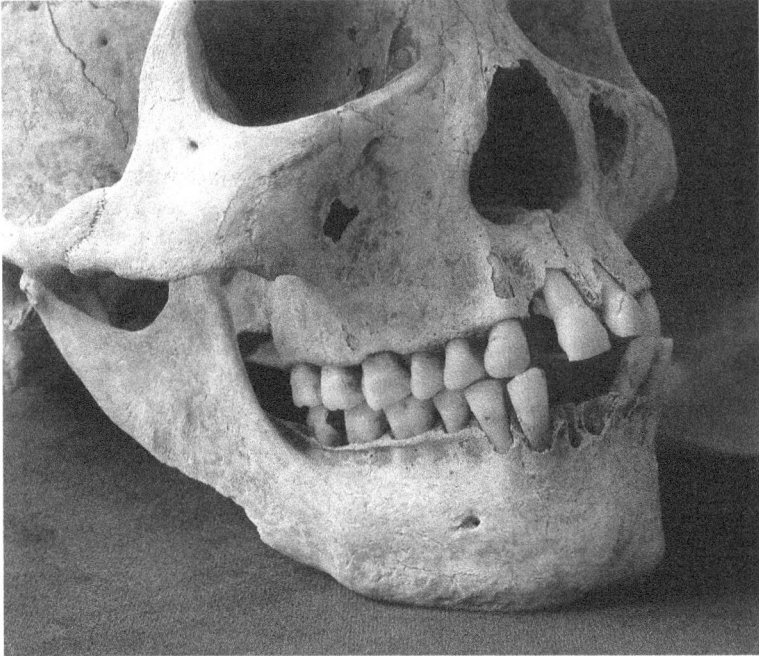

Figure 9.3a. Oblique view of 4769 v.2, showing marked prognathism and nasal guttering. (Photograph by Maia M. Langley.)

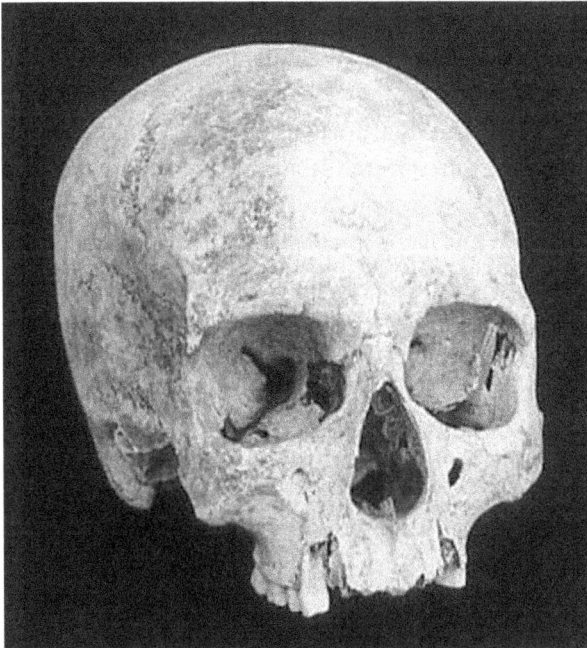

Figure 9.3b. Oblique view of an adult female cranium from Tomb 8, showing the more vertical face and sharp nasal margins usual in Europeans. (Photograph by Mary Lucas Powell.)

in table 9.1) taken from 408 African American or European American adults of known sex, age, and race in two skeletonized medical cadaver series, the Hamann-Todd collection[1] and the Terry collection,[2] and 150 Native American adults in the Archaic archaeological skeletal series from Indian Knoll,[3] as representative of the respective races. Figure 9.4 shows Giles and Elliot's scattergram of discriminant function scores for adult females in their samples with the scores calculated for the African Queen (AQ) and for eight other adult females from Torre de Palma (TP) added for comparison. Individual 4769 v.2's score lies near the very top of the "Negro" region of the plot, whereas the other Torre de Palma females cluster together inside the "White" region.

Figure 9.5 charts the distribution of the nine Torre de Palma female scores; the African Queen's score lies far outside the range of the other female scores. These results confirm our visual interpretation of her craniofacial morphology as being very *different* from that of the other adult females from this site.

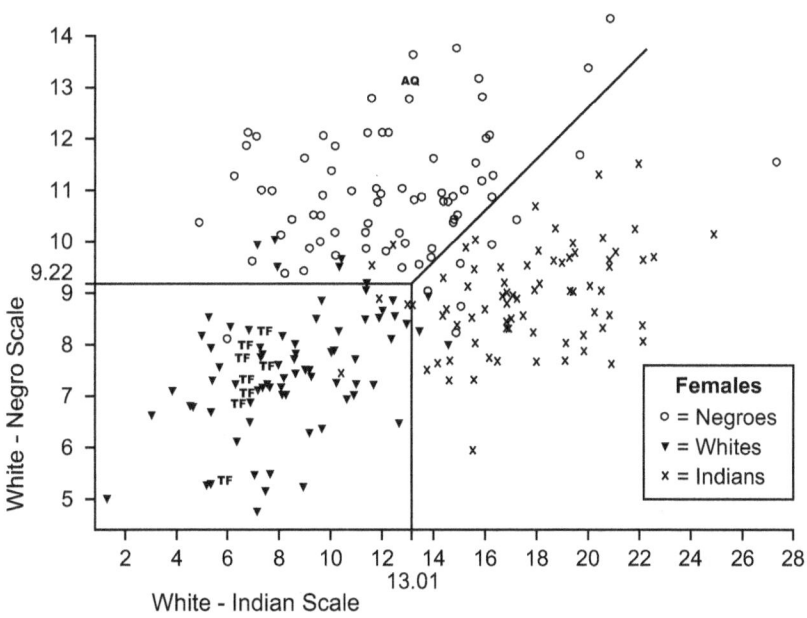

Figure 9.4. Scattergram of the Giles and Elliott (1962) female discriminant function scores, with scores for 4769 v.2 (AQ) and other females from Torre de Palma (TF) added. "White," "Negro," and "Indian" were standard descriptive terms used by physical anthropologists for the "three broad racial categories" examined by Giles and Elliott in this study. Today the term "Negro" would be replaced by "black." Their "Indian" sample consisted of the Indian Knoll Archaic series from Kentucky, which is not representative of prehistoric Amerindians or of modern Native Americans as a whole.

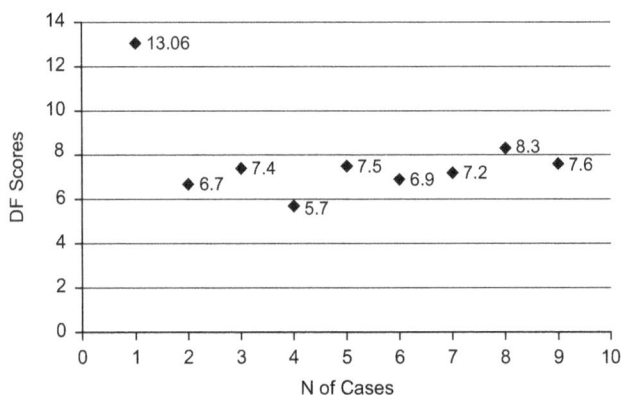

Figure 9.5. Scattergram of discriminant function (DF) scores for the African Queen and other Torre de Palma adult females. The African Queen's score (13.06) appears at the extreme upper left corner of the chart.

Comparison of cranial metric data from 4769 v.2 with data from other females from Torre de Palma reveals that this individual displays a relatively longer, lower cranial vault than is typical in this mesocranic population (table 9.1). Her cranial index of 70.4 (calculated as maximum cranial breadth 132 mm × 100/ maximum length of 187.5 mm) places her firmly in the dolichocranic (narrow or long-headed) category (Bass 1987: 69). By contrast, the mean cranial index calculated for the other eight Torre de Palma females is 77.04 (brachycranic).

FORDISC 3.0 is an interactive program developed by forensic anthropologists Stephen D. Ousley and Richard L. Jantz in order to compare skeletal measurements from an unknown individual to a database of known-race individuals using discriminate function analysis. The database includes older cadaver collections in the United States such as the Hamann-Todd collection, as well as data gathered through recent forensic cases in the United States (Ousley and Jantz 2005). FORDISC 3.0 also allows for individual comparisons with the craniometric data from populations around the globe that are included in the database generated by Harvard anthropologist William White Howells (1908–2005). For each comparison of an "unknown" sample with sample data from appropriate reference populations, FORDISC 3.0 calculates the posterior probability (a parameter in Bayesian statistics expressed as a percentage) that a positive match between the unknown sample and the reference population is an accurate reflection of the biological ancestry relationship between the two populations represented, based on the available biological criteria for comparison.

The cranial measurements of the nine Torre de Palma adult females were entered into the program and compared to "White females" and "Black females."

Eight measurements were used in this analysis: maximum cranial length, maximum cranial breadth, bizygomatic breadth, basion-bregma height, cranial base length, basion-prosthion length, upper facial height, and nasal breadth. Cranial angles were calculated in FORDISC 3.0 and were used in the final analysis. Cranium 4769 v.2 was classified as "black" with a posterior probability of 100 percent, and the eight other females were classified as "white" with posterior probabilities of 95 percent or better. These very high figures (100 and 95 percent, respectively) calculated for the posterior probabilities strongly support the assessment of African ancestry for 4769 v.2 and European ancestry for the other eight Torre de Palma females in this study.

Next, we compared Individual 4769 v.2 to several African groups in the Howells database: Bushman, Dogon, Egypt, Teita, and Zulu. None of these samples represent the West African populations who were most strongly represented among the enslaved Africans transported to Portugal (Lowe 2005), so it is not surprising that 4769 v.2 is not strikingly similar to any of the groups sampled: the closest match is with Zulu females (posterior probability = 52.7 percent). A possible explanation for this significantly lower posterior probability value is that 4769 v.2 was more similar in her biological ancestry to the American "Black" sample, many of whom undoubtedly had some degree of European admixture.

Individual 4769 v.2 was also compared to all of the female samples in the Howells database, including samples from North America and Asia. She was most similar to indigenous Australian females (posterior probability = 36.6 percent). There is no historical support for a scenario linking rural Portugal with Australia; hence the balance of the FORDISC 3.0 analysis indicates that 4769 v.2 was of African descent.

Dental Morphology and the Question of the Missing Maxillary Lateral Incisors

Dental morphology provides an independent source of information on ancestry. Individual 4769 v.2 (see figure 9.6) has large maxillary central incisors with remnants of a well-developed tuberculum dentale (an extra lingual cusp on the upper permanent incisors or canines) still visible on the right despite heavy wear, features we expect to see in persons of African ancestry. There is no Carabelli's cusp (an extra lingual cusp on the mesial-lingual cusp [protocone] of the upper permanent first molars), a European feature the absence of which is not surprising in Portugal (Edgar 2005) given the frequent admixture of non-European genes over the past 2,000 years (Earle and Lowe 2005). On the other hand, there is considerable distal molar reduction (the second and third molars are progressively smaller, relative to the first molar), a feature that is surprising in someone of African ancestry. Reduced cusp number in third molars is reported in only 20 percent of West Africans (Hellman 1928). A system using dental traits for forensic determination of African versus European ancestry (Edgar 2005) gives a somewhat mixed picture of Individual 4769 v.2. Two pairs of character states in the mandibular premolars yield Bayesian posterior probabilities of 93 percent and 86 percent for African ancestry: (1) lower anterior premolar cusp variation present with lower first molar deflecting wrinkle present, and (2) lower anterior premolar cusp variation present and lower posterior premolar cusp variation present. If we follow Edgar's advice and limit ourselves to trait combinations with probabilities in excess of 85 percent, no other pairs of traits are relevant, although many scores point to European ancestry. It is possible, as stated earlier, that this individual is of mixed African and European ancestry, but these analytical techniques do not allow this determination.

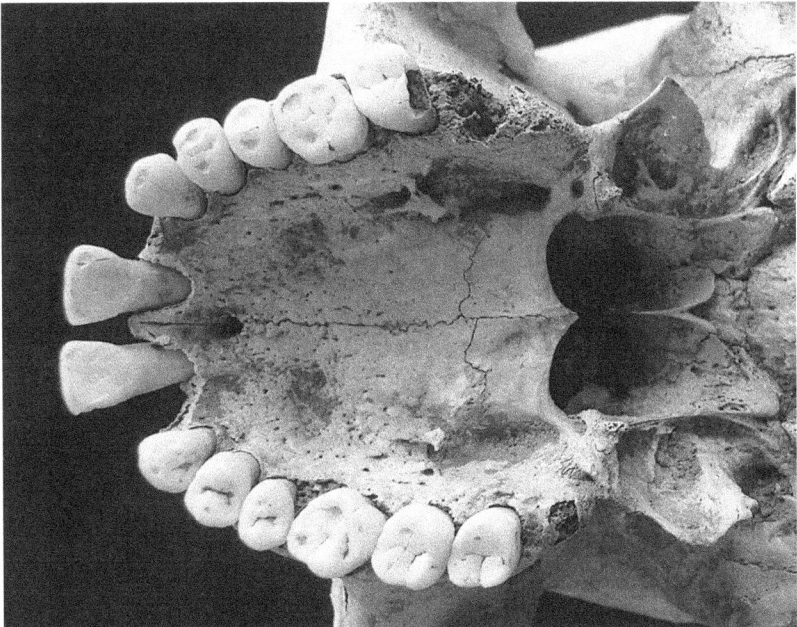

Figure 9.6. Occlusal view of maxilla showing bilateral missing lateral incisors. Note the oblique wear on the lingual aspects of the central incisors and the lingual accessory cusp (tuberculum dentale) on the canines. (Photograph by Maia M. Langley.)

Dental Modification

Dental modification is a useful marker of African birth as distinguished from African ancestry (Handler 1994). For this reason, the evidence for dental modification in this burial is particularly interesting. Individual 4769 v.2 is missing both her maxillary lateral incisors (see figure 9.6). The alveolar bone where the tooth sockets would have been visible is completely healed over, and there are no visible root remnants. There are no caries, decalcified patches, or erosions on the adjacent teeth that would point to caries as an explanation for the absent teeth. The absence of wear facets suggests that the lateral incisors had been absent for many years, as does the condition of the alveolar bone. While agenesis of the lateral incisors is fairly common, people with agenesis have small central incisors and canines, and the remaining teeth are retracted, not procumbent as hers are (Woodworth et al. 1985).

Dental modification is widespread among African populations, and there is an enormous literature on patterns of avulsion, chipping and filing, age and sex associations, and cultural meanings. There appears to be no comprehensive review of this information, and most reports are anecdotal. By far the most common patterns reported are avulsion of all maxillary incisors, a v-shaped notch between the upper central incisors, and tooth pointing (Jones 1992). Few authors report frequencies, but the practice was nearly universal in some ethnic groups, and patterns were to some extent ethnic markers (de Almeida 1953). We have discovered no reports of the specific pattern that we see in Individual 4769 v.2—avulsion of the upper lateral incisors but not of the central incisors. However, archaeological discoveries of modified dentitions are known from regions in which the practice no longer exists (Haour and Pearson 2005), and patterns have been discovered in fairly recent archaeological contexts that are not documented in ethnographic or medical studies of descendant groups (Brabant 1974). It is not surprising that dental modification practices have changed under the pressure of Islamic and Christian missionization, slavery, and colonial exploitation; hence we do not consider the lack of modern documentation for this novel pattern to be an impediment to our interpretation.

The central incisors show pronounced wear on the lingual surfaces that suggests use of the teeth as tools or for specialized food processing. Strikingly similar wear has been reported in crania from Senegal, in which it was attributed to foods introduced during the colonial period (Irish and Turner 1997). Marked lingual surface wear has also been reported in individuals from Renaissance Cyprus, where it is attributed to flax or silk processing (Harper 2006).

Ancestry versus Anomaly

This unusual person raises interesting issues regarding the interpretation of unusual morphology. In his 1866 "Observations on an Ethnic Classification of Idiots," Langdon Down proposed Ethiopian, Malay, and American types in addition to his eponymous Mongolian syndrome (Down 1866). Is it possible that this was a person with a developmental syndrome? The continuing controversy over the Flores hominid points to the importance of paying equal attention to ancestry and dysmorphology in evaluating unusual remains.

Sagittal synostosis (premature fusion of the sagittal suture between the two parietal bones) might account for the dolichocranic appearance of Individual 4769 v.2, but there is no closure of the sagittal suture visible ectocranially. Childhood closure of the sagittal suture can result in a long, narrow cranial vault with a sharp ridge along the closed suture. The medical term that describes this condition, "scaphocephaly," comes from the Greek *skaphe* (boat) and *kephale* (head), from the supposed resemblance of the ridged vault to the keel of an upturned boat. The vault is filled with soil so that the endocranial surfaces cannot be observed. Stewart (1982) has pointed out the relatively high frequency of scaphocephaly in African crania, and this may be related to the tendency of these populations toward dolichocephaly. However, we would not expect to see prognathism in a narrow-vaulted European with scaphocephaly.

Endemic cretinism, a condition characterized by retarded physical growth and mental development due to thyroid insufficiency in infancy, was once common in parts of the Iberian Peninsula as a consequence of limited soil iodine in interior regions, as well as the iodine-binding propensities of certain staple foods, most notably chestnuts (Fernandez 1990). Cretinism is associated with distinctive skull proportions including microcephaly, prognathism, flat nasal bridge, and wide nose; these features are accompanied by an abnormally small, broad (brachycephalic) cranial vault and hypoplastic facial bones, the result of deficient cranial growth. There is no evidence for microcephaly in 4769 v.2 when her cranial measurements are compared with the other females from Torre de Palma (table 9.1).

Statistical comparison provides a more open-ended approach to the issue of anomaly versus ancestry; our colleagues Rick Ward and Paul Jamison have proposed discordant Z-scores as a diagnostic criterion for facial dysmorphology. A bony, site-specific version of the Craniofacial Variability Index (Ward et al. 1998) for 4769 v.2 produces low, concordant Z-scores, suggesting that she was not dysmorphic.

Ancient DNA

Using standard ancient DNA methods and precautions (Kaestle and Horsburgh 2002), we successfully extracted and amplified approximately 175 base pairs (nt 16038–16213) of the first hypervariable region of the mitochondrial genome from 0.1 g of dentin sampled from the left maxillary first molar. Compared to the Cambridge Reference Sequence (Anderson et al. 1981), the 4769 v.2 sequence for this region contained transitions at positions 16111 and 16124. These mutations are consistent with 4769 v.2 belonging to mitochondrial haplogroup L3, a haplogroup of African origin (Watson et al. 1996). A BLAST search of 4769 v.2's sequence against the National Center for Biotechnology Information's Genbank public database (Benson et al. 2008) resulted in 100 percent matches with seven sequences of either African or likely African (for example, Cuban) origin (U94015, AY210602, DQ517651, EU649825, EU649835, EU597512, and EU092735). Unfortunately, we were neither able to replicate this result from a second extraction attempt nor to expand the sequenced region to obtain greater phylogenetic specificity. We decided not to resample, preferring to conserve the enamel morphology and lab resources. We therefore regard these results as suggestive of an African origin for 4769 v.2 (which is fully consistent with the cranial and dental findings described above), but not conclusive according to the strict standards for verification of ancient sequence (Kaestle and Horsburgh 2002).

Chronology and Context

A sample of bone from the mandible and a phalanx of 4769 v.2 was sent to Beta Analytical Laboratories for radiocarbon dating. The results indicate that she died sometime between A.D. 1469 and 1648 (2 Sigma, calibrated for eastern Portugal using the calibration program developed by the Portuguese archaeologist Monge Soares). Radiocarbon dating of mortar samples from the eastern portion of the church at Torre de Palma indicates that construction was begun in the early fifth century A.D., and the adjacent western basilica and cruciform baptistery were added during the following centuries (Huffstott 1998; Hale et al. 1999–2000; Langley 2006). The eastern portion of the church was abandoned around the end of the first millennium A.D., but the western portion remained in use until at least the sixteenth century, according to ecclesiastical documents (Soares, Curvo e Lima, 1758, in Langley et al. 2007) and to the identification of sixteenth-century coins in two burials of children in the western basilica

(Huffstott 1999/2000). Indeed, at the time of the site's discovery in 1947, the low ruined eastern apse wall of the ancient church was still known locally as the Ermidas de São Domingos (Langley et al. 2007). Although most of the materials that were collected from the first MNA excavations were clearly marked with designations such as "Cemiterio," "Capela," or "Cemiterio ao pe das Ermidas" and assigned to specific sepulturas, the later stages of the MNA excavations were focused on the eastern area of the church. This individual's MNA catalog number (4769 v.2) was the last one entered for human remains for the entire Torre de Palma collection, which strongly suggests that it was recovered from the last MNA excavation campaign (and probably its final days) at this site.

Discussion

In the early fifteenth century Portuguese explorers began charting the west coast of Africa, making frequent landfalls and establishing trading connections. A regrettable consequence of this exploration was the appearance of numerous enslaved sub-Saharan Africans in Portugal, whose numbers steadily increased over the next two centuries (Lowe 2005). In death as in life, these people were often treated with great disrespect, as attested by historical accounts (Earle and Lowe 2005) and the recent excavation of a sixteenth–seventeenth-century slave cemetery at Lagos, a city on the southwest coast of Portugal that was a major port for ships involved in west African exploration and commerce (Neves et al. 2009).

Saunders's (1982) fascinating study of black African slaves and freedmen in fifteenth–sixteenth-century Portugal describes in detail the numerous occupations followed by black Africans in both urban and rural locations throughout Iberia. One possible scenario to explain the presence of the Black African woman known to us as the African Queen at the site of Torre de Palma is that she was employed in some capacity (either enslaved or free) at the large Herdade de Torre de Palma, perhaps as a domestic worker at the Monte or an agricultural laborer elsewhere on the vast estate. The marked lingual wear on the maxillary central incisors may identify her as a textile worker or seamstress (Harper 2006).

Enslaved Africans brought to Portugal were "Christianized" as a matter of course (Saunders 1982; Earle and Lowe 2005) and were frequently buried in sanctified ground. In Lisbon and Evora, for example, religious confraternities associated with São Domingos (Saint Dominic) were responsible for the charitable burial of both enslaved and free black Africans (Saunders 1982). The association of our subject with a locality remembered to the present day as a hermitage of the Dominican missionary order may be no accident. We will never know whether our African Queen was enslaved or a free "woman of color," or how she came to Portugal. But at the end of her life she was regarded by the people around her as worthy of Christian burial, and was interred on the grounds of the old Ermidas de São Domingos, a place of honor and respect, regardless of the social and economic circumstances of her earthly journey.

Just as the African Queen was a surprise because of her cranial morphology, her late date was also somewhat unexpected. Black Africans appeared in Europe during the Roman Empire (Leach et al. 2010), and we thought it possible that she dated from the era of the villas. We began this study expecting that the Basilica burials represented an early medieval rural elite contemporary with the construction of the earlier basilica. Instead, the African Queen shows us that the locale continued to be used as a cemetery after the churches were no longer being renovated or were in ruins. Torre de Palma thus presents an exceptional example of long-term continuity in local use of sacred ground as cemetery space. It seems unlikely that the late burials were high-status persons, and we suspect that the elite dead of this time were buried in some active church in the surrounding towns.

The identification of 4769 v.2 as an individual with some degree of sub-Saharan ancestry is ironic, given the fact that Manuel Heleno, the director of the MNA excavations at Torre de Palma for almost two decades, had written his doctoral dissertation in 1933 on the history of African slaves in Portugal (Heleno 1933). Had he looked closely at this distinctive skull in the MNA *vitrine*, he might have recognized 4769 v.2 as a remarkable example of this history. In contrast to other regions in the African diaspora, slave and free blacks in Portugal were not confined to a limited range of occupations or markedly separated from the remainder of society (Saunders 1982; Earle and Lowe 2005). The diverse roles documented in historical sources tempt us to speculate about our subject's social identity: Was she the bride in a marriage arranged to cement business ties between Portuguese and Gold Coast traders? The child of a Wolof recruited for his equestrian skills? A Dominican religious or lay sister? A priest's or land-owner's concubine? An embroiderer or seamstress famous for her craft? Such women did exist in late medieval Portugal, and one of them may have lived out her life at Torre de Palma. The stable carbon isotope ratio (12C/13C) obtained from a bone sample from the African Queen is slightly less negative than the majority of the ratios available for the other Torre de Palma adults, but it does not suggest that her diet differed greatly from that of other adults buried here.

It is perhaps parsimonious to see her as a slave attached to the Monte and given a Christian burial. She is important because we have very little archaeological evidence of Africans in Portugal. Historical sources give us names of owners, a few names of slaves and freedmen, and locations of the ghettos where they lived, but their lives, deaths, and burials have been lost to view.

Acknowledgments

I (MLP) would like to thank Stephanie Maloney (the director of the University of Louisville Torre de Palma Archaeological Project) for inviting me to join the project team in 1996, and John Hale (University of Louisville) for his initial identification of the "African Queen." We thank Luis Raposo, the director of the Museu Nacional de Arqueologia in Lisbon, for permission to remove bone and tooth samples from this very interesting individual in the Museu's Torre de Palma collection, for the purpose of radiocarbon dating and other analyses. We thank Ana Luisa Santos (Universidade de Coimbra) and Carolan Wood (University of Toronto) for contributing useful information regarding the identification of ancestry from skeletal data. We thank Rui Boaventura (MNA) for photography and Mark Schurr (Notre Dame University) for stable carbon isotope data. Funds for ancient DNA analysis were provided by Indiana University.

Notes

1. The Hamann-Todd collection was assembled (1893–1938) by two professors of anatomy, Carl August Hamann and T. Wingate Todd, in the Western Reserve University School of Medicine (now known as Case-Western University) in Cleveland. It represents European Americans and African Americans who died in the Cleveland area during the very end of the nineteenth century and the first four decades of the twentieth century. This collection is presently curated by the Department of Physical Anthropology at the Cleveland Museum of Natural History.

2. The Terry collection was assembled (1910–1967) by Robert J. Terry, professor in the Anatomy Department in the Washington University Medical School, St. Louis, and by his successor, Mildred Trotter. It represents European Americans and African Americans who died in the St. Louis area. This collection is now curated in the Department of Anthropology, National Museum of Natural History, Smithsonian Institution, Washington, D.C.

3. This Late Archaic archaeological site was excavated (1937–1941) under the direction of William S. Webb, Department of Anthropology, University of Kentucky, Lexington. The human skeletal collection is curated at the W. S. Webb Museum of Anthropology at that university.

References Cited

Anderson S., A. T. Bankier, B. G. Barrell, M. H. de Bruijn, A. R. Coulson, J. Drouin, I. C. Eperon, D. P. Nierlich, B. A. Roe, F. Sanger, P. H. Schreier, A. J. Smith, R. Staden, and I. G. Young
1981   Sequence and Organization of the Human Mitochondrial Genome. *Nature* 290(5806): 457–65.

Angel, J. Lawrence, and Jennifer Olsen Kelley
1990   Inversion of the Posterior Edge of the Jaw Ramus: New Race Trait. In *Skeletal Attribution of Race*, edited by G. W. Gill and S. Rhine, pp. 33–39. Anthropological Papers No. 4. Maxwell Museum of Anthropology, Albuquerque, N.Mex.

Bass, William M.
1987   *Human Osteology: A Laboratory and Field Manual.* Missouri Archaeological Society, Columbia.

Benson, D. A., I. Karsch-Mizrachi, D. J. Lipman, J. Ostell, and D. L. Wheeler
2008   Genbank. *Nucleic Acids Research* 36 (Database Issue): D25–30.

Brabant, H.
1974   Remarques sur la Denture du Crâne du Roi Cyirima II Rujugira (Afrique Central). *Bulletin du Groupement Européen pour la Recherche Scientifique en Stomatologie et Odontologie* 17(2): 99–103.

Brooks, Sheilagh, Richard H. Brooks, and Diane France
1990   Alveolar Prognathism Contour, an Aspect of Racial Identification. In *Skeletal Attribution of Race*, edited by G. W. Gill and S. Rhine, pp. 41–46. Anthropological Papers No. 4. Maxwell Museum of Anthropology, Albuquerque, N.Mex.

Brues, Alice M.
1990   The Once and Future Diagnosis of Race. In *Skeletal Attribution of Race*, edited by G. W. Gill and S. Rhine, pp. 1–7. Anthropological Papers No. 4. Maxwell Museum of Anthropology, Albuquerque, N.Mex.

Byers, Steven N.
2002   *Introduction to Forensic Anthropology: A Textbook.* Allyn & Bacon, Boston.

de Almeida, Reinaldo
1953   Mutilações Dentárias nos Negros da Lunda. *Anais do Instituto de Medicina Tropical (Lisboa)* 10(4 Part 2): 3601–39.

Down, J. Langdon H.
1866   Observations on an Ethnic Classification of Idiots. *London Hospital Clinical Lectures and Reports* 3: 259–62. Reprinted in *Down's Syndrome (Mongolism): A Reference Bibliography*, edited by Rudolf F. Vollman. U.S. National Institutes of Health, Bethesda, Md., 1969.

Earle, T. F., and Kate Lowe
2005   *Black Africans in Renaissance Europe.* Cambridge University Press, Cambridge.

Edgar, Heather J. H.
2005   Prediction of Race Using Characteristics of Dental Morphology. *Journal of Forensic Science* 50(2): 269–73.

Fernandez, Renate Lellep
1990   *A Simple Matter of Salt: An Ethnography of Nutritional Deficiency in Spain.* University of California Press, Berkeley.

Giles, Eugene, and Orville Elliott

1962 Race Identification from Cranial Measurements. *Journal of Forensic Sciences* 7(2): 147–57.

Hale, John R., Åsa Ringbom, Alf Lindroos, and Jan Heinemeier

1999–2000 A Datação por Radiocarbono de Argamassas, Fazendo Uso da Técnica AMS (Espectrometria de Massa com Acelerador). *A Cidade—Revista Cultural de Portalegre* 13/14: 145–56. Edições Colibri, Lisbon.

Handler, Jerome S.

1994 Determining African Birth from Skeletal Remains: A Note on Tooth Mutilation. *Historical Archaeology* 28(3): 113–19.

Haour, A., and J. A. Pearson

2005 An Instance of Dental Modification on a Human Skeleton from Niger, West Africa. *Oxford Journal of Archaeology* 24(4): 427–33.

Harper, Nathan

2006 Industrial Wear from Venetian Period Cyprus. In *Supplement to the Paleopathology Newsletter: Program and Abstracts, XVI European Meeting of the Paleopathology Association, Santorini, Greece.* Paleopathology Association, Lexington, Ky.

Heleno, Manuel

1933 *Os Escravos em Portugal.* Vol. 1. Tip. da Emprêsa do Anuário Comercial, Lisbon.

1962 A "villa" Lusitano-romana de Torre de Palma (Monforte). *O Arqueólogo Português* (2a Série) 4: 313–38.

Hellman, Milo

1928 Racial Characters in Human Dentition. *Proceedings of the American Philosophical Society* 67: 157–74.

Huffstott, John S.

1998 Votive(?) Use of Coins in Fourth-century Lusitania: The Builders' Deposit in the Torre de Palma Basilica. *Revista Portuguesa de Arqueologica* 1 (1): 221–26.

1999/2000 Moedas das Escavações Promovidas pela Universidade de Louisville em Torre de Palma, 1983–99. *A Cidade—Revista Cultural de Portalegre* 13/14: 121–28. Edições Colibri, Lisbon.

Irish, Joel D., and Christy G. Turner II

1997 Brief Communication: First Evidence of LSAMAT in Non-Native Americans: Historic Senegalese from West Africa. *American Journal of Physical Anthropology* 102 (1): 141–46.

Jones, Alan

1992 Tooth Mutilation in Angola. *British Dental Journal* 173(5): 177–78.

Kaestle, Frederika, and K. Ann Horsburgh

2002 Ancient DNA in Anthropology: Methods, Applications, and Ethics. *Yearbook of Physical Anthropology* 45: 92–130.

Krogman, Wilton Marion

1962 *The Human Skeleton in Forensic Medicine.* Charles C. Thomas, Springfield, Ill.

Langley, Maia

2006 Est in Agris, a Spatial Analysis of Roman *Uillae* in the Region of Monforte, Alto Alentejo, Portugal. *Revista Portuguesa de Arqueologia* 9(2): 317–28. IPA, Lisbon.

Langley, Maia, Rui Mataloto, Rui Boaventura, and David Gonçalves

2007   A Ocupação da Idade do Ferro de Torre de Palma: "Escavando Nos Fundos" do Museu Nacional de Arqueologia. *O Arqueologo Português* 25(Serie 4): 229–90.

Leach, S., H. Eckhardt, C. Chenery, G. Muldner, and M. Lewis

2010   A Lady of York: Migration, Ethnicity, and Identity in Roman Britain. *Antiquity* 84(323): 131–45.

Lowe, Kate

2005   Introduction: The Black African Presence in Renaissance Europe. In *Black Africans in Renaissance Europe*, edited by Kate J. P. Lowe and T. F. Earle, pp. 1–14. Cambridge University Press, Cambridge.

Maloney, Stephanie J., and John R. Hale

1996   The Villa of Torre de Palma (Alto Alentejo). *Journal of Roman Archaeology* 9: 275–94.

Neves, Maria João, Sofia Wasterlain, and Maria Teresa Ferreira

2009   Dental Modification in a 16th/17th Century Sample of African Slaves Found at Lagos (Portugal): Pathological Consequences of Intentional Chipping. Paper presented at the Third Paleopathology Association Meeting in South America (PAMinSA III), Necochea, Argentina.

Ousley, Stephen D., and Richard L. Jantz

2005   FORDISC 3.0: Personal Computer Forensic Discriminant Functions. Electronic document, http://web.utk.edu/~fac/fordisc.shtml.

Saunders, A. C. de C. M.

1982   *A Social History of Black Slaves and Freedmen in Portugal (1441-1555).* Cambridge University Press, Cambridge.

Stewart, T. Dale

1982   La scaphocéphalie chez les Noirs: Une variété de déformation pathologique de la tête. *Bulletins et Mémoires de la Société d'Anthropologie de Paris* 9 (Série 13): 267–69.

Ward, Richard E., Paul L. Jamison, and Leslie G. Farkas

1998   Craniofacial Variability Index: A Simple Measure of Normal and Abnormal Variation in the Head and Face. *American Journal of Medical Genetics* 80(3): 232–40.

Watson, Elizabeth, Karin Bauer, Rashid Aman, Gunter Weiss, Arndt von Haesseler, and Svante Pääbo

1996   mtDNA Sequence Diversity in Africa. *American Journal of Human Genetics* 59: 437–41.

Woodworth, D. A., P. M. Sinclair, and R. G. Alexander

1985   Bilateral Congenital Absence of Maxillary Lateral Incisors: A Craniofacial and Dental Cast Analysis. *American Journal of Orthodontics* 87(4): 280–93.

THREE ❖ Craftsmen and Artisans

10 ◈ Sew Long?

The Osteobiography of a Woman from Medieval Polis, Cyprus

Brenda J. Baker, Claire E. Terhune, and Amy Papalexandrou

Individual Profile

Site: Polis Chrysochous (Roman Arsinoë)
Location: In and around the town of Polis Chrysochous, on the northwest coast, Republic of Cyprus
Cultural Affiliation: Christian (Late Antique/Medieval)
Date: 7th–11th centuries A.D., based on stratigraphic and ceramic evidence
Feature: Burial 2005-2
Location of Grave: Trench E.F2.m10, 12 m south of the E.F2 basilica (designations refer to the Princeton site grid consisting of 10 m units)
Burial and Grave Type: Single primary inhumation in extended, supine position; subsurface pit defined by several large rocks along its perimeter and covered with unworked limestone slabs
Associated Materials: In direct association with the skeleton: a bone needle, iron nail, and ceramic bottle base; additional artifacts in grave fill: a small, ovoid stone with pecking evident on one surface
Preservation and Completeness: Good preservation, with fragmentation of some skeletal elements—particularly articular surfaces and cranium—and some reconstruction of long bones
Age at Death and Basis of Estimate: 30–39 years, based on auricular surface and dental attrition
Sex and Basis of Determination: Female, based on cranial and pelvic morphology
Conditions Observed: Malocclusion and wear on the anterior dentition suggesting use of the teeth to hold material and to draw thread; rugose muscle attachments and facet development on hand bones consistent with occupational stress attributed to tailors; alterations to the legs indicate habitual kneeling or squatting
Specialized Analysis: None to date
Excavated: 2005, Princeton University Expedition to Polis Chrysochous, directed by William A. P. Childs, Princeton University
Archaeological Report: Childs 1988
Current Disposition: Curated in Polis, Cyprus

Mortuary practices of the early medieval period (mid- to late first millennium A.D.) in Cyprus are known from only a handful of sites. At Polis Chrysochous, excavations conducted by Princeton University since the mid-1980s have uncovered over 200 burials clustered in and around two medium-size, early Christian basilicas at the north edge of the modern town, within a five-minute walk of each other. Both basilicas date to the late fifth or early sixth century. The presence of multiple churches within the same settlement is not unusual for the Late Antique/Byzantine period.

The church to the north, in the E.G0 project area, was conceived as a cemetery basilica, with ossuary pits (subterranean facilities that contained commingled remains of multiple individuals) lining its north and east walls. The basilica to the south, in the project area designated E.F2, is the more standard type, with three aisles terminated by apses and preceded by a narthex to the west. This building was not outfitted with ossuary pits, presumably because of its location in the town center, where burials would have been initially discouraged. The area was densely inhabited with a network of streets, workshops, and a system of water lines and drainage channels dating to the Roman period. Following construction of the E.F2 basilica, however, graves were eventually dug into the floor of the main church, the south portico, and the narthex. At the same time, the grounds to the east and south of this church were eventually co-opted for use as a cemetery for the local population. The basilica seems to have been active, with intermittent periods of decline or abandonment, until the eleventh century, when it fell completely out of use.

The location of graves in relation to the E.F2 basilica and the types and presence of grave goods indicate differences in high- and low-status interments. For example, three interior tombs lining the south wall of the south aisle are large, deep, and carefully built, with a smooth coating of mortar-plaster lining on the inside walls. One of these tombs was covered with large marble slabs. The middle tomb contained a coin dating to the fifth or sixth century along with a large, bronze pectoral cross. The placement (near the sanctuary) and construction of these tombs and the quality of the grave goods indicate they are high-status burials. Less elaborate graves excavated in the 1980s seem to be clustered in the area south and east of the basilica in the cemetery outside of the building (see Buck 1993). Because these graves are typically simple subsurface pits with few or no lining stones that are infrequently covered by slabs, their occupants are assumed to be of lower status than individuals buried in cist tombs to the west or in favored locations inside the church.

During the 2005 field season, a grave in this lower-status area was excavated 12 m south of the E.F2 basilica (figures 10.1, 10.2). This area has been

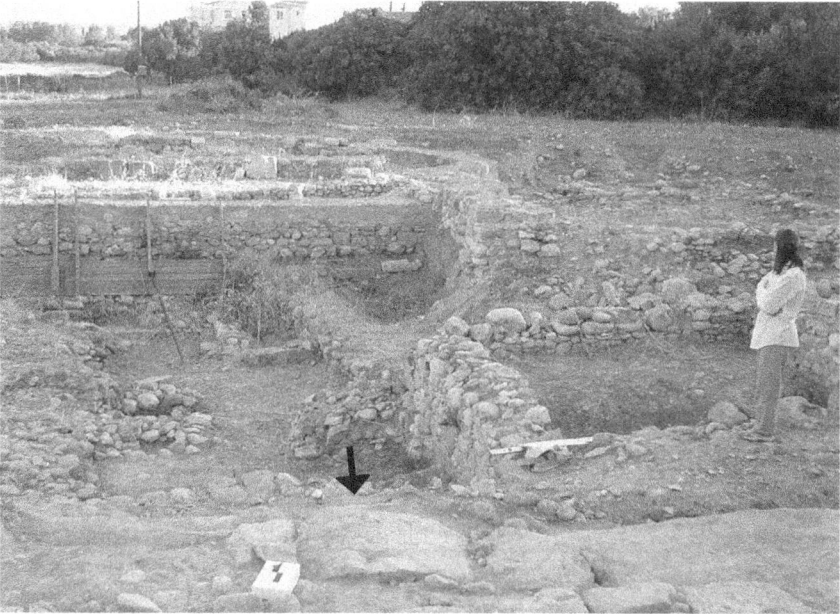

Figure 10.1. Location of grave (black arrow) with the basilica in the background (view to the north). (Photograph by Claire E. Terhune.)

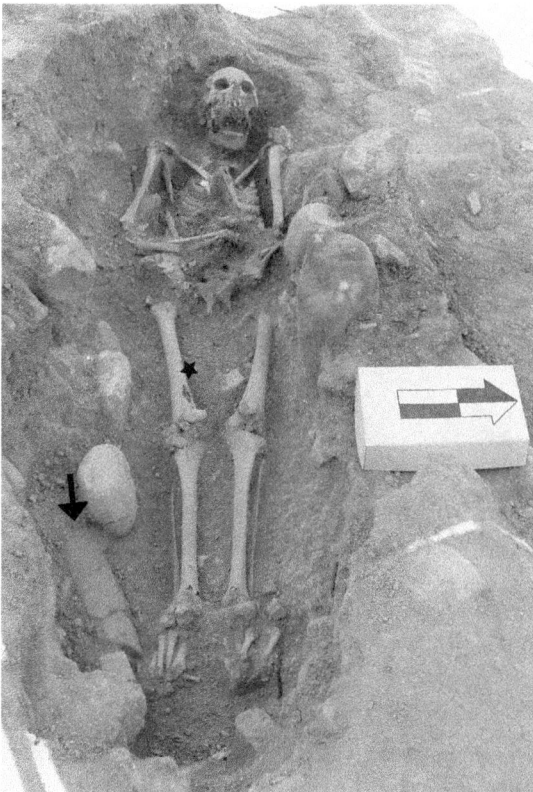

Figure 10.2. The seamstress's skeleton in situ, showing the outline of the grave and the Roman pipe (arrow). The location of the bone needle is indicated by the star on the medial side of the right femur. (Photograph by Brenda J. Baker.)

reconstructed by Childs (2008) as a hub of Roman workshops prior to the basilica's construction. The body, that of a woman who died in her thirties, was placed in a subsurface pit covered with unworked limestone slabs. The pit cut into a late Roman drainage pipe, and her body was placed beside it. Thus, by the time of interment (in the seventh to eleventh centuries A.D.), the water system in this area was apparently no longer in use. In keeping with other graves in the vicinity and in comparison to other burials within and around the E.F2 basilica, this grave was relatively simple. The paucity of grave goods (for example, high-status items like jewelry or coins) also suggests a lower-status individual. Gaps permitted soil to accumulate in the grave, which was occupied by a large number of snails just under the slabs. Root disturbance was also noted, with one root extending through the medullary cavity of the right humerus.

Artifacts found in the grave include a bone needle next to the right femur and a small, rounded ground stone, damaged on one aspect, in the fill above the skeleton (figure 10.3). These grave inclusions suggested the possibility that this individual sewed and/or worked with textiles, leather, or perhaps nets. Our subsequent analysis of her skeleton was directed toward investigating the hypothesis that this woman was a seamstress.

The skeletal analysis conducted in July 2006 identified a series of activity-related changes that supported this initial hypothesis. These alterations are discussed in the context of previous ethnographic and bioarchaeological studies of

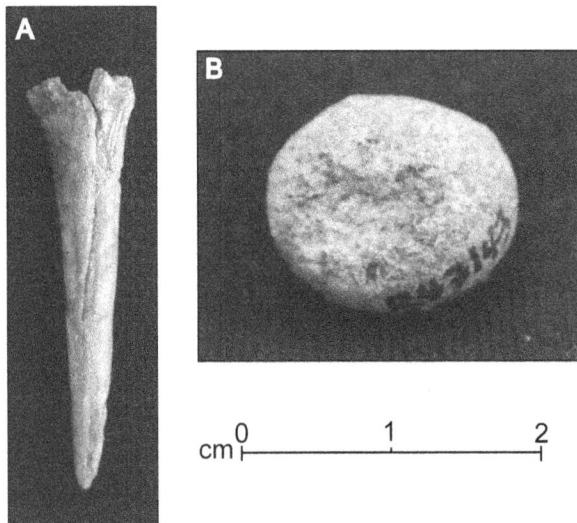

Figure 10.3. The bone needle recovered from the seamstress's grave (A) and the small ground stone (B). (Photographs by Brenda J. Baker.)

occupational stresses (e.g., Wells 1967; Merbs 1983; Kennedy 1989). Further research on the grave goods informs this discussion. We conclude this chapter by comparing the pattern of activity-related skeletal changes with evidence from other medieval sites in Cyprus (and elsewhere). For ease of communication, we refer to this individual as a seamstress, a term defined as "a woman who is expert at sewing, esp. one who makes her living by sewing" (Merriam-Webster 1988), though we imply only that she sewed regularly over her lifetime and did not necessarily practice sewing as an occupation.

Skeletal Analysis

During cleaning and inventory of the seamstress's skeletal remains in 2005, we observed several grooves on the distolingual interproximal surfaces of both maxillary lateral incisors (the area between the second upper incisors and canine teeth). Two grooves are located on the distal margin of the left lateral

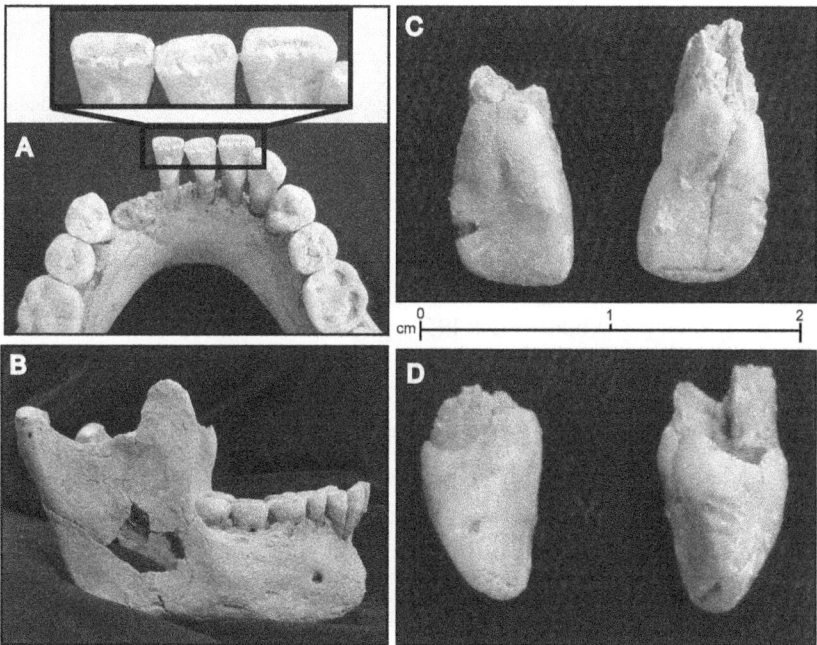

Figure 10.4. Modifications to the seamstress's dentition, showing (A) the occlusal wear and anterior-posterior striations (inset) on the mandibular incisors, (B) the projection of the anterior mandibular dentition, (C) a posterior (lingual) view, and (D) a distal view of the grooves on the maxillary lateral incisors (C and D to scale). (Photographs by Brenda J. Baker.)

incisor, while three smaller striations are present on the right (figure 10.4). These grooves are all less than 1.0 mm wide, indicating repetitive use of these teeth, most likely for drawing thread or fiber alongside them. Further analysis in 2006 revealed a suite of dental and skeletal alterations consistent with the hypothesis that this individual was a seamstress (table 10.1).

In addition to the multiple grooves initially observed on the maxillary lateral incisors, dental pathology includes anterior-posterior (labial-lingual) notches and anterior projection of the mandibular incisors, with alveolar resorption and heavy occlusal wear (figure 10.4). The malocclusion and wear suggest that she held and pulled material with her front teeth (Ronchese 1948; Merbs 1983), while the striations suggest holding or cutting thread (Ronchese 1948) or that she may have held pins with these teeth. There are no matching striations on the maxillary central incisors, probably due to malocclusion of her anterior teeth. The slight osteoarthritis of the articular surfaces of both mandibular condyles is also consistent with use of the anterior teeth as tools (Merbs 1983).

In the infracranial skeleton (figure 10.5), muscle attachments are more developed on the metacarpals of this woman's right hand than her left, a condition known as "seamstress's fingers" (Merbs 1983; Kennedy 1989). Her right clavicle is more robust than the left, with osteoarthritis of the articular facets for the sternum and first rib and much greater development of the attachment for the costoclavicular ligament. These changes are consistent with occupational stresses attributed to tailors (e.g., Lane 1888; Merbs 1983; Kennedy 1989). Morphological signs on the bones of the legs and feet indicate habitual squatting or kneeling. The development of an accessory facet above the adductor tubercle in the area of attachment for the gastrocnemius muscle on the distal femur is known as Charles's facet and arises from stresses of a squatting posture (Charles 1893–1894; Klaatsch 1900; Kostick 1963). The distal tibiae were damaged postmortem, but squatting facets are evident on both tali (Thomson 1889, 1890; Das 1959; Singh 1959; Kostick 1963). Facets on the dorsal surfaces of both the right and left first metatarsals and on the proximal toe phalanges reflect habitual hyperextension of the metatarsophalangeal joints associated with regular kneeling (Ubelaker 1978, 1979). Additional development of muscle attachments and facetlike articular extensions in the feet (table 10.1) are also related to these activities.

Osteoarthritis is mild in this woman, but she has more than would be expected for an individual in her thirties. Along with the temporomandibular joint and right clavicle, arthritic changes affect the right wrist, middle of the spine, both hip joints, right ankle and lateral portion of the foot, and the left knee.

Table 10.1. Skeletal alterations and related activities

Skeletal Changes	Occupational Activity
Labio-lingual striations on occlusal surfaces of mandibular incisors (Figure 10.4A)	Holding and cutting thread
Anterior projection of mandibular incisors with alveolar resorption and heavy occlusal wear (Figure 10.4B)	Increased use of the anterior teeth for holding items while working
Disto-lingual grooves on distal interproximal surfaces of maxillary I2s (Figure 10.4C–D)	Pulling thread between incisors and canines
Slight porosity to articular surfaces of R and L mandibular condyles	Osteoarthritis of the TMJ while holding objects in teeth
Robust R clavicle with degeneration of sternal end along articulations with sternum and first rib (Figure 10.5A)	Hand sewing
R metacarpals more robust with more pronounced muscle markings (Figure 10.5B)	Seamstress's fingers
Increased rugosity of the L ischial tuberosity	Inflammation from long periods of sitting
Charles's facet present above the medial condyle of the R distal femur (Figure 10.5D)	Squatting
Facetlike extension of dorsal aspect of R navicular, possibly related to squatting facets present on the tali	Squatting
Rugose and enlarged muscle attachments on the plantar surface of the medial tubercles on both calcanei	Flexion of the foot at the lateral four metatarsophalangeal joints, as associated with kneeling
Anterior extension of the trochlear articular surface onto the necks of both tali (Figure10.5C)	Squatting facets
Facets on the dorsal surfaces of both first metatarsals and first proximal phalanges at the metatarsophalangeal joint (Figure 10.5E)	Hyperextension at the metatarsophalangeal joints associated with kneeling with toes bent at approximately 90 degrees

Lipping and porosity of the bodies and neural arches of at least three midthoracic vertebrae, both scapular glenoid fossae, distal margin of the R hamate, lunate surfaces of the acetabulum, distal articular surface of the R fibula, corresponding articular facets of the R 4th and 5th metatarsals, and lateral articular facet of L patella. These changes are due to osteoarthritis.

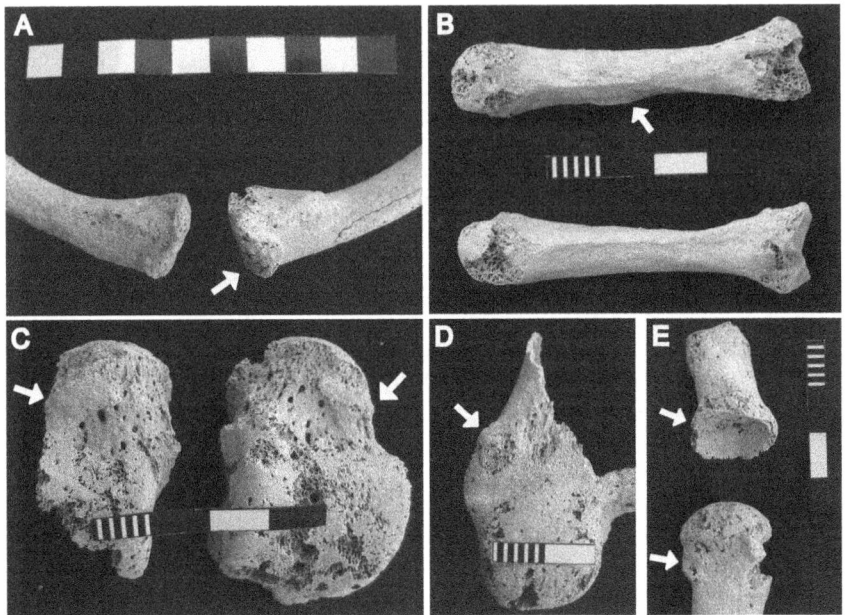

Figure 10.5. Markers of occupational stress on the seamstress's infracranial skeleton includes (A) osteoarthritic changes to the sternal ends of both clavicles, (B) strong muscle markings on the right second metacarpal (arrow) compared to the left second metacarpal, (C) extension of the articular facets onto the necks of both tali, (D) Charles's facet on the right distal femur, and (E) extension of the articular surfaces on the left first metatarsal and first proximal phalanx. (Photographs by Brenda J. Baker.)

Artifact Analysis

The bone needle found along the inside of the woman's right thigh was made from the modified dorsal spine of a large fish, such as catfish, similar to those found at other sites in Europe and North Africa (Irving 1992). These long, pointed bones have fossae (indentations) or small foramina (holes) that may be enlarged for use as a needle. While short and stout compared to needles used in fine sewing (for example, embroidery), such a needle would be useful for working with heavy or coarse material. The fact that this bone has clearly had its opening enlarged and is heavily polished (see figure 10.3) indicates that it was, in fact, used as a tool and is not simply a cast-off fish bone (see Irving 1992 for comparisons of unmodified spines and those modified for use as tools).

The small, ovoid ground stone is approximately 1.7 cm long and is chipped on only one surface, indicating that it was held between the fingers in a certain way. Photographs shown to an archaeologist who specializes in the study of ground stone tools from prehistoric Cyprus provided additional information

(Laura Swantek, personal communication 2007). The use wear shows that the stone was a percussion tool similar to an expedient (that is, unshaped prior to use) hammerstone. The size and shape of the stone allow it to fit comfortably between the fingertips of one hand, suggesting it was used for delicate work like striking an implement with a fine edge, such as a needle or small awl. It may have been used as a kind of thimble to push or hammer a needle through thick material like animal hide, or more likely in conjunction with a metal or bone awl to puncture holes in animal hide through which a needle and thread could easily pass. In current practice, a metal thimble is used in sewing to push needles through thick fabric like denim or canvas, much as this stone may have been used by the woman with whom it was buried.

Interpretations and Implications

Both skeletal and artifactual analyses support the hypothesis that this woman practiced some type of sewing activity on a regular basis. Participants in textile production have been identified previously in Cyprus from the Venetian period (fifteenth to sixteenth centuries) at Malloura by Harper (2005, 2006). The dental grooves, notches, and wear on these individuals are similar to those found on the teeth of the woman from Polis. Harper (2005, 2006) related the dental wear pattern to the use of the mouth in spinning cotton or flax. Erdal (2008) reports occlusal grooves in the dentition of women from the tenth-century Anatolian site of Kovuklukaya, but the grooves run transversely across their teeth, rather than from front to back or interproximally as in the Cypriot cases here. Based on ethnographic research, Erdal (2008) concluded that these Anatolian women used their mouths to wet fibers when spinning yarn into cord, resulting in a completely different pattern of dental wear from that found in the woman from Polis, and again reinforcing the suggestion that she practiced a type of activity that was related to sewing with needle and thread. The short, stout needle and small hammerstone accompanying her in death indicate that she often worked with coarse, possibly heavy material such as canvas or leather.

The observation of dental wear and additional skeletal indicators in this individual from Polis provide evidence for sewing heavy or coarse material as early as A.D. 650–1100. It appears that this work may have been performed largely by women, based on our identification of the woman from Polis and by the later evidence from the fifteenth and sixteenth centuries at Malloura, where at least two affected individuals were females (Harper 2005, 2006). Systematic study of the skeletal remains from the long-term Princeton project at Polis was initiated in 2005, and much work remains, including the further investigation of the sex ratio and status of individuals with similar patterns of activity-related stressors.

Conclusion

The detailed analysis and contextualization of this skeleton not only indicates the activity in which this woman may have been involved, but also contributes information on Cypriot society that would be lost if subsumed in reports emphasizing only population data. As such, it provides a deeper biocultural understanding of the site and society. This woman's burial reveals a personal account of life and death in the past that underscores the contribution bioarchaeologists and physical anthropologists can make to large-scale archaeological projects. With the increased necessity to convey our research to the public, this woman's story is one to which people today can relate.

Acknowledgments

We thank William A. P. Childs, director of the Princeton University Archaeological Expedition to Polis, Cyprus, for support of this work, and the Department of Antiquities of Cyprus and then-director Pavlos Florentzos for their cooperation. Alexandros Koupparis, the expedition foreman, facilitated the fieldwork. Justin Goering, supervisor of the trench in which the burial was located, assisted with excavation of the seamstress.

References Cited

Buck, Stacey A.
1993   Life on the Edge of the Empire: Demography and Health in Byzantine Cyprus. Master's thesis, Department of Anthropology, Arizona State University.

Charles, R. Havelock
1893–1894   The Influence of Function, as Exemplified in the Morphology of the Lower Extremity of the Panjabi. *Journal of Anatomy and Physiology* 28: 1–18.

Childs, William A. P.
1988   First Preliminary Report on the Excavations at Polis Chrysochous by Princeton University. *Nicosia: Report of the Department of Antiquities, Cyprus* (1988), Nicosia: 121–30.
2008   Polis Chrysochous: Princeton University's Excavations of Ancient Marion and Arsinoe. *Near Eastern Archaeology* 71: 64–75.

Das, A. C.
1959   Squatting Facets on the Talus in U.P. (Uttar Pradesh) Subjects. *Journal of Anatomy and Society India* 8: 90–92.

Erdal, Y. S.
2008   Occlusal Grooves in Anterior Dentition among Kovuklukaya Inhabitants (Sinop, Northern Anatolia, 10th century A.D.). *International Journal of Osteoarchaeology* 18(2): 152–66.

Harper, Nathan K.
2005   Specialized Dental Wear from Venetian Period Cyprus. Poster presented at the 71st Annual Meeting of the Society for American Archaeology, Salt Lake City.

2006   Industrial Dental Wear from Venetian Period Cyprus. Poster presented at the 16th European Meeting of the Paleopathology Association, Santorini, Greece.

Irving, Brian G.

1992   The Pectoral Fin Spines of European Catfish *Siliuris glanis*; Cultural Artifacts or Food Remains? *International Journal of Osteoarchaeology* 2: 189–97.

Kennedy, Kenneth A. R.

1989   Skeletal Markers of Occupational Stress. In *Reconstruction of Life from the Skeleton*, edited by M. Y. Iscan and K. A. R. Kennedy, pp. 129–60. Alan R. Liss, New York.

Klaatsch, Hermann

1900   Die wichtigsten Variationen am Skelet der freien unteren Extremität des Menschen und ihre Bedeutung für das Abstammungsproblem. *Ergebnisse der Anatomie und Entwicklungsgeschichte* 10: 599–719.

Kostick, E. L.

1963   Facets and Imprints on the Upper and Lower Extremities of Femora from a Western Nigerian Population. *Journal of Anatomy* 97: 393–402.

Lane, W. Arbuthnot

1888   The Anatomy and Physiology of the Shoemaker. *Journal of Anatomy and Physiology* 22: 593–628.

Merbs, Charles F.

1983   *Patterns of Activity-Induced Pathology in a Canadian Inuit Population*. National Museum of Man Mercury Series, Archaeology Survey of Canada No. 119. National Museums of Canada, Ottawa.

Merriam-Webster

1988   S.v. "seamstress." *Webster's New World Dictionary of American English*. 3rd College Ed. Simon & Schuster, New York.

Ronchese, Francesco

1948   *Occupational Marks and Other Physical Signs: A Guide to Personal Identification*. Grune and Stratton, New York.

Singh, Inderbir

1959   Squatting Facets on the Talus and Tibia in Indians. *Journal of Anatomy* 93: 540–50.

Thomson, Arthur

1889   The Influence of Posture on the Form of the Articular Surfaces of the Tibia and Astragalus in the Different Races of Man and the Higher Apes. *Journal of Anatomy and Physiology* 23: 616–39.

1890   Additional Note on the Influence of Posture on the Form of the Articular Surfaces of the Tibia and Astragalus in the Different Races of Man and the Higher Apes. *Journal of Anatomy and Physiology* 24: 210–17.

Ubelaker, Douglas H.

1978   *Human Skeletal Remains: Excavation, Analysis, Interpretation*. Aldine, Chicago.

1979   Skeletal Evidence for Kneeling in Prehistoric Ecuador. *American Journal of Physical Anthropology* 51(4): 679–85.

Wells, Calvin

1967   Weaver, Tailor or Shoemaker? An Osteological Detective story. *Medical and Biological Illustration* 17: 39–47.

11 ◆ A Master Artisan?

TRIBUTE TO THE FOUNDER OF A TEOTIHUACÁN
APARTMENT COMPOUND

Rebecca Storey and Randolph J. Widmer

Individual Profile

Site: Tlajinga 33 Apartment Compound (S3W1:33)
Location: Teotihuacán, Valley of Mexico, 25 miles northeast of Mexico City
Cultural Affiliation: Pre-Columbian Central Mexican Highlander
Date: A.D. 250–300, Tlamimilolpa period, based on Teotihuacán ceramic chronology
Location of Grave: Under a shrine structure in the earliest principal patio in the compound
Burial and Grave Type: Burial 57—a single primary inhumation, seated and tightly flexed in a rectangular pit cut 1.25 m into the volcanic tuff bedrock (tepetate)
Associated Materials: Three ceramic outcurving bowls, one ceramic olla, three marine shell fragments, 10 small shell ornaments, 4,000+ painted and drilled small gastropod shell beads, a headdress/mask of two shell disks in rattlesnake form and two shell filigree disks, two greenstone beads
Preservation and Completeness: Most of skeleton present but skeletal elements broken and brittle; cranium fragmentary; long bones reconstructed
Age at Death and Basis of Estimate: 50–59, based on auricular surface morphology and dental wear
Sex and Basis of Determination: Male, based on morphology of pelvis and cranium
Conditions Observed: Active infection in the foot
Specialized Analysis: None
Excavated: 1980, Tlajinga 33 Project, directed by William Sanders, Rebecca Storey, and Randolph J. Widmer
Archaeological Report: Storey 1992
Current Disposition: Curated at the Teotihuacán Archaeological Laboratory, Teotihuacán, Mexico

---

Teotihuacán, in the central highland basin of Mexico, was one of the largest cities in the world during its florescence from ca. 100 B.C. to A.D. 600, and certainly the most influential in Mesoamerica during that time. Teotihuacán grew and nucleated rapidly, and by the A.D. 200s had some of the largest and best-integrated public architecture in Mesoamerica (Cowgill 1997). Structures like the Pyramid of the Sun and the 5 km long "Street of the Dead" remain some of the most impressive constructions of pre-Columbian Mesoamerica.

The impressive public architecture is just one element in the complex, planned layout for the city. The Teotihuacán Mapping Project shows the regular street grids in the ancient city, and the structures and main streets characterized by a uniform orientation (Millon 1981). The residential structures, called apartment compounds, have well-defined outer boundaries and multiple apartments inside. These compounds were probably formed by related families, usually (but not always) through male lineages (Spence 1994). There are obvious status differences among various compounds, although the exact proportions of different status residences are not yet clear (Cowgill 2003).

Some residences were clustered in districts. One of these is the Tlajinga district, located in the southern part of the city. The compounds here are more dispersed, are of relatively low status, and appear to have been the focus of ceramic production (Cowgill 1997). The apartment compounds are the principal unit for production of goods and crafts, as there are very few nonresidential craft areas. The lack of residences in the surrounding agricultural fields suggests that farmers also lived in compounds at Teotihuacán. In addition to apartments and open-air activity areas, each compound had a principal patio that was the focus of compoundwide rituals, especially those for ancestor veneration (Headrick 2007).

Tlajinga 33 (S3W1:33 on the Teotihuacán map) was founded during the Early Tlamimilolpa period, between about A.D. 250 and 300 (figure 11.1). Specialized ceramic production, the work of many family members, took place here during the later phases of occupation, and we hoped that the excavation would tell us what the Tlajinga 33 residents did before they became ceramic specialists. The work on this earlier component of occupation revealed that for the first 100–150 years of the compound, the residents specialized in lapidary work using both exotic and common materials, such as shell, greenstone, slate, and travertine (Widmer 1991).

In pre-Columbian Mesoamerica, burials were generally placed under and around residences. A total of 206 individuals were recovered from Tlajinga 33, although there were only 68 in actual burial contexts; the rest were found in disturbed, secondary contexts (Storey 1992). Important individuals from a

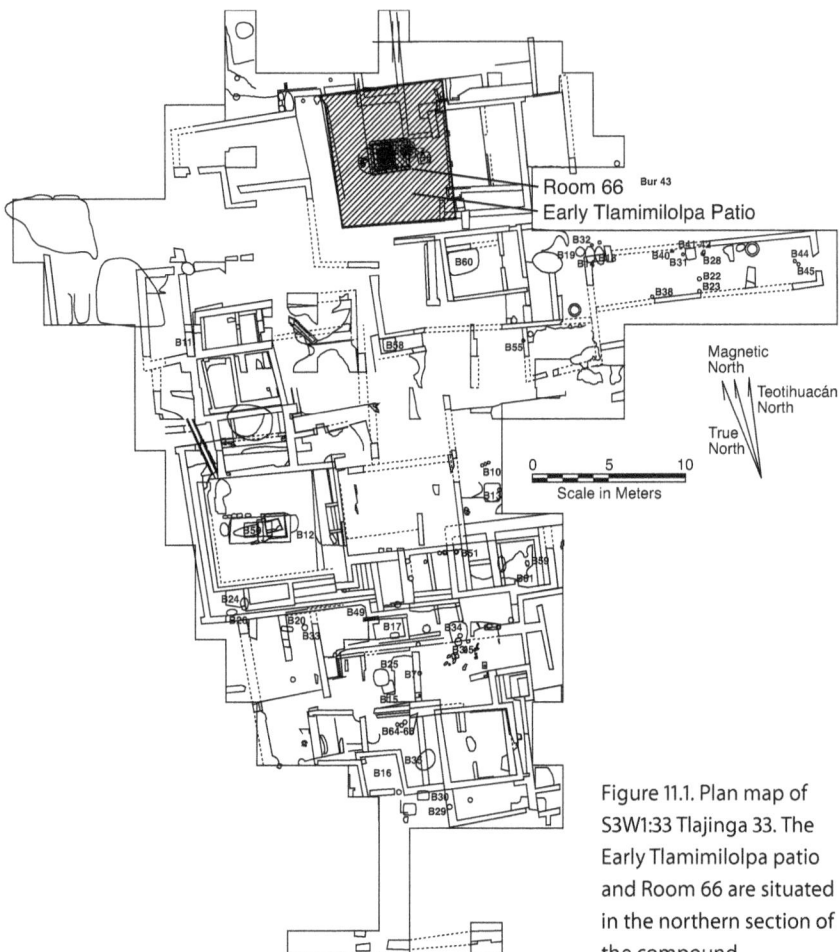

Figure 11.1. Plan map of S3W1:33 Tlajinga 33. The Early Tlamimilolpa patio and Room 66 are situated in the northern section of the compound.

compound were accorded burial in the principal patios under altars. The pre-Columbian Mesoamericans often had elaborate rituals marking "dedication" and "termination" events, as well as special mortuary treatment for the founders of places (Mock 1998). Even the lower-status apartment compounds hold one or a few rich graves, especially from early in their histories, which may be those of founders (Cowgill 1997; Headrick 2007).

Burial 57, the most elaborate burial at Tlajinga 33, was found in the principal patio dating to the Early Tlamimilolpa period. Who was this individual among the residents of this modest apartment compound? To understand his role, we need to take a very detailed look at the archaeological context of his grave, as well as his osteobiography. It is the architectural history of his burial location that indicates his importance.

The Archaeological and Architectural Context of Burial 57

The reconstruction of events surrounding the interment of Burial 57 can be summarized as follows:

1. The compound is constructed during the Early Tlamimilolpa. The principal patio with Room 66, a shrine room, is in the northeast corner.
2. The shrine room is used to display a Huehueteotl (Old Fire God) incense burner and probably the bundled body of Burial 57 after his death.
3. Burial 56 is interred in the center of the shrine room, and the room continues in use.
4. After some time, it is decided to ritually terminate the patio, temple, and shrine room, probably because a new central patio was being constructed.
5. Burial 57 is interred, the shrine room razed, and the Huehueteotl (Old Fire God) incense burner ritually "killed" and buried.
6. Even though terminated, there are memorials for the continued veneration of the shrine rooms and its contents.

The cobblestoned Early Tlamimilolpa principal patio was the only one with a shrine room instead of just an altar. This room (Room 66), about 4 m² in area, was centrally located in the patio. The shrine room and temple are on a line that is 91° west of Teotihuacán North (15.5° east of true north). This line bisects the temple, shrine room, and Feature 18, which is situated just to the west of the shrine room (figure 11.2). This is not an accidental layout, as this has been clearly identified as a standardized Teotihuacán angle (Millon 1973: 38), and indicates that construction of Tlajinga 33 conformed at this time to the overall plan of the city. Remnants of wall scars on all but the east side indicate that access to the room was from the east. The floor of the shrine room, countersunk 12 cm below the patio paving, consisted of cobblestones in the western two-thirds of the room, while the eastern one-third of the room appears to have been bare *tepetate* bedrock, perhaps cut and shaped to create a prepared floor (see figures 11.3, 11.4).

It is impossible to determine the original height of the Room 66 walls because the wall scars terminate at the level of the patio surface. It is likely that Room 66 was walled and completely roofed over, with a separate altar in the eastern third of the room. This is suggested by the low, platformlike ledge of *tepetate*, which could have served as the base of an altar.

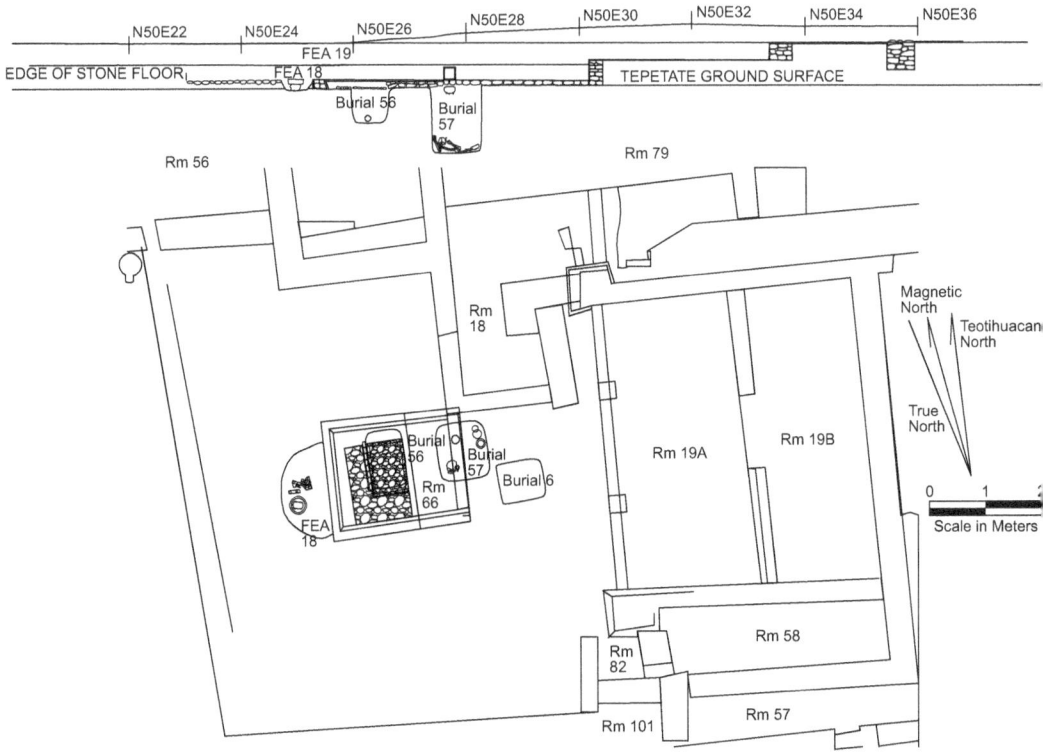

Figure 11.2. Plan map of the Early Tlamimilolpa patio and temple complex with profile above.

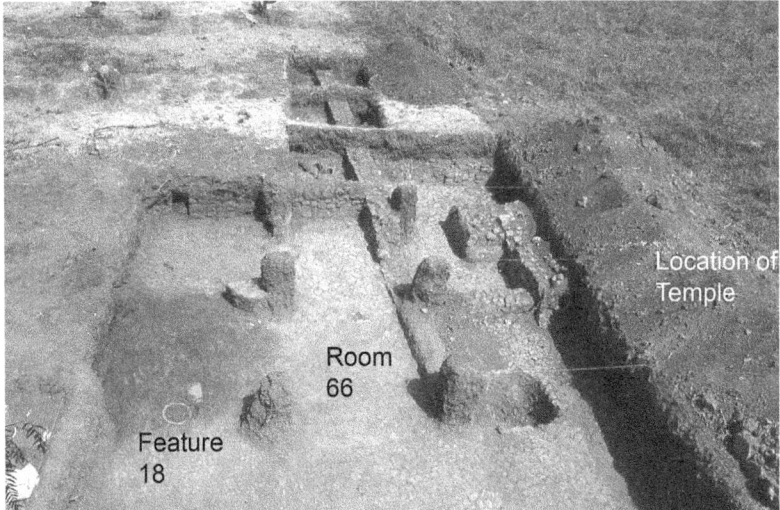

Figure 11.3. Photograph of the Early Tlamimilolpa patio and temple complex showing unexcavated Room 66 and Feature 18.

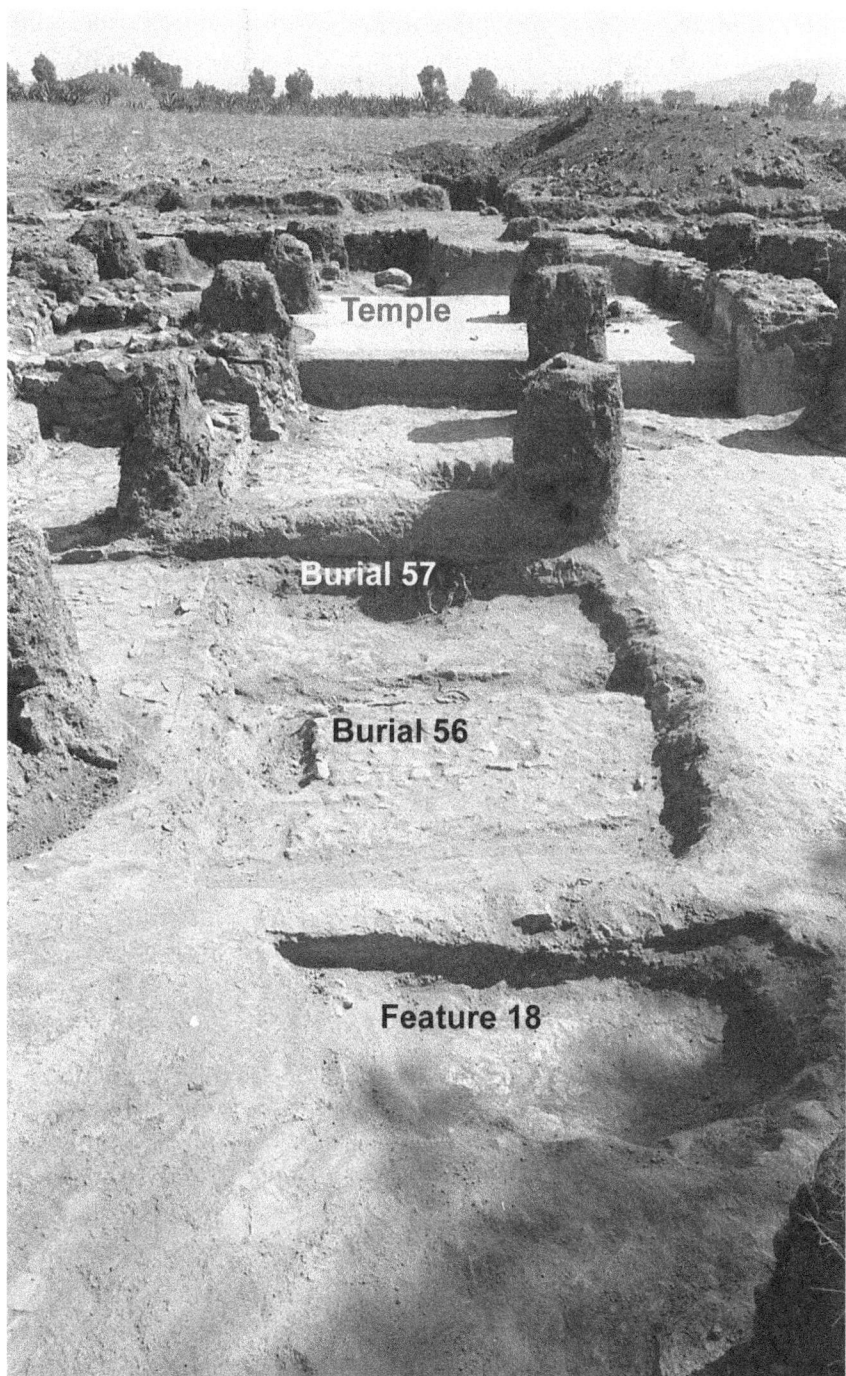

Figure 11.4. Room 66 containing Burials 56 and 57, with the temple east of the Room 66 and Feature 18 west of Room 66.

The shrine room opened onto the largest Early Tlamimilolpa structure at the compound at the east edge of this principal patio that was the locus of ritual activity. This eastern building is interpreted as a temple (figure 11.4). It has only a single platform level, unlike other temples, which have staircases and multiple platform levels. This building does have a spacious portico and scars for central pillars very similar to other buildings identified as temples. It might be that the height of the platform is a function of the economic status of the compound rather than the ritual context.

Sometime during the Early Tlamimilolpa, Burial 56 was interred in a pit dug 58 cm into the *tepetate* in the center of the shrine room. The cobblestone floor was replaced over the pit (evidenced by the visible repair lines of stone), indicating continuing function of the room. Given his privileged location of interment, Burial 56 should have been a high-status individual, and so the offerings indicate. This 40- to 49-year-old male was tightly flexed, placed on his back, and accompanied by a ceramic offering of 32 vessels, the largest among the Tlajinga burials recovered and almost double the number in the next largest group of ceramic offerings. In addition, his body was accompanied by one obsidian blade and several long-distance trade goods: three complete, unmodified Caribbean seashells (an immature *Turbinella angulata*, a *Strombus raminus*, and an *Oliva cf. reticularis*), and one drilled serpentine bead. The bead was in his mouth, a common location for greenstone beads for Tlajinga burials from the Tlamimilolpa phase. There was also a lump of white substance, probably chalk, by his left shoulder.

Later (but still during the Early Tlamimilolpa), Burial 57 was interred at the eastern entrance of the shrine room in a burial pit 80 × 80 cm, which was excavated 1.25 m into the *tepetate* (figure 11.5). The pit was partially in the patio and partially in the shrine room. This was part of a deliberate and elaborate termination ritual for the shrine room and the patio. We can only speculate about the reason for the termination ritual, but the later central patios and altars for the compound are to the southwest, more central to the construction of those periods. The residents probably decided to change the location of the ritually important central patio. After the placement of the individual in the bottom, the pit was filled and carefully covered with cobbles in the patio area. Room 66 was razed to the level of the patio surface, and then a square pillar, perhaps from the architecture of the room, was placed across the sealed burial pit. A ceramic vessel offering was placed in the upper fill of the burial pit directly underneath the pillar. Inside the room, the pit was sealed with fragments of stuccoed square pillars and stucco rubble, presumably from the shrine room.

Also at this time, the grave of Burial 56 was opened along its eastern and

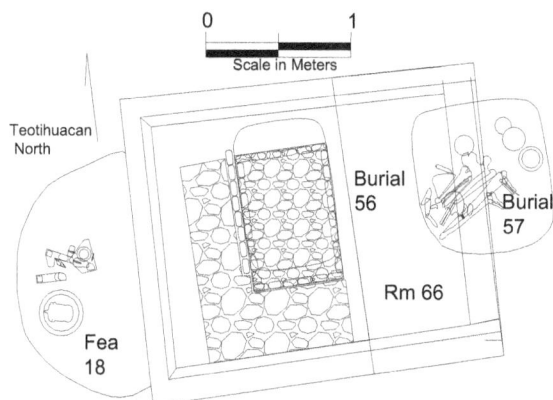

Figure 11.5. Plan map of Burials 56 and 57 and Feature 18.

northern margin, and five of the ceramic vessels and two of the marine shells were placed at a higher level than the other offerings. The disturbed cobblestone floor was not repaired, and the artifacts were alone at the top of the pit, in fill clearly above the level of the burial. Apparently at this time, the entire shrine room was razed and filled in to form a floor now flush with the rest of the cobblestone patio. Just beyond the west wall of the shrine room was the Feature 18 Huehueteotl (Old Fire God) incense burner and associated artifacts.

The Huehueteotl incense burner (figure 11.6), with the bowl on the head, is a depiction of one of the main deities of the Central Mexican pantheon and is often found at Teotihuacán. The origin of this deity has deep roots in the area; rituals involving Huehueteotl were one of the integrating practices leading up to the regional domination of Teotihuacán (Carballo 2007). During Teotihuacán times, the incense burners were used in domestic rituals (Carballo 2007).

The Huehueteotl incense burner was placed in a broad, shallow pit excavated into the *tepetate*, and positioned so that the rim of the censer bowl was even with the surrounding cobblestone paving of the patio. The face was oriented to 78° west of Teotihuacán North, and its left and right arm and leg supports were broken off and placed to the north. Between the two support pieces was a horse conch (*Pleuroplocus gigantae*) marine shell. The back was broken off from the head and bowl of the incense burner, but was not recovered in the excavation.

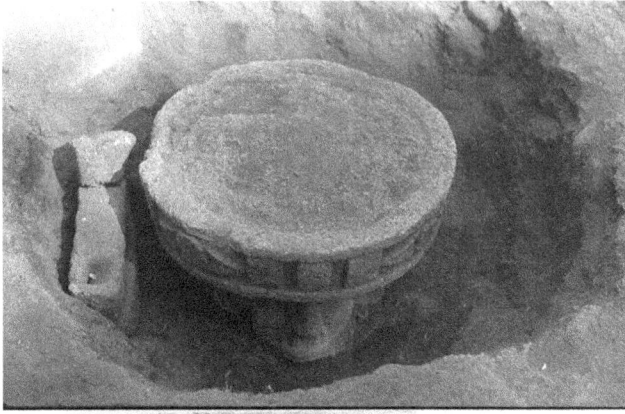

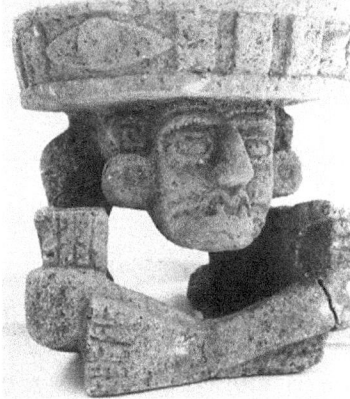

Figure 11.6. View of Feature 18 stone Huehueteotl (Old Fire God) incense burner in situ and reconstructed.

Five centimeters to the north of the censer arms was a flagging stone, and under this was a small olla (a ceramic jarlike vessel) with little fill inside. The stone functioned as a lid, so the olla could be used for continuous rituals. We know that the olla predated the interment of the censer because the center of the olla is on that 91° line that bisects the temple, shrine room, and also the skull of Burial 57. Four tiny unifacial hafted darts fabricated from obsidian blades were placed around the olla, three in a cruciform pattern that does not correlate with Teotihuacán North. These darts were probably used for self-sacrificial bloodletting into the olla, as a form of ancestor veneration. Such bloodletting or autosacrifice was common in Prehispanic Mesoamerica and at Teotihuacán (Headrick 2007).

The destruction of the Huehueteotl incense burner was probably deliberate and not simply to facilitate its placement flush with the patio, as the pit simply could have been excavated deeper to achieve the same result. Its destruction was ritual in nature, probably meant to desanctify the incense burner by "killing." We believe that these items were originally in the shrine room, and that the destruction and ultimate position of the incense burner are related to the room's new function as a kind of memorial to the room and the burials, since the incense burner's bowl could still have been used to burn offerings long after the termination ritual.

The interment of Burial 57 appears to be pivotal to this entire sequence of ritual events and reconstruction of the ritual space. As discussed below, Burial 57 was a bundle burial and probably was on display in the shrine room prior to the death and interment of Burial 56. Only when the shrine room was razed and terminated as a ritual space was the bundle burial finally interred. However, the incense burner's bowl, the lid over the olla, and the shrine room with its recumbent pillar remained visible, probably as a memorial to the individuals who were interred there.

The Burial Furniture and Display of Burial 57

Burial 57, without a doubt, is the highest-ranked individual at this time and for all phases of the compound. The offerings with this individual are distinctive (figures 11.7, 11.8). There are only four ceramic vessels, one of which was interred subsequent to the original interment, but this burial also contains the most elaborate shell artifacts at Tlajinga. Shell was a valued item in Teotihuacán, especially marine shell as it had to come through long-distance trade. There were over 4,000 small, drilled gastropod shells ranging in length from 6 to 14 mm of two marine species: *Olivella nivea*, the more common of the two, and *Nitadella ocellata*. Many of these shells, probably part of an elaborate collar, still had red paint on them.

On Burial 57's skull was a headdress consisting of a pair of large ring-shaped rattlesnakes made from shell, representing goggles signifying the Rain God. These goggles are often associated with warriors (Headrick 2007). The shell is that of a nacreous bivalve, probably a freshwater mussel (*Unionidea*). Two thin nacreous shell disks decorated with a delicate excised slot pattern were located nearby and probably integrated in some fashion with the goggles.

Additional shell artifacts include four thin tapering cut pieces of *Spondylus* sp. (Pacific thorny oyster). These are 12 mm long and taper to a point from a width of 6 mm. One of these has a clearly defined band of red paint that bisects the long axis of the artifact 4 mm from the distal end. These were descriptively called "false teeth" because of their shape. However, they may actually have been incorporated into some sort of perishable funerary mask that represented the face of the individual sewn on the shroud just below the Rain God goggles.

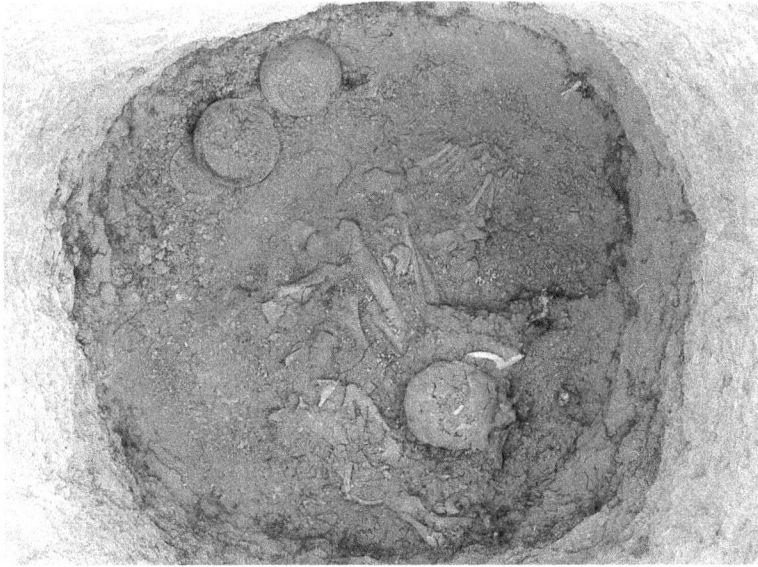

Figure 11.7. Burial 57 in situ with one rattlesnake headdress clearly visible and the small shells, appearing as white specks, distributed around the body.

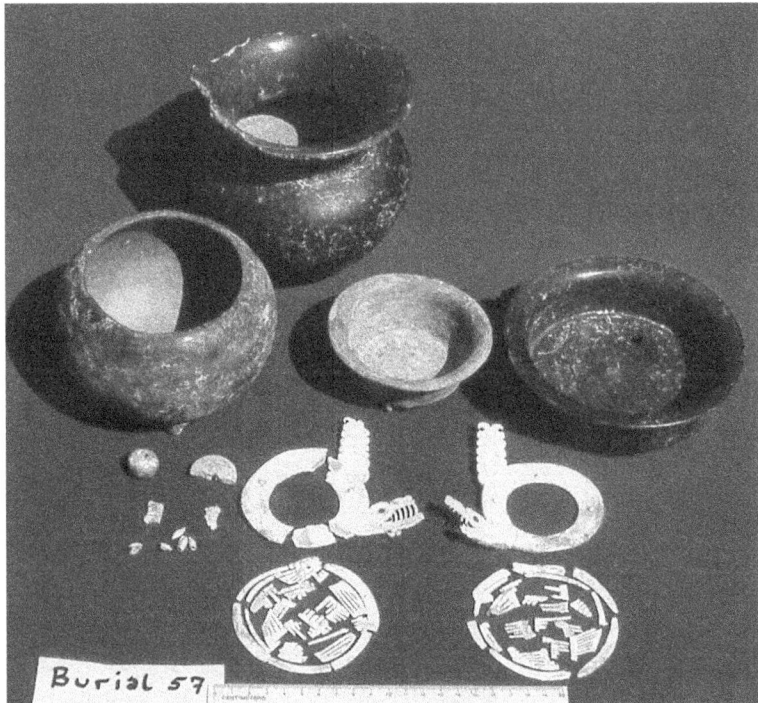

Burial 57

Figure 11.8. Photograph of Burial 57 grave offerings. The shell headdress is in the front with a sample of small shells and the jade beads to the left.

Two flower/crown-shaped cut *Spondylus* artifacts with traces of yellow and red paint on them were found. It is suggested that these served as fasteners for the bead cloak or the burial shroud. Four fragments of *Oliva* shell, with their spires cut off and then ground to form tinklers or pendants, were also associated with the burial. Interestingly, three of these appear to have been intentionally broken and might have actually been offerings associated with the termination ritual. A large, drilled jadeite bead had been placed in his mouth, and lumps of yellow pigment and a greenish substance (copal?) were found in the pit near the body. A complete avian eggshell was also recovered from the burial fill; its color and thickness suggest a quail egg. The quantity of offerings was smaller than for Burial 56, but these are definitely more elaborate and are dominated by valuable materials for lapidaries.

There can be little doubt that the body was wrapped in a cloth and represented a mortuary bundle, a common treatment in Teotihuacán (Headrick 2007). The body was tightly flexed and seated in the pit. The goggle headdress, false teeth, and shell collar were probably sewn onto the cloth wrapping the corpse. These bundles, with the shell bead collars and Rain God goggles, are depicted in the iconography at Teotihuacán (Headrick 2007: 56–57). The shell artifacts were probably made in this compound and belonged to this man. Their placement on the mortuary bundle would ensure that he was clearly identified while displayed in the shrine room.

The Burial 57 Osteobiography

The skeleton of Burial 57 was fairly complete but very brittle due to root activity. This was a robust male, probably 50–59 years at death. The sex estimation was based on the morphology of the pelvis and cranium, while aging was done by auricular surface morphology and dental wear (based on standard methods in Buikstra and Ubelaker 1994). While this is not very old by modern standards, only 12 individuals in the Tlajinga skeletal sample were older than age 50 at death. Burial 57 was one of the older individuals, although not the oldest, found in a formal burial in the compound.

Among health indicators preserved on a skeleton, some record stresses and events during the adult years and others preserve evidence of stress during childhood. Most of the skeletal features that reflect adult health suggest that Burial 57 was in good health at the time of death. He had no dental caries, and all of his teeth were present except for the maxillary left canine. His skeleton revealed no evidence of healed broken bones or weapon injury, and little evidence of osteoarthritis except in the elbows and shoulders. Thus there is no clear evidence that the goggles indicate he was a warrior. The osteoarthritis might be linked to the lapidary specialization, which involved the arms and hands for cutting and polishing, but osteoarthritis cannot be so simply interpreted (Jurmain 1999).

There was a well-healed, localized area of periosteal reaction on the left femur, and a systemic (not localized) periosteal reaction on the left fibula and the metatarsals of the feet, which ranged from partly healed to still active at the time of death. These "nonspecific" reactions on the surface of the bone usually indicate a bacterial infection and may be complications of some other illness or a result of trauma to the soft tissue (Larsen 1997). Such infections are difficult to diagnose, but this one was widespread and may have contributed to the death of this individual.

Burial 57 had no evidence of the healed porosity on his cranium that would indicate childhood anemia or scurvy, but three episodes of physiological stress sufficient to interfere with normal growth during childhood are documented by dental hypoplasias of the teeth. These are dents or pits in the enamel of multiple teeth, indicating thinner or disturbed enamel formed when the individual was severely stressed. The approximate ages at which these defects formed are 2–2 ½, 3 ½–4, and 4–4 ½ years. Hypoplasias are nonspecific growth arrest indicators; they can be caused by many different illnesses or periods of malnutrition or trauma. Three is a high number, just above the average frequency of 2.7 hypoplasia-causing episodes in the Tlajinga 33 residents. This suggests that he may have experienced and survived recurrent bouts of illness during childhood and had episodes of illness as an adult, including one at the time of death.

Social Status

His burial context and the accompanying grave goods indicate that Burial 57 was an elite individual, but we want to know whether his high status was achieved as a result of his adult contributions to the compound or if he was a member of a cadet branch of an elite lineage that was sent to found a new compound, as suggested by Headrick (2007). His skeleton has several characteristics that suggest that Burial 57 was born into status. Poor childhood nutrition, health, and environmental circumstances may cause stunting and influence adult stature (Larsen 1997). However, at 175 cm (5 feet 10 inches) Burial 57 was the tallest individual in Tlajinga for all time periods. In comparison, Burial 56 was of average stature for Tlajinga males, 163 cm (5 feet 4 inches). Burial 57 managed to reach that height in spite of the physiological stress episodes that caused the enamel hypoplasias, which indicates both a strong constitution and probably a high-quality diet and care during childhood. His lack of caries rules out a diet dominated by sugars and starches. He managed to live to an old age with 31 teeth, in spite of severe childhood stress. His central maxillary incisors have artificial grooves on the distal edges. This type of dental modification is found on only two other individuals in the compound, including Burial 56. Such treatment was only given to certain individuals and may be proof of the ascribed elite status of this individual.

Conclusion

The complexity of the mortuary treatment and the valuable materials placed with Burial 57 argue that this individual was an important person. Teotihuacán imported raw materials, like marine shell, and used its artisans to work them, rather than bringing in finished products (Cowgill 1997). The headdress and other shell artifacts, including the shell collar, were probably manufactured at Tlajinga 33, a compound of lapidary craftsmen. But no one else in the compound was buried with anything so fine. Who, then, was this individual?

The elaborate ritual that attended his burial seems to indicate that he was the founder of the compound. One apparent contradiction to this interpretation is that Burial 56 was interred first, but the offerings with Burial 56 are not as valuable in terms of their raw material, nor do they show the degree of lapidary skill as the shell work found with Burial 57. Mortuary bundles (tightly wrapped corpses) were important in Mesoamerica and Teotihuacán, and the bundles of important individuals were often publicly displayed for a time (Headrick 2007). We hypothesize that Burial 57's mortuary bundle was displayed in the shrine room before and during the time of the interment of Burial 56. The founder, perhaps the master artisan and a warrior as suggested by the Rain God goggles and his headdress, was venerated for some time, and then given final disposition in an elaborate "termination" funeral event. The shells were on the bundle cloth and the headdress sewn on the outside, so that there could be no question among the living as to who was being venerated and why. The destroyed shrine room and the buried incense burner would remind later generations of Tlajinga 33 residents of this ancestor and founder.

References Cited

Buikstra, Jane E., and Douglas H. Ubelaker (editors)
1994   *Standards for Data Collection from Human Skeletal Remains.* Arkansas Archeological Survey Research Series No. 44. Arkansas Archeological Survey, Fayetteville.

Carballo, David M.

2007   Effigy Vessels, Religious Integration, and the Origins of the Central Mexican Pantheon. *Ancient Mesoamerica* 18: 53–67.

Cowgill, George L.

1997   State and Society at Teotihuacan, Mexico. *Annual Review of Anthropology* 26: 129–61.

2003   Teotihuacan: Cosmic Glories and Mundane Needs. In *The Social Construction of Ancient Cities*, edited by M. L. Smith, pp. 37–55. Smithsonian Institution Press, Washington, D.C.

Headrick, Annabeth

2007   *The Teotihuacan Trinity: The Sociopolitical Structure of an Ancient Mesoamerican City*. University of Texas Press, Austin.

Jurmain, Robert

1999   *Stories from the Skeleton: Behavioral Reconstruction in Human Osteology*. Gordon and Breach, Amsterdam.

Larsen, Clark S.

1997   *Bioarchaeology: Interpreting Behavior from the Human Skeleton*. Cambridge University Press, Cambridge.

Millon, Rene

1973   *Urbanization at Teotihuacan: The Teotihuacan Map*, Vol. 1, Part 1. University of Texas Press, Austin.

1981   Teotihuacan: City, State, and Civilization. In *Supplement to the Handbook of Middle American Indians*, Vol. 1, *Archaeology*, edited by J. A. Sabloff, pp. 198–243. University of Texas Press, Austin.

Mock, Shirley (editor)

1998   *The Sowing and the Dawning: Termination, Dedication, and Transformation in the Archaeological and Ethnographic Record of Mesoamerica*. University of New Mexico Press, Albuquerque.

Spence, Michael W.

1994   Human Skeletal Material from Teotihuacan. In *Mortuary Practices and Skeletal Remains at Teotihuacan*, edited by M. Sempowski and M. Spence, pp. 315–445. University of Utah Press, Salt Lake City.

Storey, Rebecca

1992   *Life and Death in the Ancient City of Teotihuacan: A Modern Paleodemographic Synthesis*. University of Alabama Press, Tuscaloosa.

Widmer, Randolph J.

1991   Lapidary Craft Specialization at Teotihuacan: Implications for Community Structure at 33:S3W1 and Economic Organization in the City. *Ancient Mesoamerica* 2: 131–41.

12 ◆ Vulcan

Skilled Village Craftsman of Ban Chiang, Thailand

Michele Toomay Douglas and Michael Pietrusewsky

Individual Profile

Site: Ban Chiang

Location: Udon Thani Province, northeast Thailand

Cultural Affiliation: Ban Chiang Cultural Tradition

Date: Upper Early Period Burial Phase V, ca. 1700–900 B.C. (^{14}C on rice temper)

Feature: BC Burial 23

Location of Grave: Square C5, south quadrants, layer 11, Distance Below Datum Point 1.73 m (skull), orientation northwest 322°

Burial and Grave Type: Supine, extended primary inhumation

Associated Materials: Ceramic pot; four bronze bangles around the left forearm; cache of 30 small clay pellets; socketed bronze adze head

Preservation and Completeness: Good to excellent preservation, but only one limb bone is complete; portions of the face and the right temporal bone missing, as are most of the right femur, most of both fibulae, and parts of both feet; left ulna and radius exhibit a greenish stain from the copper-base bangles; slight green-blue staining on the labial enamel of the maxillary canines and incisors

Age at Death and Basis of Estimate: 45–50 years, based on auricular surface morphology, dental wear, cranial suture fusion

Sex and Basis of Determination: Male, based on cranial and os coxae morphologies

Conditions Observed: Healed coarse porosity of the superior cranial vault; dental wear to the pulp on molars and maxillary incisors, dentin exposure in remaining teeth; enamel hypoplasias; slight to moderate calculus; reactive bone growth on internal borders of left lower ribs; osseous lesions in right glenoid fossa, right first proximal hand phalanx, and right fourth metatarsal

Specialized Analysis: Carbon and nitrogen isotopes from bone apatite and collagen; oxygen, carbon, and strontium isotopes from tooth dentin; radiographs of cranium, left ribs, left scapula, and humeral head, right first proximal hand phalanx, left tibia

Excavated: 1974 by the University of Pennsylvania Museum and the Thai Fine Arts Department, under the direction of Chester Gorman and Pisit Charoenwongsa

Archaeological Report: Gorman and Charoenwongsa 1976 (original chronology); White 1982, 1986 (revised chronology)

Current Disposition: On loan to and curated by the Department of Anthropology, University of Hawai'i–Mānoa

The history of the Ban Chiang project and the story of this collaborative archaeological excavation, one of the first in Southeast Asia, are vital to understanding the site, each of the individuals buried there, and their contributions to the prehistory of the region. The osteobiography of Vulcan documents a talented member of an ancient society and reflects a culture in transition.

The predominant issues in archaeological research in Southeast Asia include the historical and biological relationships of the inhabitants, origins of intensified wet-rice agriculture, and origins of complex societies. All of these issues center around two models—the agricultural expansion theory, which proposes that colonizing immigrants brought agriculture to the indigenous people (e.g., Bayard 1996; Higham 1996; Bellwood 2005), and the continuity model, which posits that the ideas for agriculture originated or were adopted in situ (e.g., Bulbeck 1982; Hanihara 1993; Pietrusewsky 2006). These issues and models evolved from early archaeological excavations in Thailand, including Ban Kao, Non Nok Tha, and Ban Chiang (Higham 1989).

Ban Chiang is a modern village on the Khorat Plateau in Udon Thani Province, northeastern Thailand, which came to international attention in the early 1970s when looting revealed a heretofore unknown rich cultural prehistory beneath the village (White 1982). The joint program of the University of Pennsylvania and the Thai Fine Arts Department first excavated in 1974 in the yard of a private home, a locale named "BC" (figure 12.1), which had minimal disturbance from looters (Gorman and Charoengwasa 1976). The second excavation, in 1975, was conducted in the middle of a road (*soi* in Thai). The prehistoric deposits at this site, designated Ban Chiang Eastern Soi, or BCES, were relatively undisturbed by looting. The beautiful red-on-buff pottery found at Ban Chiang and evidence of early metallurgy moved the region from a "cultural backwater" to the frontline of investigations on the origins and dissemination of rice agriculture and metallurgy.

However, the untimely and unfortunate death of Chester Gorman in 1981 temporarily stopped the project. Physical anthropologist Michael Pietrusewsky (1980) was the only participant to complete his analysis. Subsequently, Joyce White took up the enormous task of analysis, reporting, and fund-raising for this important archaeological site (White 1986, 1988, 1990, 2008). The Ban Chiang Project has led to much valuable research on topics such as biological distance relationships in skeletal populations from Southeast Asia and Oceania (Pietrusewsky 1978, 1981, 1982, 1984, 2006), ethnoecology (White 1995b), metallurgy (White and Pigott 1996), and paleopalynology (White et al. 2004). Earlier and subsequent excavations at the village unearthed additional human skeletal remains, some of which are preserved in situ at the Ban Chiang Museum.

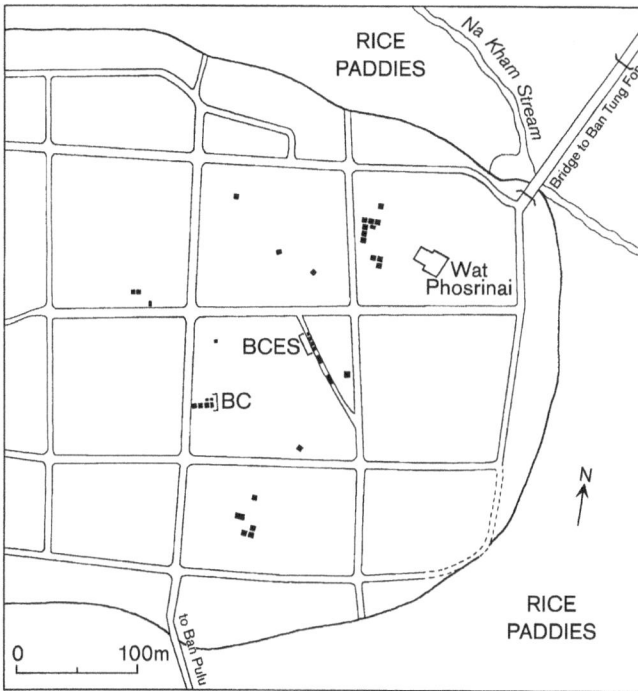

Figure 12.1. The village of Ban Chiang, northeast Thailand, showing the excavation locales.

A second, more detailed examination of the Ban Chiang skeletal series was published by Pietrusewsky and Douglas (2002), though without benefit of the archaeological report.

Designated a UNESCO World Heritage Site in 1992,[1] Ban Chiang contin-ues to be a very important archaeological site and human skeletal collection, providing a glimpse of lifeways during the early metal and metal periods of Southeast Asia.

Cultural Background

Ban Chiang is a mortuary and occupation site with mixed usage including habi-tation and occupation activities. Three periods identified in the Ban Chiang excavations (Early, Middle, and Late) are divided into 10 burial phases (table 12.1). Vulcan lived during the Early period, which defines the "Ban Chiang Cul-tural Tradition" described as small communities of hunter/gatherer/cultivators who moved from the lowlands out onto the alluvial plateau around 4000 B.C. These people utilized the wild resources of the forest and river, in addition to cultivating wild rice and domesticated pigs, dogs, chickens, and cattle. Village life included a pottery tradition and houses constructed on stilts. Much of the material culture was organic (wood, bamboo, fiber) and thus unpreserved.

Table 12.1. Ban Chiang archaeological context

Period	No. of Burials	Burial Phase	Attributes	Working date range
Late	10	X	Wet rice agriculture using water buffalo and possibly iron plowshares	ca. 300 B.C.–A.D. 200
	5	IX		
Middle	2	VIII	Broad subsistence resources, appearance of water buffalo, iron metallurgy, gain in forests; frequent low-intensity burning suggests intensifying agriculture	ca. 900–300 B.C.
	21	VII		
	10	VI		
Upper Early	32	V	Hunter-gatherer-cultivator economy with domesticates incl. rice, bronze metallurgy, change in ceramic styles and grave orientation, transition to matrilocality	ca. 1700–900 B.C.
Lower Early	25	IV	Hunter-gatherer-cultivator economy with domesticates incl. rice, bronze in mortuary and nonmortuary contexts	ca. 2100–1700 B.C.
	14	III		
	21	II	Hunter-gatherer-cultivator economy with domesticates incl. rice, early metallurgy evident in nonmortuary contexts (ca. 2000 B.C.), slow forest recovery from Middle Holocene	
	1	I	Hunter-gatherer-cultivator economy with domesticates incl. rice	
Initial			Occupation before mortuary use of BC and BCES locales, evidence of large-scale burning indicates forest clearing	4000?–ca. 2100 B.C.

Source: Adapted from White 2008 and Pietrusewsky and Douglas 2002.
Note: Burial numbers include BC and BCES locales. New dates obtained from human bone now challange this chronology (see Higham et al., 2011).

Rice is present from the earliest levels and is found in pottery tempers (as an additive to the clay), suggesting relative abundance. Metal and metal-related artifacts are found in both burial and nonburial contexts in the Early period dating from as early as ca. 2000 B.C. (White 2008). This range of contexts suggests that metal was not reserved for rituals but was used in daily life (White 2008: 95). It is estimated that perhaps 500 people lived at Ban Chiang during Vulcan's time, with an egalitarian social structure and achieved status rather than inherited rank. Preliminary analysis of the ceramics from Ban Chiang suggests that pottery production traditions and craftsmanship are local developments (White et al. 1991). No evidence is found for a centralized authority or institutionalized conflict at this time. The concept of heterarchy has been applied to this horizontal social structure wherein it is the local village and individual relationships within and between the villages that are important rather than a vertical hierarchical structure (White 1995a).

The societies of the Ban Chiang Cultural Tradition seem likely to have followed the modern division of labor in this part of Thailand—women bear and raise the children and manage the household chores, generally gathering fruits and vegetables. Pottery production and rice field preparation, planting, and harvesting may have been a joint endeavor between the men and women. Men manage the livestock, build houses, craft objects, and hunt and gather resources from farther afield. Most people who died at Ban Chiang during the Early period were buried in supine, extended primary inhumations. Pottery vessels were placed at their heads or toward their feet. A few people were buried in the flexed position, and very young infants and fetuses were interred in beautiful funerary jars.

The Mortuary Feature

Excavation of the BC locale in 1974 began in earnest in March and continued well into July of that year; Michael Pietrusewsky was there beginning in mid-May (Michael Pietrusewsky, personal communication 2007):"The temperature and humidity levels for this time of year, the transition from the hot season to the rainy season, were oppressively high. Work at the site, although covered by a tarp, was extremely uncomfortable, especially as the excavated units descended to their lowest levels. Among the rewards of excavating under these hot, sticky conditions was finding relatively intact burials associated with a variety of grave goods. Burial 23, nicknamed "Vulcan" by the excavators, certainly was one of the most exciting discoveries to be made during that fieldwork season at Ban Chiang."

BC Burial 23 was excavated from Square C5, south quadrants, layer 11, and is dated to Early Period V, 1700–900 B.C. This burial was among the deepest grave cuts of this square (figure 12.2). As was typical of most burials at Ban Chiang then, he was placed in the grave in a supine position (on his back), arms and legs extended, with his hands by his sides. Grave goods included four bronze bangles, a partial ceramic vessel, a cache of 30 clay pellets, and a socketed bronze adze head (figure 12.3). Postdepositional disturbances (for example, postholes, pits) resulted in the loss of the right femur and left foot.

Burial 23 was nicknamed "Vulcan," after the Roman god of fire and metalworking, because of the rare occurrence of not just one but two classes of metal objects in his grave. Vulcan's grave does not bear the earliest occurrence of a metal object at Ban Chiang, but the presence of metal artifacts within a grave assemblage suggests that there was enough surplus for these items to be ritually disposed of, no longer available for use by the living. It certainly appears that this individual was a distinctive member of the ancient society because of the unique nature of the grave furniture.

Four copper-based bangles with a simple circular cross section were found at the left forearm, staining the radius and ulna green. Metal jewelry was found with only two other Early period burials, both children, who wore ankle bracelets on both legs. While today bracelets and anklets are typically thought to be worn by females, at Ban Chiang perhaps the bangles were associated with male sex or some other social attribute. Since estimating sex in children is currently problematic, no firm interpretation can be made at this time. Metal bangles found as grave goods in other contemporaneous and later sites in Thailand are not consistently distributed by age or sex (Chang 2001). Chang (2001) has argued that because many of these bangles exhibited little or no wear, they were worn only in death. Vulcan's bronze bangles are too oxidized to assess for evidence of wear.

The well-made, copper-based adze head placed above Vulcan's left shoulder was probably hafted at the time it was deposited. Examination of the 7 cm working edge reveals that when manufactured, the blade was not hammered to harden it, and the adze had received little if any use (White 1982: 40). Few of the copper-based bronze items found at Ban Chiang were suitable for work, even though some examples from the Early period show that the Ban Chiang craftsmen knew of the technique of annealing and hammering. This suggests that many of the copper-based items in graves were made specifically for burial (Elizabeth Hamilton, personal communication 2007). So this was not a favorite tool of the deceased but rather represents a significant expenditure of time, raw material, and skill in his honor. The artifact suggests that Vulcan was good

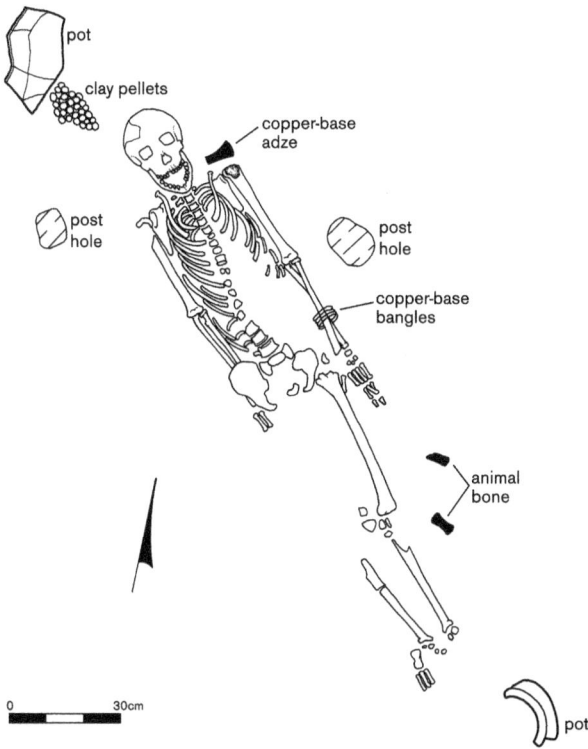

Figure 12.2. BC Burial 23 (plan view). The ceramic vessel above his head was not part of his grave furniture.

pot
clay pellets
copper-base adze
post hole
post hole
copper-base bangles
animal bone
0   30cm
pot

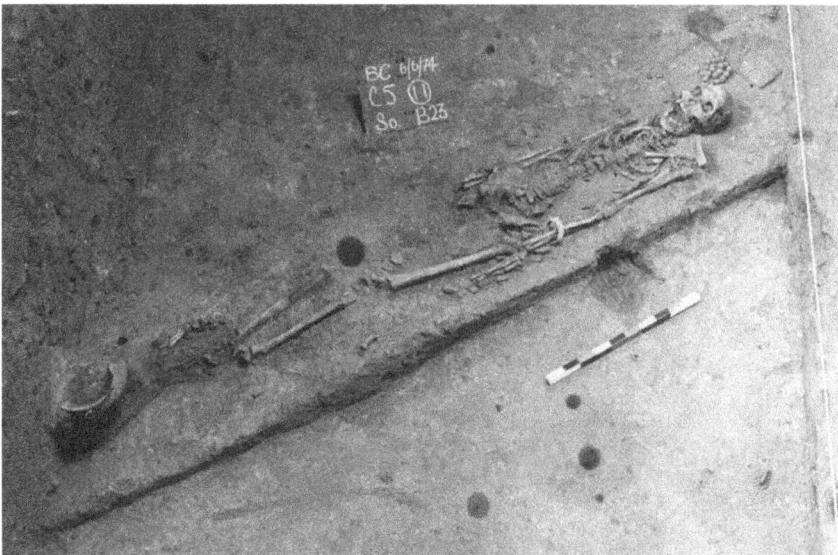

Figure 12.3. Vulcan. The grave was quite large. The right hand was palm up while the left hand was palm down. The right sciatic notch is visible and suggests male sex.

with his hands; he might have been the village metal worker, creating metal ornaments and objects for others in the village, or he might have used adzes in woodworking. Perhaps he educated the next generation in these skills.

A cache of some 30 clay pellets (about 2.0 cm average diameter), which were used as ammunition for the pellet bow, was placed to the right of his head in a small pile (White 1982: 24). The grouping of the pellets in a pile suggests that they were contained in a bag or deliberately stacked like cannonballs. The pellets are slightly larger in size than those found in nonmortuary contexts (Joyce White, personal communication 2007), suggesting they are funerary objects like the pottery vessels. The pellet bow may have been present within the grave as well, but being made of organic materials was lost to the soil. A pellet bow looks much like an archery bow but is used more like a slingshot. At the center of the bow string a small woven basket or piece of leather or fabric holds the pellet, and this is drawn back and let loose. The projectile is meant to stun an animal or bird or knock it down from the trees rather than kill it. Shooting pellets is also an effective means for herding some domestic animals, such as cattle. An implement such as this requires a great deal of practice in order to become proficient at hitting small targets. The abundant supply of pellets suggests that Vulcan was provisioned for a journey or the afterlife.

An incomplete single pottery vessel, an incised and painted, medium-size (10–25 cm maximum dimension) globular cord-marked pot, was found at Vulcan's feet. The design incised on the shoulders and painted red is a curvilinear scroll-like pattern. No wear or other signs of use are evident on the fragment. We do not know what was in this pot when it was placed in the grave, but the shape and size are comparable to vessels used to steam rice or cook soup in modern villages in Thailand (White 1982: 33).

Although fashioned specifically for the occasion, the grave goods associated with Vulcan are both decorative and utilitarian. While one might interpret these items as evidence for belief in an afterlife journey, pottery in various shapes and sizes is the only constant accoutrement in the Early period graves. Instead, these items appear to be "tools of the trade," suggesting Vulcan was a wood- or metal-working craftsman as well as a capable hunter and hinting that he would be sorely missed by his family and other villagers.

Osteobiography

Vulcan's skeleton is moderately complete (figure 12.4). The skull is missing the right temporal, portions of the face, hyoid horns, left mandibular condyle, and left mandibular central incisor. Some portions of his infracranial skeleton are

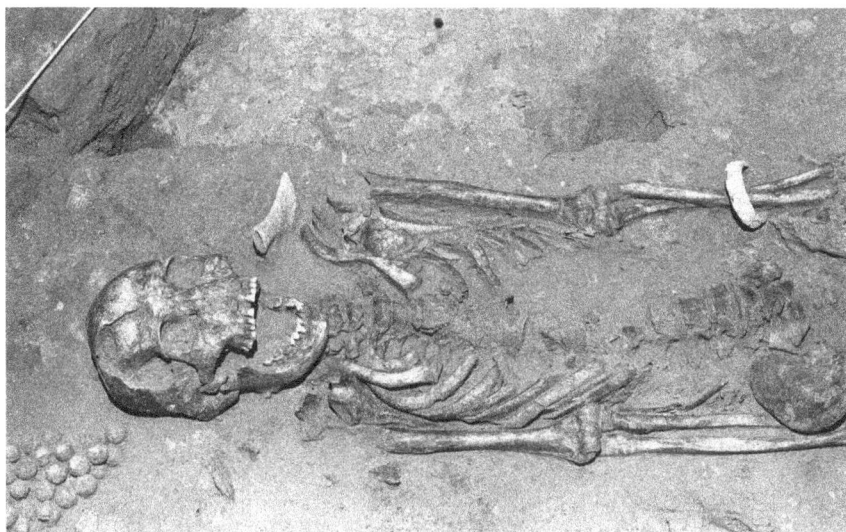

Figure 12.4. Vulcan with his bronze socketed adze head, cache of clay pellets, and four bronze bangles.

also missing: the left pelvic bone, sternum, right femur distal to the greater trochanter, left patella, left femoral head and condyles, most of the fibulae, most of the left foot bones, and most of the right foot phalanges. Preservation is good to excellent. Many parts of the skeleton are beautifully preserved but incomplete; the missing portions of the skeleton are not present as fragments and so are assumed to have been removed by later disturbances associated with continued habitation and occupational activities. The cranial vault is reconstructed, but the face could not be restored to the vault.

Sex is male based on cranial and pelvic morphologies. Age is estimated as 45–50 years. Lipping of the inferior terminus of the auricular surface and density of the surface give a score of 6, age 45–50 years. The cranial sutures that were observable indicate an age of at least 32.0 ± 8.3 years. Exposure of the pulp and dentin in the teeth and moderate osteoarthritis also support an older age estimate. The symphysis pubis and sternal end of the fourth rib are not available for observation.

Vulcan is distinguished by his age and his robust size. At 175 ± 5.0 cm, he was taller than the average man at Ban Chiang (166.8 cm), and he has a markedly large femoral head diameter (51 mm) compared to the male average (46.1 mm). Muscle markings on his skeleton attest to a very active physical life. Small linear hypoplastic pitting in the enamel of the mandibular canines are the only evidence for physiological stress, at about age 4–4½ years, but his robusticity and long life suggest this stress was transient and without long-term effects.

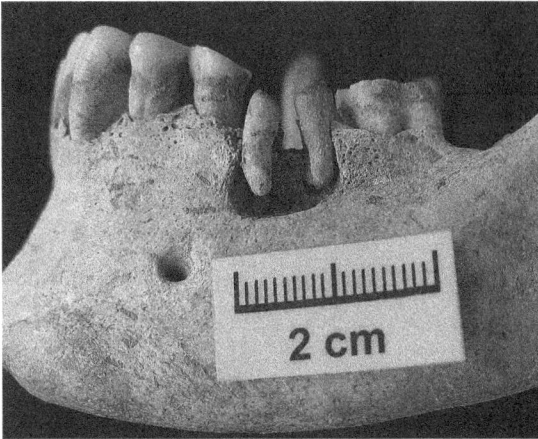

Figure 12.5. Lateral view of the left mandible showing complete loss of the first molar crown and marked vertical alveolar bone loss.

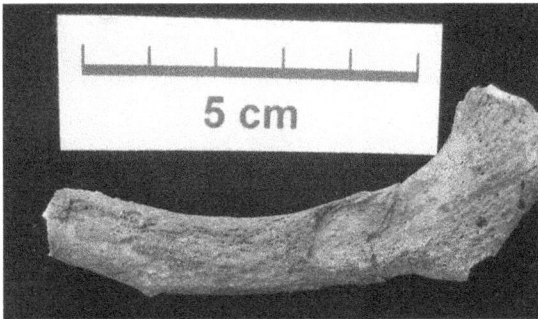

Figure 12.6. Active infection of the interior border of a lower left rib. The darker-colored area is new bone laid down on top of the old cortex.

Vulcan has nearly complete dentition. His left mandibular third molar was lost well before death (the socket is healed), while the mandibular left central incisor was lost after burial. Slight shovel-shaping of the mandibular incisors and enamel extensions in the molars are present and are common in Ban Chiang individuals.

Vulcan suffered from slight to moderate gum disease in both jaws, and this is likely the cause of small neck caries on the maxillary first and second molars. Advanced dental wear is noted, including pulp exposure in the maxillary incisors and molars of both of his jaws with dentin exposure in the remaining teeth. The left mandibular first molar crown is completely missing, probably the result of advanced attrition with exposure of the pulp cavity and subsequent massive caries (figure 12.5). The roots remain in situ in spite of advanced vertical loss of the boney socket resulting from infection. The extreme wear on the teeth suggests Vulcan used his teeth as tools, such as in pulling fibers across the teeth or in repeatedly holding something between the teeth.

Evidence of active reactive periostitis on the pleural borders of the left lower

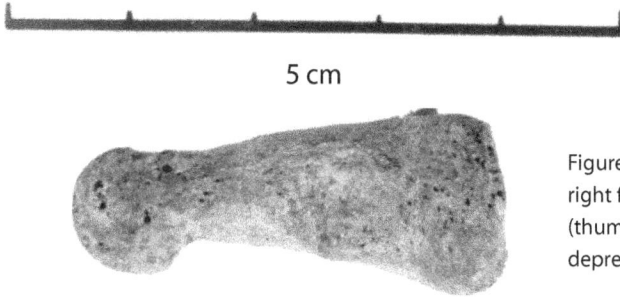

5 cm

Figure 12.7. Lateral view of the right first proximal phalanx (thumb) showing a circular depression with raised edges.

ribs (8–11, right ribs unaffected) suggests Vulcan may have died of a pulmonary infection—the illness appears to be relatively long-standing because multiple layers of reactive bone are visible (figure 12.6), with evidence of remodeling at intervals (Douglas 1996). Infection associated with his dental abscess may also have played a role in the cause of death.

Vulcan's right shoulder exhibits severe osteoarthritis with lytic erosion around the articular surfaces of both humeral head and scapula, possibly due to a secondary infection within the joint. His left side is incomplete, so we do not know if both shoulders were this severely affected. Even with the pathology affecting his right shoulder, there is little loss of robusticity in his other right arm bones.

Vulcan's right first proximal hand phalanx (thumb) appears swollen and coarse (figure 12.7). The radial side (that is, the side opposite the fingers) of the proximal shaft has a slightly depressed semicircular defect (7×8 mm) with a smooth floor, in stark contrast to the texture of the rest of the bone. No reactive bone is present.

Several factors can be used to suggest whether Vulcan was right-handed or left-handed. The placement of the adze at his left shoulder suggests he may have been left-handed. Many of the measurements of his limb bones are bilaterally symmetrical, while others (for example, the humeral minimal and midshaft circumferences and the tibial circumferences at the nutrient foramen) differ by only 1 mm, which is within the error of measurement. The tibial thickness index and platycnemic index are both greater on his right side. The right thumb lesion may be the result of pulling the string of the pellet bow. There is evidence of a slight preference for the right side, but Vulcan is quite symmetrical in physique.

Isotopic Analysis

Isotopic analysis was performed on both bone and teeth from Ban Chiang individuals, including Vulcan (Bentley et al. 2005; King 2006; King and Norr 2006).

Strontium and oxygen stable isotopes isolated from the enamel of the upper second and third molars reflect the isotopic signature of the groundwater in the particular geographic location where the individual lived when the teeth were forming—age 7–8 years for the second molar, and age 12–16 years for the third molar. In this analysis (Bentley et al. 2005), the "local" signature is determined by the clustering of individual values. Results reveal substantial variation in isotope values among the individuals at Ban Chiang, significant differences between males and females, and differences between the two locales (BC and BCES). Also noteworthy is a narrowing of the range of strontium values in females during Early Period V while the male range remains wide, suggesting a transition to matrilocality in this phase. Vulcan was found to have "exceptional" values for all three isotopes: $^{87}Sr/^{86}Sr$ (0.71070), $\delta^{18}O$ (25.2 percent), and $\delta^{13}C$ (-12.93 percent). The strontium and oxygen isotopes suggest he is nonlocal, an immigrant.

Ban Chiang skeletons were also sampled for carbon and nitrogen stable isotopes, using bone collagen and apatite, in an effort to assess diachronic dietary change (King 2006; King and Norr 2006). Small shifts in dietary resource use were found, including reduced diversity in protein sources over time and evidence (more marked in females than in males) for increasing reliance on plants grown in and/or animals grazing in more open, nonforested environments (King 2006: 210, and supported by Bentley et al. 2005: 876). The wide ranges of isotope values from Ban Chiang suggest that individual diets were extremely diverse; people took advantage of a broad selection of wild and domestic plant and animal resources. Vulcan's bone isotope values are unremarkable, falling within the cluster of the majority of Ban Chiang individuals (King 2006: 244, plotted on 143–46). Thus, although he may have been a successful hunter, he was not consuming this bounty by himself.

BC Burial 23, Vulcan, was a robust man, who died, possibly of a pulmonary infection, after a relatively long life of physical activity, including hunting and possibly crafting metal or wood. He was an immigrant, perhaps marrying into the village, who contributed valuable skills to his family and the community.

Conclusion

Vulcan lived during the Bronze Age in Thailand. Metallurgy did not transform the society or the technological repertoire; rather, it was incorporated into the traditional crafts—probably alongside other traditional raw materials like shell, wood, and bamboo. But subtle changes do occur at the Early Period IV to Early Period V transition at Ban Chiang. Strontium analysis suggests that this is the beginning of a matrilocal society, where closely clustered strontium values in women suggest they remain in their birth village, and more variable strontium values in males suggest they migrate away from their birth village. Environmental changes, evidenced by systematic low-intensity landscape burning with restoration of forests in nonfield contexts, suggest the establishment of rice paddy fields and more intensified agriculture (White et al. 2004).

Ban Chiang was excavated more than 30 years ago, two separate complete skeletal analyses have been conducted, and yet the final archaeological report is still not published. This is not only a problem for older archaeological excavations; the pressures of cultural resource management work and the Native American Graves Protection and Repatriation Act (NAGPRA) also lead to situations where skeletal analyses and reports are completed and the skeletons are reinterred even before the draft archaeological site report appears. The potential for the truly contextualized interpretation of human remains, the purpose of "bioarchaeology" (Buikstra and Beck 2006), cannot be met when the interpretation of the skeletons is made without the benefit of the full context of each burial. Certainly valuable knowledge about ancient people is available in these situations, but it is not nearly as rich as it could be.

By the grace and forethought of the Thai people, the Ban Chiang skeletal remains are curated—available for a variety of different research topics and a number of different researchers. The skeletal remains are available for the application of the most advanced techniques (for example, isotope analysis, aDNA analysis), and for reinterpretation as more and more sites in Thailand and elsewhere in Southeast Asia are excavated and additional human remains are recovered.

Since the second monograph on the Ban Chiang skeletons (Pietrusewsky and Douglas 2002) was published, a more refined dating sequence has been proposed (White 2008). Moreover, where the burials were once thought to be clustered in cemeteries, they are now thought to have been interred beneath or close to houses in the village (White 2007). The deceased are kept near the living, suggesting they are "stakeholders in descendant societies rather than passive reflectors of their own and their kin groups' status" (White 2007). This new interpretation of the archaeology has a major impact on future bioarchaeological studies. Rather than searching for biological patterns in a large assortment of graves over time and space, we *know* that certain individuals, such as those buried close to Vulcan, are related at a household level. The bioarchaeology data can be used to examine variation in morphology (metric and nonmetric traits), skeletal stress indicators, and mortuary behavior within and between households spatially and over time. Assessment of the impact of these new archaeological interpretations on the skeletal biology of Ban Chiang is possible because the raw data are available online (Pietrusewsky and Douglas 2002) and the skeletons are curated for future research.

Acknowledgments

Our thanks to Joyce White for providing needed detail for this osteobiography, for reading earlier drafts, and for her steadfast commitment to Ban Chiang archaeology. Elizabeth Hamilton addressed questions about the metal artifacts. Ardeth Abrams assisted in meeting the technical aspects of all of the illustrations. Our appreciation to an anonymous reviewer and the editors for thoughtful and helpful comments.

Note

1. See UNESCO, "Ban Chiang Archaeological Site," http://whc.unesco.org/en/list/575.

References Cited

Bayard, Donn T.
1996   Linguistics, Archaeologists, and Austronesian Origins: Comparative and Sociolinguistic Aspects of the Meacham-Bellwood Debate. *Bulletin of the Indo-Pacific Prehistory Association* 15: 71–85.
Bellwood, Peter
2005   *First Farmers: The Origins of Agricultural Societies*. Blackwell, Malden, Mass.
Bentley, R. Alexander, Michael Pietrusewsky, Michele T. Douglas, and Tim C. Atkinson
2005   Matrilocality during the Prehistoric Transition to Agriculture in Thailand? *Antiquity* 79(306): 865–81.
Buikstra, Jane E., and Lane A. Beck (editors)
2006   *Bioarchaeology: The Contextual Analysis of Human Remains*. Academic Press, New York.
Bulbeck, David
1982   A Re-evaluation of Possible Evolutionary Processes in Southeast Asia since the Late Pleistocene. *Bulletin of the Indo-Pacific Prehistory Association* 3: 1–21.
Chang, Nigel J.
2001   Personal Ornaments in Thai Prehistory: Nong Nor, Ban Lum Khao, and Noen-U-Loke. Ph.D. dissertation, University of Otago, Dunedin, New Zealand.
Douglas, Michele Toomay
1996   Paleopathology in Human Skeletal Remains from the Pre-Metal, Bronze, and Iron Ages, Northeastern Thailand. Ph.D. dissertation, Department of Anthropology, University of Hawai'i–Mānoa.

Gorman, Chester Francis, and Pisit Charoenwongsa

1976   Ban Chiang: A Mosaic of Impressions from the First Two Years. *Expedition* 18(4): 14–26.

Hanihara, Tsunehiko

1993   Population Prehistory of East Asia and the Pacific as Viewed from Craniofacial Morphology: The Basic Populations in East Asia, VII. *American Journal of Physical Anthropology* 91: 173–87.

Higham, Charles

1989   *The Archaeology of Mainland Southeast Asia*. Cambridge University Press, Cambridge.

1996   *The Bronze Age of Southeast Asia*. Cambridge University Press, Cambridge.

Higham, Charles, Thomas Higham, Roberto Ciarla, Katerina Douka, Amphan Kijngam, Fiorella Rispoli, and Michael Pietrusewsky

2011   The Origins of the Bronze Age of Southeast Asia. *Journal of World Prehistory* 24(4): 227–74.

King, Christopher A.

2006   Paleodietary Change among Pre-state Metal Age Societies in Northeast Thailand: A Stable Isotope Approach. Ph.D. dissertation, University of Hawai'i–Mānoa.

King, Christopher A., and Lynette Norr

2006   Paleodietary Change among Pre-state Metal Age Societies in Northeast Thailand: A Study Using Bone Stable Isotopes. In *Bioarchaeology of Southeast Asia*, edited by M. Oxenham and N. Tayles, pp. 241–62. Cambridge University Press, Cambridge.

Pietrusewsky, Michael

1978   A Study of Early Metal Age Crania from Ban Chiang, Northeast Thailand. *Journal of Human Evolution* 7: 383–92.

1980   The Human Remains from Ban Chiang. Manuscript on file at the University Museum, University of Pennsylvania, Philadelphia.

1981   Cranial Variation in Early Metal Age Thailand and Southeast Asia Studied by Multivariate Procedures. *Homo* 32: 1–26.

1982   The Ancient Inhabitants of Ban Chiang: The Evidence from the Human Skeletal and Dental Remains. *Expedition* 24(4): 42–50.

1984   *Metric and Non-Metric Cranial Variation in Australian Aboriginal Populations Compared with Populations from the Pacific and Asia*. Occasional Papers in Human Biology No. 3. Australian Institute of Aboriginal Studies, Canberra.

2006   A Multivariate Craniometric Study of the Prehistoric and Modern Inhabitants of Southeast Asia, East Asia, and Surrounding Regions: A Human Kaleidoscope? In *Bioarchaeology of Southeast Asia*, edited by M. Oxenham and N. Tayles, pp. 59–90. Cambridge University Press, Cambridge.

Pietrusewsky, Michael, and Michele Toomay Douglas

2002   *Ban Chiang, a Prehistoric Village Site in Northeast Thailand 1: The Human Skeletal Remains*. Thai Archaeology Monograph Series. University of Pennsylvania Museum of Archaeology and Anthropology, Philadelphia.

White, Joyce C.

1982   *Ban Chiang: Discovery of a Lost Bronze Age*. University of Pennsylvania, Philadelphia.

1986   A Revision of the Chronology of Ban Chiang and Its Implications for the Prehistory of Northeast Thailand. Ph.D. dissertation, Department of Anthropology, University of Pennsylvania.

1988   Ban Chiang and Charcoal in Hypothetical Hindsight. *Bulletin of the Indo-Pacific Prehistory Association* 8: 54–74.

1990   The Ban Chiang Chronology Revised. In *Southeast Asian Archaeology 1986: Proceedings of the First Conference of the Association of Southeast Asian Archaeologists in Western Europe*, edited by I. C. Glover et al., pp. 121–30. BAR International Series 561. British Archaeological Reports, Oxford.

1995a   Incorporating Heterarchy into Theory on Socio-Political Development: The Case from Southeast Asia. In *Heterarchy and the Analysis of Complex Societies*, edited by R. M. Ehrenreich, C. L. Crumley, and J. E. Levy, pp. 101–23. Archaeological Papers of the American Anthropological Association 6. American Anthropological Association, Arlington, Va.

1995b   Modelling the Development of Early Rice Agriculture: Ethnoecological Perspectives from Northeast Thailand. *Asian Perspectives* 34(1): 37–68.

2007   Residential Burial and the Metal Age of Thailand. Paper presented at the Society for American Archaeology 72nd Annual Meeting, Austin, Tex., April 2007.

2008   Dating Early Bronze at Ban Chiang, Thailand. In *From Homo erectus to the Living Traditions: Choice of Papers from the 11th Conference of the European Association of Southeast Asian Archaeologists: Bougon, 25th–29th September 2006*, edited by J.-P. Pautreau, A.-S. Coupey, V. Zeitoun, and E. Rambault, pp. 91–104. Siam Ratana, Chiang Mai, Thailand.

White, Joyce C., and Vincent C. Pigott

1996   From Community Raft to Regional Specialization: Intensification of Copper Production in Pre-state Thailand. In *Craft Specialization and Social Evolution: In Memory of V. Gordon Childe*, edited by B. Wailes, pp. 151–75. University Museum Monograph No. 93. University Museum of Anthropology and Archaeology, Philadelphia.

White, Joyce C., Lisa Kealhofer, and Bernard Maloney

2004   Vegetation Changes from the Late Pleistocene through the Holocene from Three Areas of Archaeological Significance in Thailand. *Quaternary International* 113(1): 111–32.

White, Joyce C., William W. Vernon, Stuart J. Fleming, William D. Glanzman, Ron G. V. Hancock, and Andrew Pelcin

1991   Preliminary Cultural Implications from Initial Studies of the Ceramic Technology at Ban Chiang. *Bulletin of the Indo-Pacific Prehistory Association* 11: 188–203.

13 ◈ Written in Stone, Written in Bone

The Osteobiography of a Bronze Age Craftsman from Alalakh

Alexis T. Boutin

Individual Profile

Site: Tell Atchana (ancient Alalakh)

Location: Hatay Province, southern Turkey

Cultural Affiliation: Ancient Syria, Late Bronze Age

Date: Ca. mid-15th to late 14th centuries B.C.E.

Feature: Square 45-72, Locus 03-3009, Pail 41, Skeleton S04-4

Location of Grave: The highest layer of burials in a crowded pit-grave cemetery on the mound's eastern slope (Area 3)

Burial and Grave Type: A single primary inhumation in a pit with an uneven floor and sloping sides; deposited on his back, with legs flexed, arms folded over chest, and head resting on the left side

Associated Materials: None

Preservation and Completeness: Fully articulated, fairly complete skull, axial elements highly fragmentary, bones of arms and upper legs fairly complete; body entered baulk at knees, so lower legs not excavated

Age at Death and Basis of Estimate: 35–50 years, based on cranial suture closure (Meindl and Lovejoy 1985) and progression of osteoarthritis (Ubelaker 1999:84–87)

Sex and Basis of Determination: Male, based on pelvic and cranial morphology (Buikstra and Ubelaker 1994) and metrics of femur (midshaft circumference) (Bass 1995) and humerus (biepicondylar width) (France 1998)

Conditions Observed: Comparatively high frequencies of dental caries and antemortem tooth loss, heavy attrition, hypercementosis, grooves on occlusal surfaces of two anterior mandibular teeth; healed fracture of left ulna; osteoarthritis and enthesopathies in upper and lower body

Specialized Analysis: None

Excavated: 2003, Expedition to Alalakh (Tell Atchana), directed by K. Aslıhan Yener, University of Chicago; since 2006 this expedition has been sponsored by the Republic of Turkey Ministry of Culture.

Archaeological Report: Yener 2010

Current Disposition: Curated in expedition depot, Tayfur Sökmen, Hatay, Turkey

Tell Atchana was first recorded as site number 136 by the Braidwoods' archaeological survey of the fertile Amuq plain, once within the cultural sphere of ancient Syria, now in the modern nation of Turkey (Braidwood and Braidwood 1960). Shortly thereafter, Sir Leonard Woolley recognized that this mound on the Orontes River was strategically located at the crossroads of major trade routes (between Anatolia and the southern Levant, and between the Mediterranean and the Euphrates River valley), making it an ideal site to investigate cultural connections between Mesopotamia, the Minoans, and the Hittites (Woolley 1937). Eight excavation seasons between 1936 and 1949 (Woolley 1953, 1955) identified Tell Atchana as Alalakh, the capital of the city-state of Mukiš during the Middle Bronze Age (MBA) and Late Bronze Age (LBA) (Mellink 1957; Klengel 1995). Archives of cuneiform tablets deriving mostly from Level VII (MBA) and Level IV (LBA) document various aspects of Alalakh's social life and highlight its connections to regional centers such as Mari and Babylon, as well as its shifting affiliation with the empires of Yamhad, Mittani, and the Hittites (Wiseman 1953). Woolley's expedition also excavated numerous burials from the MBA and LBA, although he published "only a selection of the graves" (Woolley 1955: 201), specifically the 122 burials that best aided his interpretation of the site's function and chronology (table 13.1).

Building upon seven seasons of research by the Amuq Valley Regional Project (Yener 2005, 2010), renewed excavations at Alalakh are revisiting and clarifying Woolley's stratigraphy and pottery typologies, as well as exploring new parts of the site. As the expedition's mortuary specialist and osteologist, I analyzed the burials of at least 58 people excavated in 2003 and 2004 (Boutin 2008, 2010). These recently excavated burials greatly expand the corpus of mortuary remains from Alalakh and illustrate how archaeological, osteological,

Table 13.1. Chronological framework for Middle–Late Bronze Age Alalakh

Woolley's Level	Period	Absolute dates B.C.E.
XVII–VIII	Middle Bronze IIA–IIB	Late 19th to mid-17th century
VII	MB IIB	Mid-17th to mid-16th century
VI	MB IIC	Second half of 16th century
V	Late Bronze IA	First half of 15th century
IV	LB IB–IIA	Mid-15th to late 14th century

Note: The calendar years reflect the "low" chronology demonstrated as most suitable to Alalakh's stratigraphy and ceramic typologies (Gates 1981, 1987; Heinz 1992) and followed by many scholars (e.g., Stein 1997; Bergoffen 2005).

and documentary evidence, when interpreted in a complementary and contextual fashion, can shed light on the social production of embodied personhood through mortuary practices in the ancient Near East. The analysis of Skeleton S04-4 exemplifies the utility of this approach.

Political and Biocultural Context

Ancient Syria was "the primary arena of confrontation for a succession of competing multiregional polities, including the Mitannian, Egyptian, Hittite, and Assyrian empires" (Akkermans and Schwartz 2003: 327). Mukiš, with its capital at Alalakh, was frequently involved—whether as passive witness or active instigator—in these often violent political machinations. In the MB II period, Alalakh grew to its maximum size of 22 hectares (54 acres) and became the dominant settlement on the Amuq plain (Verstraete and Wilkinson 2000: 185). Not coincidentally, it was around this time that Alalakh, along with the rest of northern Syria, became a vassal of the Amorite kingdom of Yamhad, whose seat was in Halab (modern Aleppo) (Klengel 1992: 60–64). Although the period of occupation recorded in Level VII at Alalakh ended violently—a victim of the Hittite empire's aggressive territorial expansion out of Anatolia (Bryce 1998)—the city eventually reestablished its independence with the support of Mittani, a growing regional superpower based in the Syrian Jezireh (Wilhelm 1996).

By the Late IB Bronze period (recorded archaeologically as Level IV), Alalakh had regained its political and economic cosmopolitanism, as evidenced by monumental public architecture (Matthiae 2002), elaborate private houses (McClellan 1997), and pottery imported from Cyprus and the Aegean (Crouwel and Morris 1985; Bergoffen 2005). As the royal bureaucracy grew, so did its needs for skilled and unskilled labor. To keep track of who owed it service, the palace compiled census lists that grouped adult men who were legally free subjects of Mukiš into four socioeconomic classes: *hupše*, *haniahhe*, *ehele*, and *maryanni* (von Dassow 1997: 413–34). One of the names recorded in cuneiform on a now-lost clay tablet belonged to the man whose skeletal remains I have identified as Skeleton S04-4 for the purposes of osteological analysis.

The majority of the burials recently excavated at Alalakh, including S04-4 (figure 13.1), were discovered in Excavation Area 3, which straddles the mound's eastern slope. They comprise a large pit-grave cemetery of primary, single interments close to one another. This area, which previously was dominated by the city's fortification wall, was converted to a cemetery following the destruction of Level VII. A group of burials located at higher elevations (including S04-4) seems to represent a later phase of the cemetery's use during the LBA

(Level IV). On the whole, these Area 3 burials may be illustrative of a broader pattern at Alalakh, in which the edges of the mound, particularly atop fortification and occupational zones that had been abandoned, were favored for large-scale burial. This pattern complements that observed by Woolley, whose excavations focused on the northern and western parts of the city. Excavation Area 3 was occupied continuously during the MBA and LBA. In all these areas, the vast majority of the burials were associated with domestic architecture.[1]

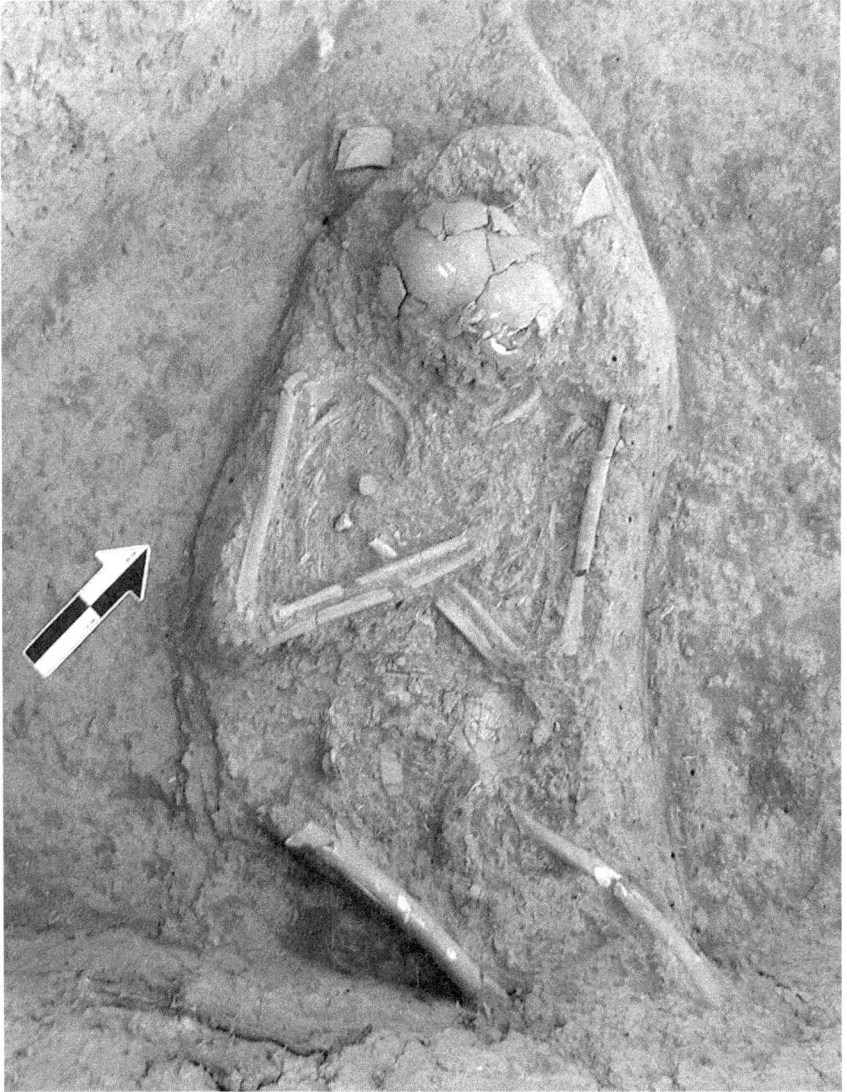

Figure 13.1. S04-4 in situ. (Photograph by Nita Lee Roberts courtesy of the Expedition to Alalakh.)

The cemetery excavated in 2003–2004 demonstrates that intramural burial was far from the only option for mortuary treatment at Alalakh, particularly in the more peripheral areas of the city and during periods of occupational transition or abandonment.

Osteobiographical Summary

Although S04-4's skeleton was distinguished by its complete articulation and comparatively good preservation, his mortuary treatment was typical of the cemetery area (the simple pit grave, the absence of grave goods, the lack of standardized orientation, the unassociated burial of a young adult male very nearby).

Masticatory and Extramasticatory Dental Modifications

S04-4's teeth have an irregular pattern of attrition, ranging from light-moderate on the M_3s to extreme (complete loss of the crown) on the anterior dentition. Four mandibular teeth and one maxillary tooth had carious lesions. On four of the five carious teeth, the lesions were interproximal (specifically, encompassing the cervical regions) or root caries, likely caused by exposure of the tooth roots (Hillson 1996: 274). Unusual grooving is evident on two anterior mandibular teeth. The right I_2 has a narrow mesio-distal groove (0.9 mm wide) on the midocclusal surface, just posterior to the pulp chamber (figure 13.2), while

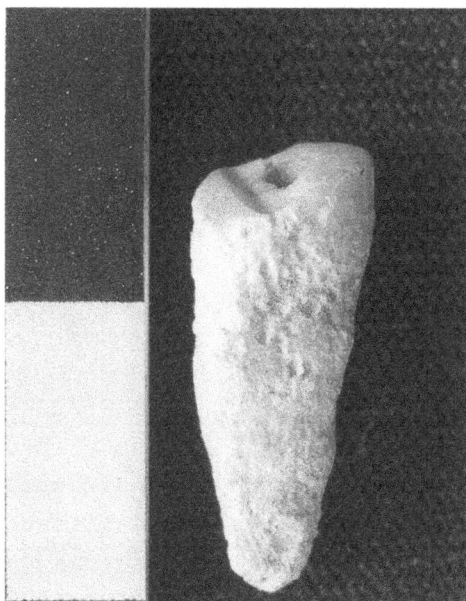

Figure 13.2. Right I_2 with mesio-distal groove. (Photograph by Alexis T. Boutin.)

the left canine has a slightly broader and flatter linguo-labial groove on the midocclusal surface, running across the pulp chamber. S04-4 lost at least seven teeth antemortem from a synergistic pulpal-alveolar disease process, which likely included very heavy attrition, extensive caries, and continuing eruption to compensate for reduction in crown height due to attrition and advancing age (Clarke and Hirsch 1991). Antemortem tooth loss seems to have preferentially affected the posterior dentition, the area that suffered most from caries. The temporomandibular joints were not sufficiently preserved to evaluate degeneration related to repetitive and forceful chewing. The attachment sites for the muscles associated with mastication (the masseteric origins of the zygomatics, zygomatic processes of the temporals, and the temporal lines) are not unusually robust, especially considering S04-4's advancing age. However, attachments for the tongue muscles (the mylohyoid lines and mental spines) are strongly marked.

S04-4's extant tooth roots exhibit generalized, slight or moderate, hypercementosis—increased thickness of the root surface caused by excess deposition and thickening of secondary cementum. These tooth roots also are shortened, ranging from slightly to severely affected. In archaeological skeletal series, these conditions have been attributed to chronic periodontal disease and nutritional stress (Corruccini et al. 1987), and to very heavy occlusal and/or pulling forces (Hylander 1977; Merbs 1983; Waters-Rist et al. 2007). In the case of S04-4, however, there does not seem to be a correlation between the severity of each tooth's attrition, hypercementosis, and root resorption. S04-4's hypercementosis and root resorption seem to reflect his advancing age, as well as the chronic pulpal-alveolar disease from which he suffered (Hillson 1986: 198; Hylander 1977: 137).

Changes to the Infracranial Skeleton

Compared to other people in the Alalakh skeletal sample, changes in S04-4's skeleton suggest that his occupation placed much heavier-than-average physical stress on his body (with the caveat that he was one of the older individuals, so there was more time for these pathologies to progress). Severe osteoarthritis is evident in his upper body. Both elbow joints exhibit extreme degeneration in the form of significant osteophyte formation, eburnation, pitting, and porosity at all sites of joint articulation (figures 13.3a, 13.3b). Severe osteoarthritis of the wrists and moderate-severe osteoarthritis of the hands and fingers is indicated by osteophyte formation and pitting of the carpals (especially on the right side), metacarpals, and phalanges. In general, S04-4's lower body, including the hip joint and the vertebral bodies, exhibits normal age-related stress responses and degeneration, in contrast to the bony responses to extremely rigorous physical activity evident in his upper body.

The distribution of S04-4's enthesopathies—the hypertrophy, rugosity, roughening, pitting, and grooving that develop at sites of tendon and ligament attachment (Kennedy 1989)—suggests some patterns of intensive, habitual activity in his upper and lower body. The upper limbs display some bilateral asymmetry: the few sites extant for comparing both right and left shoulders/ upper arms hint at more work by the left upper arm, while more evidence of

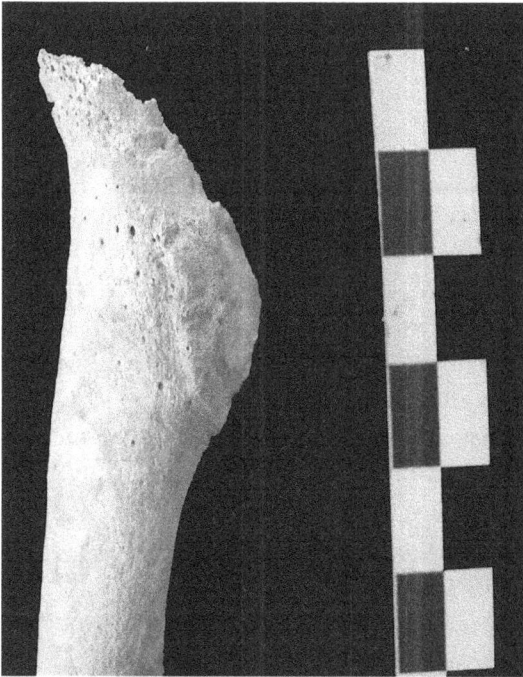

Figure 13.3a–b. Right radius showing evidence of osteoarthritis (eburnation and pitting) and enthesopathies: (a) hypertrophy and enthesophyte formation at bicipital tuberosity; (b) eburnation and pitting at proximal epiphysis. (Photograph by Alexis T. Boutin.)

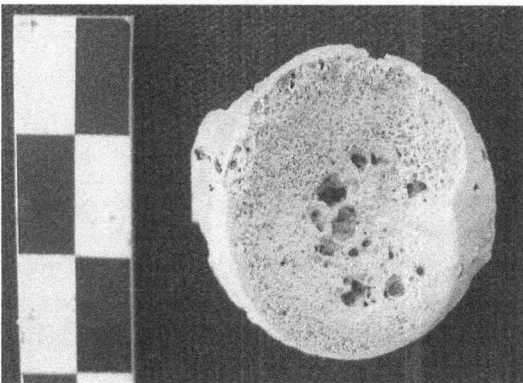

elbow/forearm work is apparent on his right side. The deltoid tuberosities of the humeri, as well as the insertions for the teres major and pectoralis major, are robust and roughened, resulting from wide-ranging movements of the shoulder joint. On the humeri, ulnae, and radii, sites of attachment for the major flexors and extensors of the elbow and wrist (such as the brachialis insertions at the ulnar tuberosities) are roughened and hypertrophied. The interosseus crests of the radii are sharp and pilastered, which could be due to pressure from adjacent muscles that aid in flexing the wrists and phalanges (Capasso et al. 1999: 118).

On the right and left femora, enthesopathies at the linea aspera and gluteal lines indicate strong adduction, extending, and rotating movements of the hip, important in maintaining balance and stability. Enthesopathies of the pectoralis major and brachialis muscle insertion sites (on the bones of the shoulder and elbow joints, respectively) and hypertrophied linea aspera on the femora together suggest the result of frequently lifting loads from the ground while in a squatting position, then carrying the loads with the forearms bent. These postures would be expected of a laborer, domestic worker, skilled tradesman, or soldier (Capasso et al. 1999: 66).

Macroscopic examination of S04-4's left ulna revealed an extra-articular fracture at the distal third of the diaphysis (figure 13.4; see Lovell 1997 for the approach to trauma analysis used here). The fracture is completely healed, although some compensatory remodeling was ongoing, which suggests that S04-4's ulnar fracture occurred at least one to two years prior to death. The lack of malunion or infection in a bone located so close to the surface of the skin indicates that the injury was well treated, by splinting and reduction. The precise type of fracture is uncertain because there was extensive remodeling and healing before he died, but the location and morphology of S04-4's fracture are consistent the type of transverse fracture labeled "parry" fractures (cf. Judd 2004: 41), which are often interpreted as evidence of interpersonal violence (Domett and Tayles 2006; Torres-Rouff and Costa Junqueira 2006; Smith 1996). However, there is no evidence of craniofacial trauma in the Alalakh skeletal series (0/141 craniofacial locations examined), and the long bone fracture rate of 0.46 percent (1/219 long bones examined, clavicle not included) is very low compared to other urban and rural Old World sites with agricultural economic bases (Djurić et al. 2006: 171–73). In fact, numerous nonviolent etiologies exist for ulnar fractures of the type observed on S04-4 (cf. Alvrus 1999: 422; Grauer and Roberts 1996; Judd 2002: 99). Given that he did not present accompanying craniofacial trauma (also characteristic of interpersonal violence), and that he seems to have regularly engaged in rigorous and even stressful physical activity, it is more likely that the cause of S04-4's forearm injury was accidental.

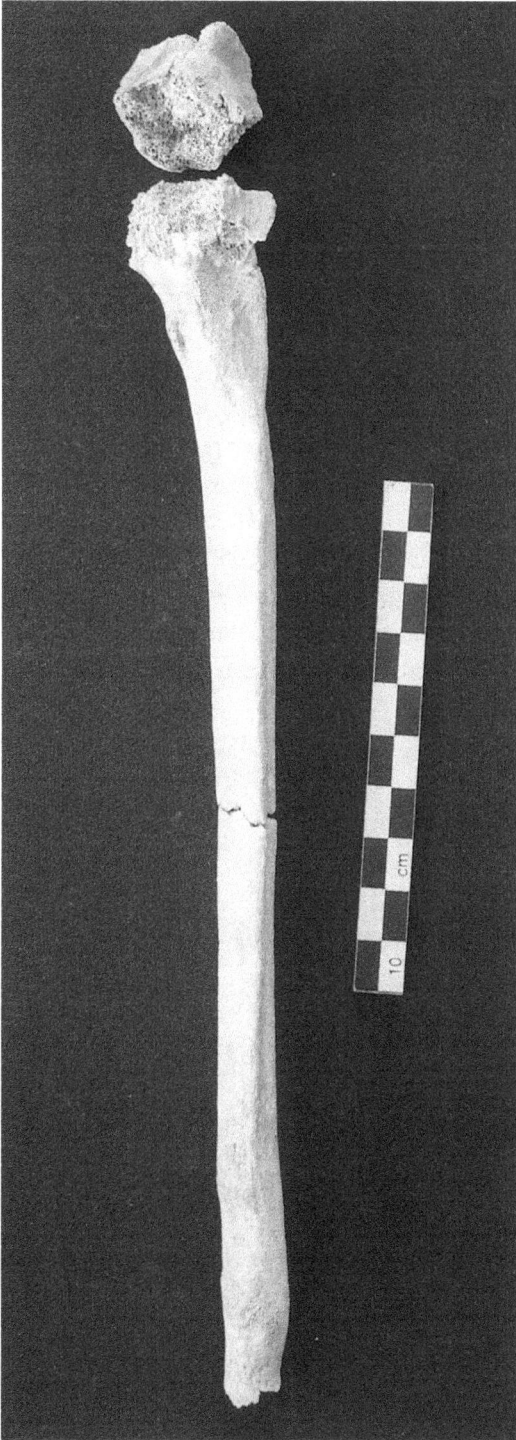

Figure 13.4. Left ulna with healed fracture.

Potential Sources of Occupational Stress

S04-4's suite of distinctive skeletal and dental signatures reflects a lifetime of arduous, and sometimes hazardous, physical labor. Thin grooving on anterior teeth has been observed in several prehistoric skeletal series from North America and Asia (Cybulski 1974; Schulz 1977; Larsen 1985; Waters-Rist et al. 2007), as well as at Neolithic sites in the Middle East (Molleson 1994; Minozzi et al. 2003). This kind of dental modification has been attributed to pulling fibrous plant materials across teeth for the production of cordage to manufacture utilitarian goods such as baskets, blankets and mats, fishnets, bags, and rope. Techniques of spinning yarn "through the mouth" are documented ethnographically in Egypt and are attested in Classical sources as well (Crowfoot 1931: 30–36). S04-4's apparently robust tongue muscles could have been regularly involved in helping manipulate the material being pulled across his heavily worn teeth. The intensive upper-body work evidenced by his enthesopathies, with lower-body involvement primarily for stabilizing purposes, also is consistent with occupations related to textile or cordage production. Ethnoarchaeological research in Iraq attests to the sometimes rigorous motions and postures involved in harvesting and preparing reeds, plaiting reed baskets and mats, weaving utilitarian

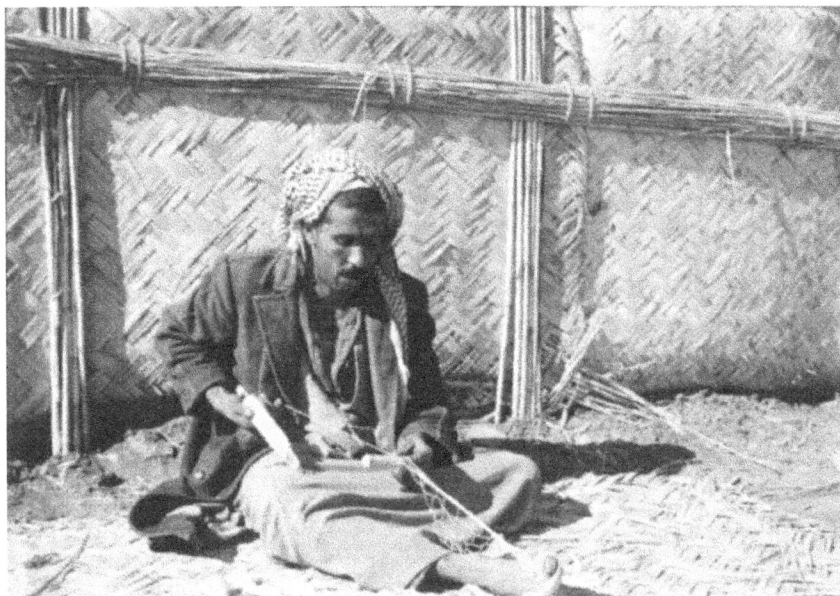

Figure 13.5. Marsh Arab fisherman making a net out of nylon cord. (Image modified from Ochsenschlager 2004, courtesy of the University of Pennsylvania Museum of Archaeology and Anthropology.)

objects by hand, and weaving tapestries on looms (figure 13.5; Ochsenschlager 2004). In fact, many textile/cordage-related occupations held by men are known from contemporary texts found at Alalakh, including weaver, headdress-maker, tapestry weaver, reed worker, spinner, and felt-maker (Dietrich and Loretz 1966, 1969). The fact that S04-4 was the only individual in the Alalakh skeletal series to exhibit either occlusal grooving or a long bone fracture suggests that his occupation may have been highly specialized or even unique.

Because muscles work cooperatively to create a range of movements, and similar movements are involved in a variety of activities (Stirland 1998), it is very difficult to attribute a specific occupation based on enthesopathies and osteoarthritis. Although additional osteological and archaeological data from S04-4 permits a multifactorial analysis, it is still risky to speculate in great detail about prehistoric contexts where the full range of quotidian and occupationally specialized bodily postures are not (and may never be) known. For the purpose of fictive osteobiographical reconstruction, I have pursued the idea that S04-4 was a reed worker.

Fictive Narrative and Osteobiography

Given the definition of osteobiography as life histories recorded in bone (Saul 1972: 8), there has been very little consideration of *how* these stories should be told. Who is telling the story? Who is the audience? How does the use of skeletal data make these stories different from other types of archaeological narratives? In response to these questions, I tell the stories from Alalakh in a nontraditional way, through osteobiographies in the format of fictive narrative, one of which is presented here (cf. Boutin 2008, 2011).

Joyce and her collaborators (2002) draw on Bakhtin's and Barthes's performance-based theories of semiotics to advocate methods of experimental writing that emphasize the dialogic nature of archaeology. They argue that (re)presenting the past through alternative media such as hypertext, fictive narrative, and actual spoken dialogue reveals the contingency, ambiguity, and collaboration that are inherent to the production of archaeological knowledge (but which are seldom apparent from the equifinality that pervades traditional archaeological writing) (Gero 1991: 126). Telling stories about the same material from multiple perspectives facilitates a view of the past that is open-ended and multivocal, and captures the plurality of lived experience (Lopiparo 2002: 74–77). As Sabloff states, narratives about the archaeological process, and how it uncovers the "richness of human experience" in past cultures, accessibly and effectively convey archaeology's relevance to the modern world, thereby helping narrow the communication gap that the academization of archaeology has created between professional archaeologists and the general public over the past century (Sabloff 1998: 871).

One of the most potent critiques of narrative modes of interpretation is that they blur fact and fiction: but can any language "adequately and fully represent the world of the past" (Pluciennik 1999: 667)? I argue that alternative and experimental media are as legitimate as any other way of (re)presenting the past. In the interests of reflexivity and full disclosure, I explicitly emphasize the fictiveness (cf. Wilkie 2003) of the osteobiographical narratives that I have written: the names, events, emotions, and thoughts described therein are products of my imagination. However, my study is based on rigorous archaeological and osteological methods and extensive research into contemporary sociohistoric contextual data from Bronze Age Syria, which are elucidated in the narratives' annotations. The use of fictive narrative discourse allows me to weave together all of these contextual sources in a holistic way that enhances and enlarges the stories told by artifacts and skeletal remains (after Schrire 1995: 5). Although these narratives are technically fictive, I believe that they carry as much interpretive weight as any other form of presentation. At the same time, they represent just one possible interpretation of these data: the dialogic nature of archaeology would not be fulfilled if responses to my interpretations do not materialize and perhaps offer alternative interpretations to continue the dialogue.

S04-4's Osteobiographical Narrative

"Do you remember your father, Ammar-Addu?[2] You, Naidu, were still suckling, and you, Tulpia, were only a boy of two cubits when death came suddenly to him.[3] He was struck by waves of suffocating heat that alternated with bone-shaking chills, and sharp pains had wracked his body.[4] But his battle with the demons of the underworld did not last long, and he was quickly and inexorably pulled into eternal sleep.[5] We had been confined to the family home for three sunsets,[6] waiting for your father's body to be released from the death grip that had frozen it.[7] The fasting period was not all that difficult for me to endure— the meager rations of barley that we received never made enough bread anyway (sometimes I think that the *ehele* receive more barley to feed their horses and cattle!).[8] But I was saddened that we could not provide your father with food and drink for his journey or for the gods who would bless him with rest and peace in the land of no return.[9] Nor could we afford to hire women to mourn, though my sisters, neighbors, and I did the best we could to maintain the waves of kneeling and bowing, weeping and wailing, that undulated into the courtyard.[10]

"Your father's life was not always marked by hardship. He received his baton and ax soon after leaving his mother's womb,[11] and his childhood was a time of peace. The gods protected him from the famine and plague that periodically struck.[12] He learned his craft from his father, who himself had been taught by the temple's master reed worker, back in the time of our ancestors when the king witnessed grand processions of deity statues floating down the river in reed boats. These days, your father kept busy at the market making everyday goods like mats, stools, buckets, and baskets[13]—and lately, these had sold so well that he no longer worried about being able to afford Naidu's dowry when the day came![14]

"Toward the end, his arms and hands ached as he harvested reeds from the riverbank and carried them in heavy bundles back to the city.[15] Even though we had scraped together the money for an *asû*[16] to fix his arm after the accident, it still throbbed deep inside the bone. When he split reeds, his tongue guided them over the few stumps of teeth remaining in his mouth. You remember, don't you Tulpia, how he was just starting to teach you the craft?[17] But no matter how hard he worked at his profession, as a *haniahhena*, he owed the palace even more labor![18] The overseers made him hoe fields, work at the granary, make mudbricks.[19] When the hand of Nergal struck your father down, his strength was spent and he could not fight it.[20]

"I remember your father best as he looked on the day of our marriage: he was somewhat shorter than other men, but well muscled and strong from years of harvesting and pounding reeds and sealing reed boats with bitumen.[21] His white hat and robes fairly shone against his black beard and tanned skin, and he stood with his hands firmly planted at his solid waist, the blue tassels of his tightly cinched belt nearly reaching the floor. I was so proud to call such a man my husband.[22] Sadly, after he had departed for the land of no return, we could not afford to bury him in such finery—your aunt helped me wrap his body in a simple, fringed swath of fabric.

"As the funeral procession trudged from our home to the cemetery on the city's edge, our bare feet moved with the cadence of the funeral dirge, kicking up puffs of dust with every step. The neighbor's husband had been kind enough to dig a simple pit for his grave—I didn't have the heart to complain that it was rather small and sloping. The men lay your father on his back as if in sleep, with his legs flexed and his arms crossed over his chest. Your uncle began chanting *šuma zakaru*: 'Ammar-addu may you stand before Šamaš and Gilgameš.' He expanded his invocation to include all of the other ancestors—his immediate relatives, his extended family, his people, his family by marriage—and asked them to protect their living offspring and to represent them before the gods of the underworld.[23] Your father looked so peaceful, and I prayed to the gods that they would let his spirit find eternal rest after all of the hard work that his body had done in the Land of the Living."

Acknowledgments

I am grateful to the current and former directorship of the Expedition to Alalakh—Murat Akar, Amir Sumaka'i Fink, David Schloen, and especially Aslıhan Yener—for granting me logistical support and access to excavation records, artifacts, and human skeletal remains. The comments of two anonymous reviewers and the volume editors aided significantly in this chapter's revision, although all mistakes remain my own. This chapter is dedicated to the memory of Stine Rossel, a superior archaeologist and an even better friend.

Notes

1. The Level I graves excavated by Woolley (1955: 204–5) may present the one significant exception. Insofar as they were dug into the ruins of private houses near the city's edge, they may have more in common with the burials excavated in 2003–2004 than with the other intramural burials. Based on Mullins's (2010) recent reassessment of Woolley's ceramic corpus, which demonstrates that Woolley's Levels IV–I should be considered one broadly coherent phase dating to the mid-fifteenth to fourteenth centuries B.C.E., Woolley's Level I graves actually could be contemporary with the LBA graves in Area 3.

2. This name appears in several Alalakh Texts (Wiseman 1953).

3. Children's age was characterized by "observable outward signs"—for example, whether they were weaned or unweaned—or by height, in terms of cubits (Roth 1987: 717).

4. It is not possible to pinpoint a specific cause of death for S04-4 or any other skeleton excavated in 2003–2004, suggesting that they were the victims of acute, infectious, and/or soft tissue diseases.

5. For the terminology associated with death and burial, see Olyan 1999; Steiner 1982.

6. The ritual mourning period lasted seven days and seven nights, after which time the mourners were supposed to achieve a state of rest and return to normal life (Pham 1999: 24).

7. Rigor mortis commences ca. 2–6 hours postmortem. It usually lasts 24–48 hours, after which the muscles relax in roughly the same order in which they stiffened (Gill-King 1997: 98).

8. Alalakh Texts 236–318 describe grain rations from the palace: barley was a dietary staple and also sometimes designated as animal fodder (Wiseman 1953: 81–93). The exclusive *ehele* group, landholders who were exempted from most royal obligations, constituted

the professional and service sector and had ties to the palace administration and nobility (von Dassow 1997: 416–17).

9. For the provision of grave goods, such as food and drink, see Tsukimoto 1985: 229–33.

10. For the performance of mourning, see Pham 1999; Levine 1993; Olyan 2004.

11. In a Mesopotamian birth incantation, male newborns are given these gifts as gendered markers signaling their "strength of heroship" (Asher-Greve 2002: 13).

12. S04-4 exhibits no cribra orbitalia (localized porous lesions on the orbital roofs) (El-Najjar et al. 1976; Stuart-Macadam 1985) or linear enamel hypoplasias (LEH) (deficiencies in enamel thickness caused by disruptions in the secretory/matrix formation phase of amelogenesis) (Goodman et al. 1980; Goodman and Armelagos 1985). These pathologies result from episodes of physiological stress suffered during childhood, including malnutrition, dietary anemia, and infectious disease. In general, frequencies of LEH in the Alalakh skeletal series were moderate-high (afflicting 63.0 percent (17/27) of individuals whose permanent teeth were observed), while those of cribra orbitalia were moderate (afflicting 31.0 percent (9/29) of individuals observed).

13. For the occupational specialization and products of reed workers, see *Chicago Assyrian Dictionary* I, 2: 494–95; van de Mieroop 1987.

14. The dowry was the daughter's share of her patrimonial inheritance, which she received at the time of her marriage. Since there are only a few records of dowry transfer, most dowries probably consisted of "movables" such as livestock, silver, or textiles (Grosz 1989: 171–72).

15. Eburnation indicates that the joints were still active at the time of death.

16. Physicians used incantations and herbal medicines as they set broken bones, lanced boils, and treated illnesses and battle wounds (Biggs 1995: 1918).

17. Unless they belonged to the upper classes, older children remained in the domestic sphere where they learned social roles and trades from their parents (Harris 2000: 18–20).

18. Reed workers belonged to the lower-status social classes (*hupše* or *haniahhe*) (Dietrich and Loretz 1969: 57). *Haniahhena*, most of whom lacked landholdings, probably subsisted as artisans, soldiers, day-laborers, or subtenants of landholders. They owed taxes, corvée labor, and military service to the palace (von Dassow 1997: 415–16).

19. At the early second millennium B.C.E. city of Isin in Mesopotamia, reed workers and other craft workers periodically had to perform these types of corvée labor (van de Mieroop 1987: 54–55).

20. Epidemics were referred to as the "hand" or "touch" of Nergal (Stol 1995: 487).

21. Humeral and femoral metrics suggest that S04-4's overall body size was somewhat smaller than average compared to other males at Alalakh. His upper body seems to have been moderately robust, and his lower body was of above-average robusticity.

22. This costume was typical of fifteenth-century Syria (Collon 1995: 510). Masculinity was signified through musculature and certain postures (Bahrani 2001: 42), and beards were gendered markers of strength and masculinity (Asher-Greve 2002: 13).

23. Šamaš and Gilgameš were the judges of the underworld (Wexler 1993: 255). For care of the family dead, see Pitard 1996; Tsukimoto 1985; van der Toorn 1996.

References Cited

Akkermans, Peter M. M. G., and Glenn M. Schwartz

2003   *The Archaeology of Syria: From Complex Hunter-Gatherers to Early Urban Societies (c. 16,000–300 B.C.)*. Cambridge University Press, Cambridge.

Alvrus, Anna

1999   Fracture Patterns among the Nubians of Semna South, Sudanese Nubia. *International Journal of Osteoarchaeology* 9: 417–29.

Asher-Greve, Julia M.

2002   Decisive Sex, Essential Gender. In *Sex and Gender in the Ancient Near East: Proceedings of the 47th Rencontre Assyriologique Internationale, Helsinki, July 2–6, 2001*, edited by S. Parpola and R. M. Whiting, pp. 11–26. Neo-Assyrian Text Corpus Project, Helsinki.

Bahrani, Zainab

2001   *Women of Babylon: Gender and Representation in Mesopotamia*. Routledge, London.

Bass, William M.

1995   *Human Osteology: A Laboratory and Field Manual*. 4th ed. Missouri Archaeological Society, Columbia.

Bergoffen, Celia J.

2005   *The Cypriot Bronze Age Pottery from Sir Leonard Woolley's Excavations at Alalakh (Tell Atchana)*. Verlag der Österreichischen Akademie der Wissenschaften, Vienna.

Biggs, Robert D.

1995   Medicine, Surgery, and Public Health in Ancient Mesopotamia. In *Civilizations of the Ancient Near East*, edited by J. M. Sasson, pp. 1911–24. Charles Scribner's Sons, New York.

Boutin, Alexis T.

2008   Embodying Life and Death: Osteobiographical Narratives from Alalakh. Ph.D. dissertation, University of Pennsylvania.

2010   The Burials. In *Tell Atchana, Ancient Alalakh*, Vol. 1, *The 2003–2004 Excavation Seasons*, edited by K. A. Yener, pp. 111–21. Koç Üniversitesi Yayınları, Istanbul.

2011   Crafting a Bioarchaeology of Personhood: Ostebiographical Narratives from Alalakh. In *Breathing New Life into the Evidence of Death: Contemporary Approaches to Bioarchaeology*, edited by A. Baadsgaard, A. T. Boutin, and J. E. Buikstra, pp. 109–133. School for Advanced Research Press, Santa Fe, N.Mex.

Braidwood, Robert J., and Linda S. Braidwood

1960   *Excavations in the Plains of Antioch I: The Earlier Assemblages, Phases A–J*. University of Chicago Oriental Institute, Chicago.

Bryce, Trevor

1998   *The Kingdom of the Hittites*. Clarendon Press, Oxford.

Buikstra, Jane E., and Douglas H. Ubelaker (editors)

1994   *Standards for Data Collection from Human Skeletal Remains*. Arkansas Archaeological Survey Research Series No. 44. Arkansas Archaeological Survey, Fayetteville.

Capasso, Luigi, Kenneth A. R. Kennedy, and Cynthia A. Wilczak

1999   *Atlas of Occupational Markers on Human Remains*. *Journal of Paleopathology*. Monographic Publication 3. Edigrafial S.p.A., Teramo.

Clarke, Nigel G., and Robert S. Hirsch

1991 Physiological, Pulpal, and Periodontal Factors Influencing Alveolar Bone. In *Advances in Dental Anthropology*, edited by M. A. Kelley and C. S. Larsen, pp. 241–66. Wiley-Liss, New York.

Collon, Dominique

1995 Clothing and Grooming in Ancient Western Asia. In *Civilizations of the Ancient Near East*, edited by J. M. Sasson, pp. 503–16. Charles Scribner's Sons, New York.

Corruccini, Robert S., Keith P. Jacobi, Jerome S. Handler, and Arthur C. Aufderheide

1987 Implications of Tooth Root Hypercementosis in a Barbados Slave Skeletal Collection. *American Journal of Physical Anthropology* 74: 179–84.

Crouwel, J. H., and C. E. Morris

1985 Mycenaean Pictorial Pottery from Tell Atchana (Alalakh). *Annual of the British School at Athens* 80: 85–98.

Crowfoot, Grace M.

1931 *Methods of Hand Spinning in Egypt and the Sudan*. F. King & Sons, Halifax, N.S.

Cybulski, Jerome S.

1974 Tooth Wear and Material Culture: Precontact Patterns in the Tsimshian Area, British Columbia. *Syesis* 7: 31–35.

Dietrich, M., and O. Loretz

1966 Die soziale Struktur von Alalah und Ugarit (I): Die Berfusbezeichnungen mit der hurritischen Endung -*huli*. *Die Welt des Orients* 3: 189–205.

1969 Die soziale Struktur von Alalah und Ugarit (II): Die sozialen Gruppen *hupšu-name, haniahhe-eku, ehele-šuzubu* und *marjanne* nach Texten aus Alalah IV. *Die Welt des Orients* 5: 57–93.

Djurić, M. P., C. A. Roberts, Z. B. Rakočević, D. D. Djonić, and A. R. Lešić

2006 Fractures in Late Medieval Skeletal Populations from Serbia. *American Journal of Physical Anthropology* 130: 167–78.

Domett, K. M., and N. Tayles

2006 Adult Fracture Patterns in Prehistoric Thailand: A Biocultural Interpretation. *International Journal of Osteoarchaeology* 16: 185–99.

El-Najjar, Mahmoud Y., Dennis J. Ryan, Christy G. Turner II, and Betsy Lozoff

1976 The Etiology of Porotic Hyperostosis among the Prehistoric and Historic Anasazi Indians of Southwestern United States. *American Journal of Physical Anthropology* 44: 477–87.

France, Diane L.

1998 Observational and Metrical Analysis of Sex in the Skeleton. In *Forensic Osteology: Advances in the Identification of Human Remains*, 2nd ed., edited by K. J. Reichs, pp. 163–86. Charles C. Thomas, Springfield, Ill.

Gates, Marie-Henriette C.

1981 *Alalakh Levels VI and V: A Chronological Reassessment*. Undena Publications, Malibu.

1987 Alalakh and Chronology Again. In *High, Middle or Low? Acts of an International Colloquium on Absolute Chronology Held at the University of Gothenburg, 20th–22nd August, 1987*, edited by Paul Åström, pp. 60–86. Paul Åströms Förlag, Gothenburg.

Gero, Joan M.

1991   Who Experienced What in Prehistory? A Narrative Explanation from Queyash, Peru. In *Processual and Postprocessual Archaeologies: Multiple Ways of Knowing the Past*, edited by R. W. Preucel, pp. 126–89. Southern Illinois University Press, Carbondale.

Gill-King, H.

1997   Chemical and Ultrastructural Aspects of Decomposition. In *Forensic Taphonomy: The Postmortem Fate of Human Remains*, edited by W. D. Haglund and M. H. Sorg, pp. 93–108. CRC Press, Boca Raton, Fla.

Goodman, Alan H., and George J. Armelagos

1985   Factors Affecting the Distribution of Enamel Hypoplasias within the Human Permanent Dentition. *American Journal of Physical Anthropology* 68: 479–93.

Goodman, Alan H., George J. Armelagos, and Jerome C. Rose

1980   Enamel Hypoplasias as Indicators of Stress in Three Prehistoric Populations from Illinois. *Human Biology* 52(3): 515–28.

Grauer, A. L., and C. A. Roberts

1996   Paleoepidemiology, Healing, and Possible Treatment of Trauma in the Medieval Cemetery Population of St. Helen-on-the-Walls, York, England. *American Journal of Physical Anthropology* 100: 531–44.

Grosz, Katarzyna

1989   Some Aspects of the Position of Women in Nuzi. In *Women's Earliest Records from Ancient Egypt and Western Asia*, edited by B. S. Lesko, pp. 167–80. Scholars Press, Atlanta.

Harris, Rivkah

2000   *Gender and Aging in Mesopotamia: The Gilgamesh Epic and Other Ancient Literature.* University of Oklahoma Press, Norman.

Heinz, Marlies

1992   *Tell Atchana/Alalakh: Die Schichten VII–XVII.* Neukirchener Verlag, Neukirchen-Vluyn, Germany.

Hillson, Simon

1986   *Teeth.* Cambridge University Press, Cambridge.

1996   *Dental Anthropology.* Cambridge University Press, Cambridge.

Hylander, William L.

1977   The Adaptive Significance of Eskimo Craniofacial Morphology. In *Orofacial Growth and Development*, edited by A. A. Dahlberg and T. M. Graber, pp. 129–69. Mouton, The Hague.

Joyce, Rosemary A., with Robert A. Preucel, Jeanne Lopiparo, Carolyn Guyer, and Michael Joyce

2002   *The Languages of Archaeology.* Blackwell, Oxford.

Judd, M.

2002   Ancient Injury Recidivism: An Example from the Kerma Period of Ancient Nubia. *International Journal of Osteoarchaeology* 12: 89–106.

2004   Trauma in the City of Kerma: Ancient versus Modern Injury Patterns. *International Journal of Osteoarchaeology* 14: 34–51.

Kennedy, Kenneth A. R.

1989   Skeletal Markers of Occupational Stress. In *Reconstruction of Life from the Skeleton*, edited by M. Y. İşcan and K. A. R. Kennedy, pp. 129–60. Alan R. Liss, New York.

Klengel, Horst

1992   *Syria: 3000 to 300 B.C.: A Handbook of Political History.* Akademie Verlag, Berlin.

1995   Mukiš. In *Reallexikon der Assyriologie und Vorderasiatischen Archäologie*, edited by D. O. Edzard, pp. 411–12. Walter de Gruyter, Berlin.

Larsen, Clark S.

1985   Dental Modifications and Tool Use in the Western Great Basin. *American Journal of Physical Anthropology* 67: 393–402.

Levine, Baruch A.

1993   Silence, Sound, and the Phenomenology of Mourning in Biblical Israel. *Journal of Ancient Near Eastern Studies* 22: 89–106.

Lopiparo, Jeanne

2002   A Second Voice: *Crafting Cosmos*. In *The Languages of Archaeology*, edited by R. A. Joyce, pp. 68–99. Blackwell, Oxford.

Lovell, Nancy C.

1997   Trauma Analysis in Paleopathology. *Yearbook of Physical Anthropology* 40: 139–70.

Matthiae, Paolo

2002   About the Formation of Old Syrian Architectural Tradition. In *Of Pots and Plans: Papers of the Archaeology and History of Mesopotamia and Syria Presented to David Oates in Honour of His 75th Birthday*, edited by L. el Gailani et al., pp. 191–209. Nabu Publications, London.

McClellan, Thomas L.

1997   Houses and Households in North Syria during the Late Bronze Age. In *Les maisons dans la Syrie antique de IIIe millénaire aux débuts de l'Islam*, edited by C. Castel, M. al-Maqdissi, and F. Villeneuve, pp. 29–59. Institut Français d'Archéologie du Proche-Orient, Beirut.

Meindl, Richard S., and C. Owen Lovejoy

1985   Ectocranial Suture Closure: A Revised Method for the Determination of Skeletal Age at Death Based on the Lateral-Anterior Sutures. *American Journal of Physical Anthropology* 68: 57–66.

Mellink, Machteld J.

1957   Review of *Alalakh: An Account of the Excavations at Tell Atchana in the Hatay, 1937–1939*, by Leonard Woolley. *American Journal of Archaeology* 61: 395–400.

Merbs, Charles F.

1983   *Patterns of Activity-Induced Pathology in a Canadian Inuit Population.* National Museums of Canada, Ottawa.

Minozzi, Simona, Giorgio Manzi, Francesca Ricci, Salvino de Lernia, and Silvana M. Borgognini Tarli

2003   Nonalimentary Tooth Use in Prehistory: An Example from Early Holocene in Central Sahara (Uan Muhaggiag, Tadrart Acacus, Libya). *American Journal of Physical Anthropology* 120: 225–32.

Molleson, Theya

1994   The Eloquent Bones of Abu Hureyra. *Scientific American* 271(2): 70–75.

Mullins, Robert A.

2010   A Comparative Analysis of the Alalakh 2003–2004 Season Pottery with Woolley's Levels. In *Tell Atchana, Ancient Alalakh*, Vol. 1, *The 2003–2004 Excavation Seasons*, edited by K. A. Yener, pp. 51–66. Koç Universitesi Yayınları, Istanbul.

Ochsenschlager, Edward L.

2004   *Iraq's Marsh Arabs in the Garden of Eden*. University of Pennsylvania Museum of Archaeology and Anthropology, Philadelphia.

Olyan, Saul M.

2004   *Biblical Mourning: Ritual and Social Dimensions*. Oxford University Press, Oxford.

Oriental Institute of the University of Chicago

1956–1999   *Chicago Assyrian Dictionary*. Oriental Institute of the University of Chicago, Chicago.

Pham, Xuan H. T.

1999   *Mourning in the Ancient Near East and the Hebrew Bible*. Sheffield Academic Press, Sheffield, U.K.

Pitard, Wayne T.

1996   Care of the Dead at Emar. In *Emar: The History, Religion, and Culture of a Syrian Town in the Late Bronze Age*, edited by M. W. Chavalas, pp. 123–40. CDL Press, Bethesda, Md.

Pluciennik, Mark

1999   Archaeological Narratives and Other Ways of Telling. *Current Anthropology* 40(5): 653–78.

Roth, Martha T.

1987   Age at Marriage and the Household: A Study of Neo-Babylonian and Neo-Assyrian Forms. *Comparative Studies in Society and History* 29(4): 715–47.

Sabloff, J. A.

1998   Distinguished Lecture in Archeology: Communication and the Future of American Archaeology. *American Anthropologist* 100(4): 869–75.

Saul, Frank P.

1972   *The Human Skeletal Remains of Altar de Sacrificios: An Osteobiographic Analysis*. Peabody Museum, Cambridge, Mass.

Schrire, Carmel

1995   *Digging through Darkness: Chronicles of an Archaeologist*. University Press of Virginia, Charlottesville.

Schulz, Peter D.

1977   Task Activity and Anterior Tooth Grooving in Prehistoric California Indians. *American Journal of Physical Anthropology* 46: 87–92.

Smith, Maria O.

1996   "Parry" Fractures and Female-Directed Interpersonal Violence: Implications from the Late Archaic Period of West Tennessee. *International Journal of Osteoarchaeology* 6: 84–91.

Stein, Diana L.

1997   Alalakh. In *The Oxford Encyclopedia of Archaeology in the Near East*, edited by E. M. Meyers, pp. 55–59. Oxford University Press, Oxford.

Steiner, Gerd

1982　Das Bedeutungsfeld "TOD" in den Sprachen des Alten Orients. *Orientalia* 51(2): 239–48.

Stirland, A. J.

1998　Musculoskeletal Evidence for Activity: Problems of Evaluation. *International Journal of Osteoarchaeology* 8: 354–62.

Stol, Marten

1995　Private Life in Ancient Mesopotamia. In *Civilizations of the Ancient Near East*, edited by J. M. Sasson, pp. 485–501. Charles Scribner's Sons, New York.

Stuart-Macadam, Patty

1985　Porotic Hyperostosis: Representative of a Childhood Condition. *American Journal of Physical Anthropology* 66: 391–98.

Torres-Rouff, Christina, and Maria Antonietta Costa Junqueira

2006　Interpersonal Violence in Prehistoric San Pedro de Atacama, Chile: Behavioral Implications of Environmental Stress. *American Journal of Physical Anthropology* 130: 60–70.

Tsukimoto, Akio

1985　*Untersuchungen zur Totenpflege (kispum) in alten Mesopotamien*. Verlag Butzon & Bercker, Kevelaer.

Ubelaker, Douglas H.

1999　*Human Skeletal Remains: Excavation, Analysis, Interpretation*. 3rd ed. Taraxacum, Washington, D.C.

van de Mieroop, Marc

1987　*Crafts in the Early Isin Period*. Department Oriëntalistiek, Leuven.

van der Toorn, Karel

1996　*Family Religion in Babylonia, Syria and Israel: Continuity and Change in the Forms of Religious Life*. Brill, Leiden.

Verstraete, J., and T. J. Wilkinson

2000　The Amuq Regional Archaeological Survey. In *The Amuq Valley Regional Project, 1995–1998*, edited by K. Aslıhan Yener et al., pp. 163–220. *American Journal of Archaeology* 104: 179–92.

von Dassow, Eva

1997　Social Stratification of Alalah under the Mittani Empire. Ph.D. dissertation, New York University.

Waters-Rist, A., V. I. Bazaliiskii, A. Weber, O. I. Goriunova, and M. A. Katzenberg

2007　Activity-Induced Dental Modification in Holocene Siberian Hunter-Gatherers. *American Journal of Physical Anthropology* 132(S44): 245.

Wexler, Robert D.

1993　The Concepts of Mortality and Immortality in Ancient Mesopotamia. Ph.D. dissertation, University of California, Los Angeles.

Wilhelm, Gernot

1996　L'Etat Actuel et les Perspectives des Etudes Hourrites. In *Mari, Ébla et les Hourrites: Dix ans de travaux*, edited by J. Durand, pp. 175–87. Éditions recherche sur les civilisations, Paris.

Wilkie, Laurie A.

2003   *The Archaeology of Mothering: An African-American Midwife's Tale*. Routledge, New York.

Wiseman, D. J.

1953   *The Alalakh Tablets*. British Institute of Archaeology at Ankara, London.

Woolley, Leonard

1937   Excavations near Antioch in 1936. *Antiquaries Journal* 17(1): 1–15.

1953   *A Forgotten Kingdom*. Penguin Books, Baltimore.

1955   *Alalakh: An Account of the Excavations at Tell Atchana in the Hatay, 1937–1949*. Society of Antiquaries, Oxford.

Yener, K. Aslıhan (editor)

2005   *The Amuq Valley Regional Projects*, Vol. 1, *Surveys in the Plain of Antioch and Orontes Delta, Turkey, 1995–2002*. Oriental Institute of the University of Chicago, Chicago.

2010   *Tell Atchana, Ancient Alalakh*, Vol. 1, *The 2003–2004 Excavation Seasons*. Koç Üniversitesi Yayınları, Istanbul.

FOUR ◈ Farm and Village

14 ◆ Life and Death of a Mother and Child in Nineteenth-Century Ontario, Canada

M. Anne Katzenberg and Shelley R. Saunders

Individual Profile

Site: Harvie Cemetery (AhHb-26)
Location: Lots 2 and 3, Concession 8, North Dumfries Township, Regional Municipality of Waterloo, Ontario
Cultural Affiliation: Canadian historic
Date: Ca. A.D. 1825–1894, based on tombstone and documentary data
Features: Burials 1 and 1a
Location of Grave: Central west edge of burial ground
Burial and Grave Type: Two single primary inhumations, fully extended, lying beside each other
Associated Materials: Some coffin nails and flat-headed screws; preserved coffin wood
Preservation and Completeness: Fair to good
Age at Death and Basis of Estimate: Mother—mean age 25 years based on pubic symphysis, rib phases, ectocranial suture closure, auricular surface morphology, histological analysis of femoral cortex; child—0.5–2.5 years, mean age 1.9 years based on dental development, occipital development, temporal development, bone lengths
Sex and Basis of Determination: Mother—female, based on pelvic morphology and femur diameters
Conditions Observed: None
Specialized Analysis: Stable isotopes of carbon and nitrogen
Excavated: 1988, McMaster University, directed by Shelley Saunders and Richard Lazenby
Archaeological Report: Saunders and Lazenby 1991
Current Disposition: Reburied in 1989

This chapter is about a woman and her child who both died of acute illness in September 1848 and who were interred in a small family cemetery in Upper Canada (part of the present-day province of Ontario). We focus on this known mother-infant pair to illustrate the value of information derived from historical contexts, for helping to understand both the lives of ordinary people and the promises and limitations of information gleaned from bones and teeth for reconstructing the lives of past people.

The Cemetery

The Harvie Cemetery (AhHb-26) was a pioneer family burial ground located on part of Lots 2 and 3, Concession 8, North Dumfries Township, in the Regional Municipality of Waterloo, Ontario (figure 14.1). In the early 1980s, when the cemetery could no longer be maintained, the tombstones were donated to Doon Heritage Crossroads, a regional pioneer village designed to highlight local history (figure 14.2). The original graves were left intact but without markers above ground. In 1988 the landowner indicated his intention to disinter the cemetery, and after talks with the archaeology division of the regional municipality, he agreed to allow an archaeological excavation. The excavation was conducted under the archaeology division's license (#88-25) by Shelley Saunders and graduate student Richard Lazenby from McMaster University. Although the location of the cemetery was known, the locations of the individual burials were not. A rough sketch of 13 known burials drawn up in 1981 at the time of donation of the tombstones to the Ontario Pioneer Community Foundation proved to be of little value in locating burial plots.

The excavation of the cemetery was conducted over approximately three weeks in November 1988, under less than ideal weather conditions. Machine grading of topsoil up to 3 feet in depth revealed two shallow grave shafts. The high gravel content of the cemetery knoll hindered identification of the remaining burials by standard archaeological methods. The locations of remaining burials were detected by shovel shining and by the expected placements next to those grave shafts already detected. Burials were recovered from various depths as a result of irregular topography as well as varying depths of the coffins. In general, burials were oriented west–southwest (head) to east–northeast (feet).

Fifteen individuals ranging in age from newborn to 98 years of age were recovered from 14 graves. Three of the recovered individuals were incomplete: one cranium was removed by machine activity; the right humerus of another individual was missing, presumably due to rodent activity; and a third burial was also disturbed by heavy equipment. Nine out of 14 grave excavations revealed coffin wood (Janusas 1991).

It was possible to transcribe much of the information on the tombstones that had been in the cemetery. Upon completion of analysis of the skeletal remains, individuals were matched with information from the tombstones on sex, age at death, and identification. All but two adults and two juvenile individuals were identified with respect to the information on the tombstones.

Historical Background

The small family cemetery was used between 1825 and 1894 by settlers to Upper Canada, which originally comprised the southern part of the present-day province of Ontario, along the upper reaches of the St. Lawrence River and the north shores of Lakes Erie and Ontario. The settlers were originally from Scotland and lived from 1810 to 1817 in New York State. Tempted by the offer of good land, they moved to Upper Canada, where they bought and cleared land for farming. Most of what is known about this particular family comes from letters and census records, including marriage lists, wills, and newspaper obituaries. In the 1830s there were several epidemics of cholera that began in large population centers such as Montreal and Toronto and spread to the surrounding rural areas. One such epidemic reached the village of Galt, not far from the Harvie property, in 1834 and killed almost one-fifth of the population (Saunders 1991). The date of death is unknown for several of the individuals buried in the cemetery, so it is possible that some died of cholera.

We focus on a mother, SC, whose gravestone notes "died Sept. 12, 1848 aged 25 years, 9 months and 4 days," and her daughter, JC, "who died Sept. 1st, 1848, aged 1 year, 10 months and 8 days." RC, the husband of SC and father of JC, died in the previous year (1847). Genealogical information from a family descendant indicates that SC and her daughter died of a fever. The remains of these individuals were examined for evidence of disease or trauma (Keenleyside and Clark-Wilson 1991), and stable isotope analysis was carried out to determine diet and to look for evidence of breast-feeding (Katzenberg 1991).

Stable isotope analysis was done on the preserved collagen present in the bones. Collagen, a structural protein, records the isotopic signature of carbon and nitrogen in food. Bone is remodeled throughout life, and collagen reflects the diet for a period of several years, depending on the age of the individual. During infancy and childhood, when the bones are growing rapidly and undergoing considerable remodeling, collagen records the diet for several years.

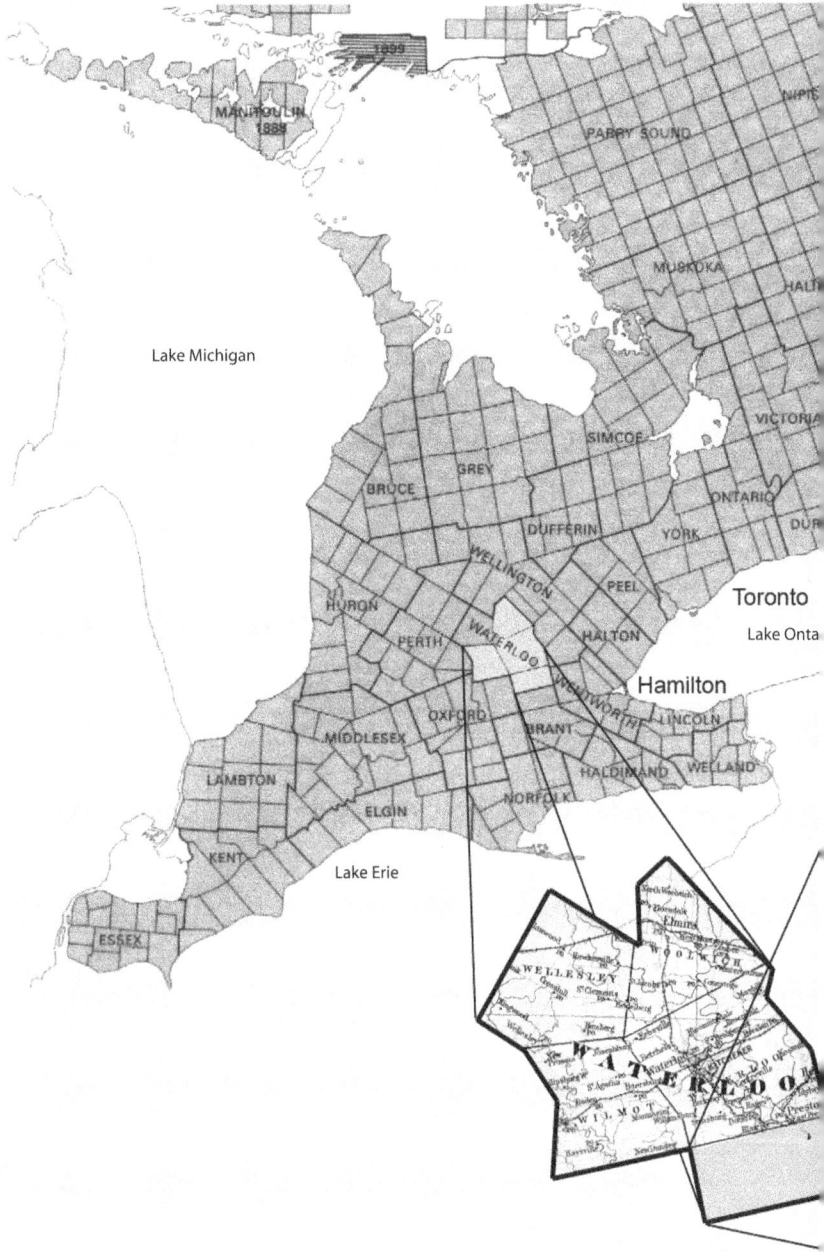

Lake Michigan

MANITOULIN
1888

1899

PARRY SOUND

NIPI

MUSKOKA

HALI

SIMCOE

VICTORIA

GREY

BRUCE

ONTARIO

DUFFERIN

YORK

DUR

WELLINGTON

PEEL

HURON

PERTH

WATERLOO

HALTON

Toronto

Lake Onta

OXFORD

WENTWORTH

Hamilton

MIDDLESEX

BRANT

LINCOLN

LAMBTON

HALDIMAND

WELLAND

ELGIN

NORFOLK

KENT

Lake Erie

ESSEX

North Woolwich
Bamberg
Elmira

WOOLWICH

WELLESLEY
St Clements

WATERLOO

WILMOT

NewDundee

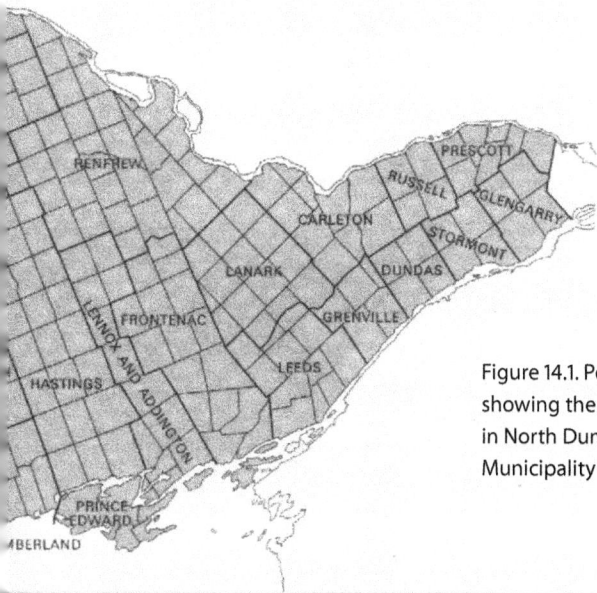

Figure 14.1. Political map of southern Ontario showing the location of the Harvie Cemetery in North Dumfries Township in the Regional Municipality of Waterloo.

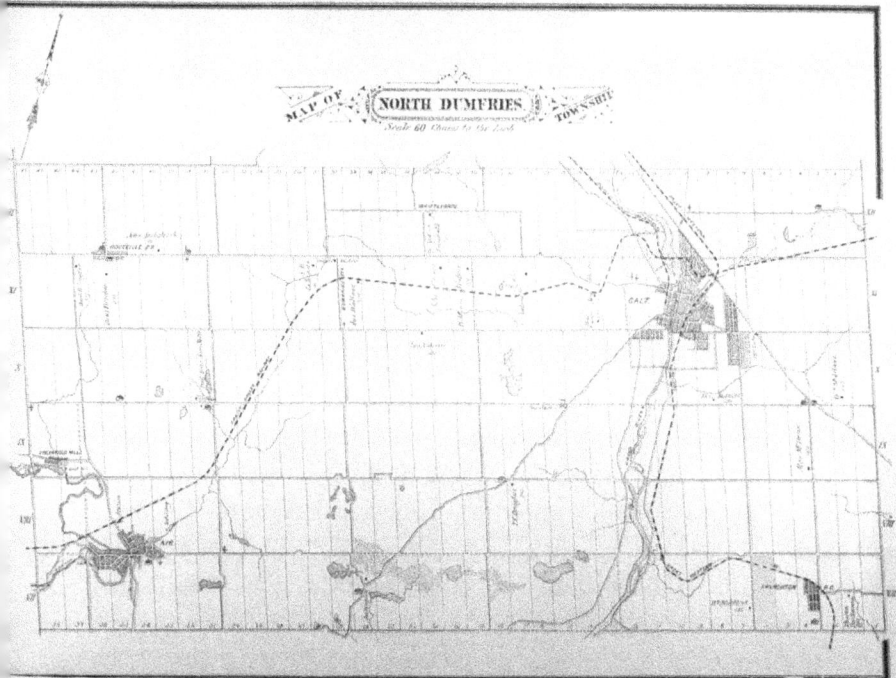

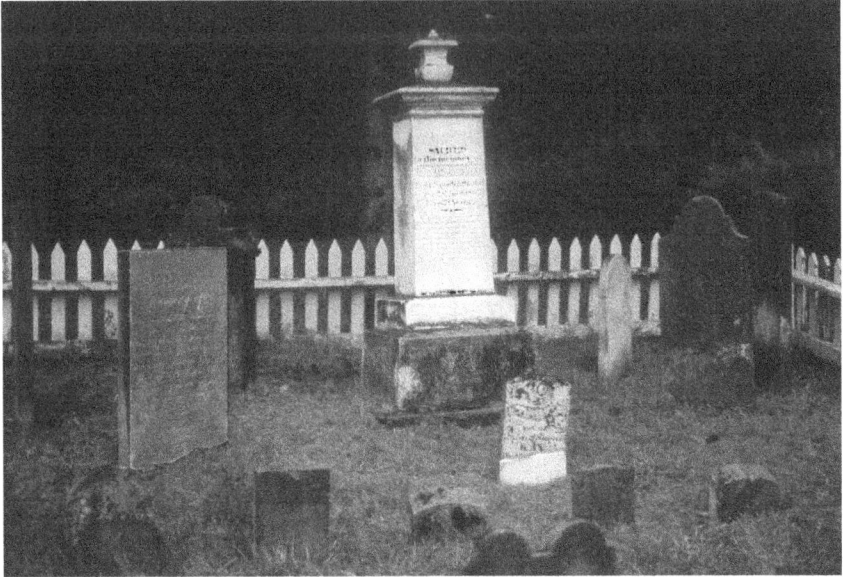

Figure 14.2. Tombstones from the Harvie Cemetery and moved to Doon Heritage Village, Kitchner, Ontario, in 1981. (Photograph originally appeared in Saunders and Lazenby 1991. Reprinted with permission of Copetown Press.)

In adults, where bone has ceased growing in length and where turnover has slowed, collagen records diet for 10 to 15 years (Stenhouse and Baxter 1979).

Stable isotopes of carbon vary depending on the types of plants consumed and on ingestion of marine or terrestrial foods. Specifically, certain grasses such as corn, millet, and sorghum convert atmospheric carbon dioxide to energy by way of a different photosynthetic pathway in comparison to most other plants from temperate regions (trees, shrubs, and other temperate plants). This difference results in a higher ratio of ^{13}C to ^{12}C in maize than in crops such as wheat or barley. Differences in the source carbon between marine and terrestrial environments result in foods from the marine environment having a higher ratio of ^{13}C to ^{12}C than foods from terrestrial environments. (For a more detailed explanation of these principles, see Katzenberg 2008.) Stable isotope ratios are expressed using delta (δ) notation where $\delta^{13}C$ is equal to the ratio of $^{13}C/^{12}C$ in a sample, relative to that same ratio in a standard substance, minus one and multiplied by 1,000. The resulting figure is expressed as $\delta^{13}C$ and for all terrestrial samples is a negative number. Similarly, $\delta^{15}N$ is the ratio of $^{15}N/^{14}N$ in a sample relative to that same ratio in a standard substance, minus one and multiplied by 1,000. Most terrestrial samples have more ^{15}N than the standard and are positive numbers.

Stable isotopes of nitrogen vary depending on the relative importance of meat and plants in the diet. There is a trophic level effect whereby with each step in the food chain, the ratio of ^{15}N to ^{14}N increases. This same principle applies to babies who are consuming mothers' milk (essentially mothers' tissue). Stable nitrogen isotopes have been used to estimate the duration of breast-feeding and the timing of weaning in past populations (Fogel et al. 1989; Katzenberg et al. 1993; Schurr 1998).

Collagen was extracted from a small sample of bone from each individual from the cemetery using the method of Longin (1971). This method removes the mineral component of bone and brings the collagen into solution. The initial isotope analysis, carried out in 1990, was done on a VG Prism II mass spectrometer. More recently, in 2006, the samples were reanalyzed on a Finnegan Mat Delta+XL mass spectrometer in order to have a complete set of data for stable nitrogen isotopes. Previous analyses, requiring a larger sample size, did not provide results for $\delta^{15}N$ for two individuals from the sample, whereas subsequent analyses provide nitrogen isotope data for all individuals.

Nitrogen Isotopes and Weaning

Fogel and colleagues (1989) were the first to demonstrate that the trophic level effect of nursing was revealed with stable nitrogen isotopes. Using hair and fingernails from modern mothers and their nursing infants, Fogel and colleagues showed that while nursing, $\delta^{15}N$ increased in infant protein, then decreased as infants were weaned. Subsequently, a number of other researchers (Katzenberg 1993; Katzenberg and Pfeiffer 1995; Schurr 1998; Mays et al. 2002) found similar patterns in archaeological samples using bone collagen as the source of protein. Problems identified by these researchers include the lag time between diet and collagen deposition and turnover during the rapid growth characteristic of early childhood, and the lack of information on cause of death.

Results from the Present Study

In the present case, we have stable isotope data from the same tissue that would be analyzed in archaeological contexts (bone collagen) as well as known identity, age at death, and an acute cause of death (rapid and therefore unlikely to alter stable isotope ratios due to physiological causes). The data are presented in table 14.1. Focusing on SC, the mother, and JC, the baby aged 1 year, 10 months (figure 14.3), there is a 1.9 percent difference in $\delta^{15}N$. Note that in table 14.1 the father and mother are identical for $\delta^{15}N$. There is more variation in $\delta^{13}C$, with

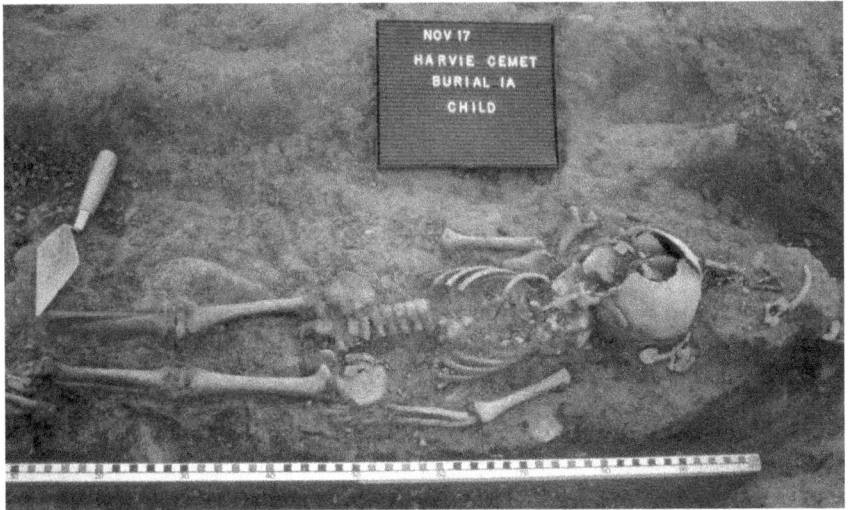

Figure 14.3. In situ photograph from the excavation of the child (JC).

the baby more depleted in the heavier isotope (^{13}C) than either parent, contrary to most studies, which show a small trophic level enrichment for δ^{13}C. For example, Fuller and colleagues (2006) suggest that δ^{13}C decreases sooner than δ^{15}N in infant collagen, and perhaps tracks the introduction of other foods.

Another mother-infant pair from the same cemetery demonstrates the lack of the trophic level effect in δ^{15}N when nursing did not occur. In that case, JH and her newborn, BH, died in childbirth. δ^{15}N for mother and baby are within the range of analytical error while δ^{13}C varies, with the infant more depleted in the heavier isotope.

Table 14.1. Stable isotope data for selected individuals from the Harvie Cemetery

Individual	δ13C%	δ15N%	Age at death	Sex	Cause of death	Date of death
Father (RC)	-18.6	12.0	31 years	M	Unknown	1847
Mother (SC)	-18.3	12.0	25 years	F	Fever	Sept. 12, 1848
Child (JC)	-18.9	13.9	1 year 10 months	F	Fever	Sept. 1, 1848
Mother (JH)	-18.4	11.8	31 years	F	Childbirth	1828
Infant (BH)	-18.9	12.0	Neonate	M		1828

Note: Analytical error is ± 0.1 percent for carbon and ± 0.2 percent for nitrogen.

Evidence for Disease and Injury

Neither the mother, SC, nor the child, JC, shows any skeletal indication of disease or injury. In eastern Canada, there were waves of epidemic diseases that started at major ports where immigrants arrived from Great Britain. There was a series of cholera epidemics in the 1830s, normally beginning in May or June and carrying on through the summer months. Frightened citizens fled the cities, spreading the disease into the surrounding areas. In 1847, the time of large-scale migration from Ireland during the potato famine, there was an epidemic of typhus that reached Quebec, Montreal, and Toronto (Godfrey 1968). Cholera reached Kingston, Ontario, in June 1849. Acute infectious diseases such as cholera rarely leave any marks on bones or teeth, so in the absence of historical information, they would not be detected as potential causes of death. Even with historical information, we are not certain of the specific acute infection that took the lives of SC and JC.

The husband of SC and father of JC (RC) did reveal skeletal evidence of a life of hard work (analysis by Keenleyside and Clark-Wilson 1991). He showed signs of osteoarthritis in several joints (jaw, elbow, hip, and wrist), healed fractures of two bones of the left foot, and a healed skull fracture. He also had evidence of back problems in the form of disk herniation (Schmorl's nodes) and arthritic changes (osteophytes and joint changes). Farming life in rural Ontario was physically demanding. The loss of one's husband would have meant the loss of crops, firewood, income, and security.

Discussion

This mother-infant pair from a historical context provides a window into variables that cannot be known in prehistoric cemeteries. For example, there is evidence from recent demographic studies for a greater risk of death among individuals who have recently lost a spouse (Johnson et al. 2000). Because of the historical information provided from tombstones/coffin plates, we know that RC died the year before SC and JC. The same condition that may only cause illness can be fatal in recently widowed individuals. Such hidden heterogeneity with respect to risk was discussed with reference to skeletal samples in the classic paper by Wood and colleagues (1992). SC undoubtedly had support from family members living next door, and these individuals were relatively wealthy, so we cannot know for certain how significant the loss of the husband and father were to the deaths of SC and JC. The point is that we would not be aware of this factor in a cemetery of unmarked graves lacking entirely in historic information.

Similarly, it is not always possible to link mothers and children in prehistoric cemeteries. Mothers who die during or shortly after childbirth are often buried with their infants, but mothers and older children may not die at the same time, and may not be buried together. Here again, the historical context allows us to know the relationship between SC and JC. So the analysis of stable isotopes of nitrogen tells us that the young child had continued to nurse up to or shortly before the time of death, since the $\delta^{15}N$ of the child's collagen is elevated by 1.9 percent relative to that of the mother.

In terms of the methods that we use to reconstruct life from prehistoric skeletal remains, the study of this mother-infant pair confirms the trophic level effect of nursing on nitrogen isotope ratios. However, the infection that led to the death of the mother and child left no marks on their skeletons. Nor were there any other indictors of sickness or injury that might suggest increased susceptibility to death.

Overall, the analysis of the individuals from this small family cemetery tells us much about life for the early Scottish immigrants to southern Ontario, and, by extension, other European settlers to Upper Canada. We know that JC was breast-fed for at least the first year and several months of her short life, and we suspect that for SC, the stress resulting from the loss of her husband in the previous year, followed by the loss of her young daughter, exacerbated her illness and led to her death. This was despite the presumed support of neighboring family members.

Life for early immigrants to Upper Canada was challenging. For this mother and her child, subsequent exposure to "fever" was fatal to both of them. In this small sample of 15 burials, five individuals died between birth and two years of age with another dying at six years of age. On the other hand, some of those who immigrated to Canada enjoyed considerable longevity. One woman lived to 98 years, while three men lived to the age of 71. The death of a mother and her child, within days of each other, provides a window into the lives of ordinary people during the early history of Upper Canada. At the same time, it provides an opportunity to view a useful indicator of infant care in the past, nitrogen isotopes, in bone collagen from individuals of known identity, age, and cause of death. Along with another mother-infant pair from the same cemetery, the contrast in $\delta^{15}N$ between an infant who nursed and one who did not is striking and informative.

Acknowledgments

The authors gratefully acknowledge the individuals who worked on the excavation and analysis of this cemetery. Stable isotope analyses were carried out in the Isotope Science Laboratory, University of Calgary, and run by Steve Taylor. We thank Ann L. W. Stodder and Ann M. Palkovich for their invitation to participate in the American Association of Physical Anthropologists session on the bioarchaeology of individuals and the subsequent edited volume. We also thank George Milner, discussant for the session, for his insightful comments regarding hidden risks for morbidity and mortality.

References Cited

Fogel, Marilyn, Noreen Tuross, and Douglas W. Owsley
1989   Nitrogen Isotope Tracers of Human Lactation in Modern and Archaeological Populations. In *Annual Report of the Director, Geophysical Laboratory, Carnegie Institution, 1988–1989*, pp. 111–17. Carnegie Institution, Washington, D.C.
Fuller, B. T., J. L. Fuller, D. A. Harris, and R. E. M. Hedges
2006   Detection of Breastfeeding and Weaning in Modern Human Infants with Carbon and Nitrogen Stable Isotope Ratios. *American Journal of Physical Anthropology* 129: 279–93.
Godfrey, C. M.
1968   *The Cholera Epidemics in Upper Canada 1822–1886*. Seccombe House, Toronto.
Janusas, Scarlett E.
1991   Background to the Excavations. In *The Links That Bind: The Harvie Family Nineteenth Century Burying Ground*, edited by Shelley R. Saunders and Richard Lazenby, pp. 5–9. Occasional Papers in Northeastern Archaeology No. 5. Copetown Press, Dundas, Ont.
Johnson, Norman J., Eric Backlund, Paul D. Sorlie, and Catherine A. Loveless
2000   Marital Status and Mortality: The National Longitudinal Mortality Study. *Annals of Epidemiology* 10(4): 224–38.
Katzenberg, M. Anne
1991   Stable Isotope Analysis of Remains from the Harvie Family. In *The Links That Bind: The Harvie Family Nineteenth Century Burying Ground*, edited by Shelley R. Saunders and Richard Lazenby, pp. 65–69. Occasional Papers in Northeastern Archaeology No. 5. Copetown Press, Dundas, Ont.
1993   Age Differences and Population Variation in Stable Isotope Values from Ontario, Canada. In *Prehistoric Human Bone: Archaeology at the Molecular Level*, edited by Joseph B. Lambert and Gisela Grupe, pp. 39–62. Springer-Verlag, Berlin.
2008   Stable Isotope Analysis: A Tool for Studying Past Diet, Demography and Life History. In *Biological Anthropology of the Human Skeleton*, 2nd ed., edited by M. Anne Katzenberg and Shelley R. Saunders, pp. 413–41. John Wiley & Sons, New York.

Katzenberg, M. Anne, and Susan Pfeiffer

1995   Nitrogen Isotope Evidence for Weaning Age in a Nineteenth Century Canadian Skeletal Sample. In *Bodies of Evidence*, edited by Anne L. Grauer, pp. 221–35. John Wiley & Sons, New York.

Katzenberg, M. Anne, Shelley R. Saunders, and William R. Fitzgerald

1993   Age Differences in Stable Carbon and Nitrogen Isotope Ratios in a Population of Prehistoric Horticulturalists. *American Journal of Physical Anthropology* 90: 267–81.

Keenleyside, Anne, and Elizabeth Clark-Wilson

1991   Skeletal Pathology. In *The Links That Bind: The Harvie Family Nineteenth Century Burying Ground*, edited by Shelley R. Saunders and Richard Lazenby, pp. 29–40. Occasional Papers in Northeastern Archaeology No. 5. Copetown Press, Dundas, Ont.

Longin, R.

1971   New Method of Collagen Extraction for Radiocarbon Dating. *Nature* 230: 241–42.

Mays, S. A., M. P. Richards, and B. T. Fuller

2002   Bone Stable Isotope Evidence for Infant Feeding in Mediaeval England. *Antiquity* 76: 654–56.

Saunders, Shelley R.

1991   Historical Background. In *The Links That Bind: The Harvie Family Nineteenth Century Burying Ground*, edited by Shelley R. Saunders and Richard Lazenby, pp. 11–20. Occasional Papers in Northeastern Archaeology No. 5. Copetown Press, Dundas, Ont.

Saunders, Shelley R., and Richard Lazenby (editors)

1991   *The Links That Bind: The Harvie Family Nineteenth Century Burying Ground*. Occasional Papers in Northeastern Archaeology No. 5. Copetown Press, Dundas, Ont.

Schurr, Mark R.

1998   Using Stable Nitrogen-Isotopes to Study Weaning Behaviour in Past Populations. *World Archaeology* 30(2): 327–42.

Stenhouse, M. J., and M. S. Baxter

1979   The Uptake of Bomb 14C in Humans. In *Radiocarbon Dating*, edited by R. Berger and H. E. Suess, pp. 324–41. University of California Press, Berkeley.

Wood, James W., George R. Milner, Henry C. Harpending, and Kenneth M. Weiss

1992   The Osteological Paradox: Problems of Inferring Prehistoric Health from Skeletal Samples. *Current Anthropology* 33(4): 343–70.

15 ◈ Thumbprints of a Midwife

BIRTH AND INFANT DEATH IN AN
ANCIENT PUEBLO COMMUNITY

Charles F. Merbs

Individual Profile

Site: Nuvakwewtaqa, Chavez Pass (35°47′N, 111°8′W)
Location: Coconino National Forest, 40 miles southeast of Flagstaff, Arizona
Cultural Affiliation: Sinagua (Clear Creek phase)
Date: Ca. A.D. 1350, based on radiocarbon and tree-ring dating
Feature: Pueblo 1, Feature 5
Location of Grave: In the floor of a room in the pueblo
Burial and Grave Type: A single primary inhumation, extended on back, in a shallow pit filled with trash-laden fill dirt
Associated Materials: None
Preservation and Completeness: Excellent preservation, several skeletal elements fractured postmortem, some bones not recovered
Age at Death and Basis of Estimate: 3–6 weeks, based on general development of the skeleton
Sex and Basis of Determination: Unknown
Conditions Observed: Partially healed rib fractures attributed to birth trauma
Specialized Analysis: Radiography
Excavated: 1981, Chavez Pass Project, directed by Fred Plog and Charles F. Merbs, Arizona State University
Archaeological Report: Brown 1990
Current Disposition: Curated at Arizona State University

This study explores the hazards of childbirth and infancy in a prehistoric Puebloan settlement. The focus of the study is a skeleton found buried in the floor of a room in Pueblo I at the site of Nuvakwewtaqa at Chavez Pass in north-central Arizona. An unusual feature of this skeleton is a series of partially healed rib fractures on the dorsal side of the thorax. The likely cause of these fractures is child abuse or birth trauma.

The Site

Nuvakwewtaqa is located at Chavez Pass in the Coconino National Forest in north-central Arizona, approximately 65 km (40 miles) southeast of Flagstaff (figure 15.1). The pass forms a natural corridor between the Little Colorado River basin to the north and higher, heavily forested plateaus to the south. An ancient aboriginal trail and trade route followed this natural access route (Fewkes 1904: 121), but presently the area is rather remote, accessible only by unpaved Forest Service roads. Nuvakwewtaqa, located on the west side of the pass, is the largest of numerous sites clustered in proximity to the pass. It consists of three major ruin complexes: Pueblos 1 and 2, located together on a south ridge (figure 15.2), and Pueblo 3, on a separated north ridge. Nuvakwewtaqa is in an

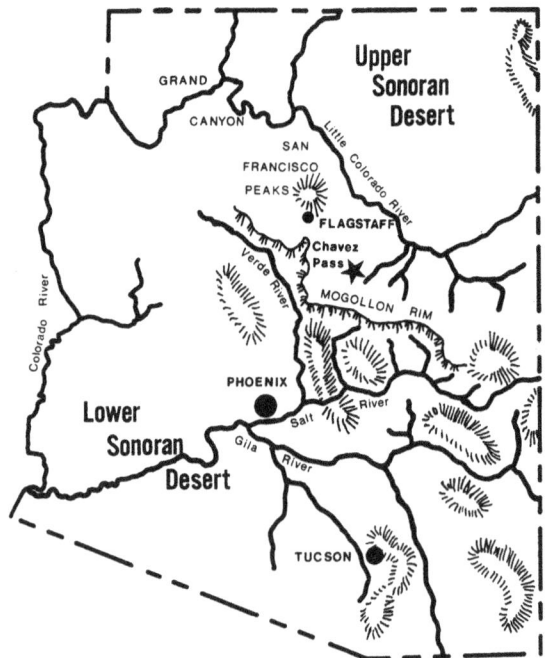

Figure 15.1. Location of Nuvakwewtaqa.

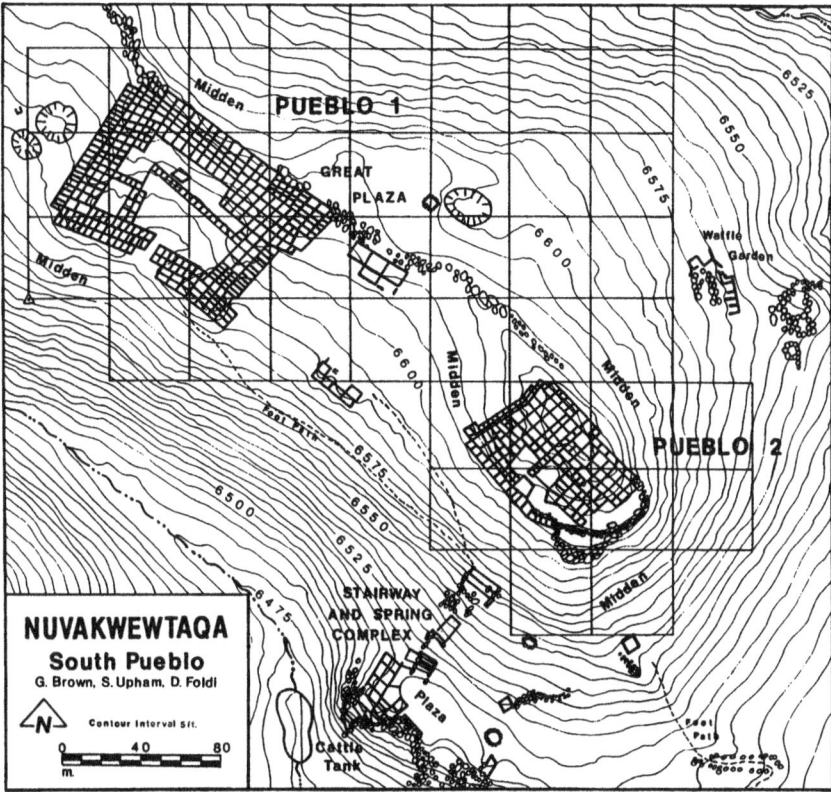

Figure 15.2. Map of South Pueblo, Nuvakwewtaqa.

overlap area of several cultural traditions (Anasazi, Mogollon, and Sinagua), but it fits most comfortably in the Sinagua tradition and is affiliated with the Clear Creek phase of Sinagua, A.D. 1300–1450) (Brown 1990).

The Burial

The heaviest concentration of burials at the site was in the extensive midden areas to the north of Pueblos 1 and 2, but several were found in the central plaza area and in the floors of rooms. The room containing the infant skeleton being considered here was located in the northeast corner of Pueblo 1. Although ^{14}C dates are available for three different levels of the room, the dates are confusing, and two appear unreliable (Coinman 1990). One, a charcoal scattering, produced a date of A.D. 790±65 and likely represents wood that was already very old before it was collected and burned. Another charcoal scatter, this one actually located below the first, produced a modern date, and is attributed to some kind of contamination. The third date, A.D. 1356±107, was obtained from carbonized maize found in close proximity to the burial and appears reliable. The bones themselves were not dated. A piece of ponderosa pine, likely used at one time as a roof support for the burial room, produced a tree-ring date of A.D. 1325. Since the tree-ring date came from below the infant burial and the carbonized maize date from slightly above the burial, we can date this interment to approximately A.D. 1350.

The burial room had been abandoned at some point and filled with debris-laden soil, so only the tops of the stone walls were exposed at the time of excavation. Approximately 3 m below the modern surface a plastered living floor was encountered. A small pit dug into this floor (figure 15.3) contained the skeleton of an infant, a few weeks beyond newborn in age, lying on its back in extended position. No identifiable grave goods were included with the body. The skeleton was carefully removed from the pit, but little attention was paid to it at the time because another living surface was quickly encountered beneath the initial floor layer. This lower surface, found to be the original floor of the room, had two graves dug into it. The one encountered first, located directly below the infant burial, contained three skeletons and three ceramic pots. Only one skeleton, about a year in age, appeared undisturbed, extended on its back, and the three

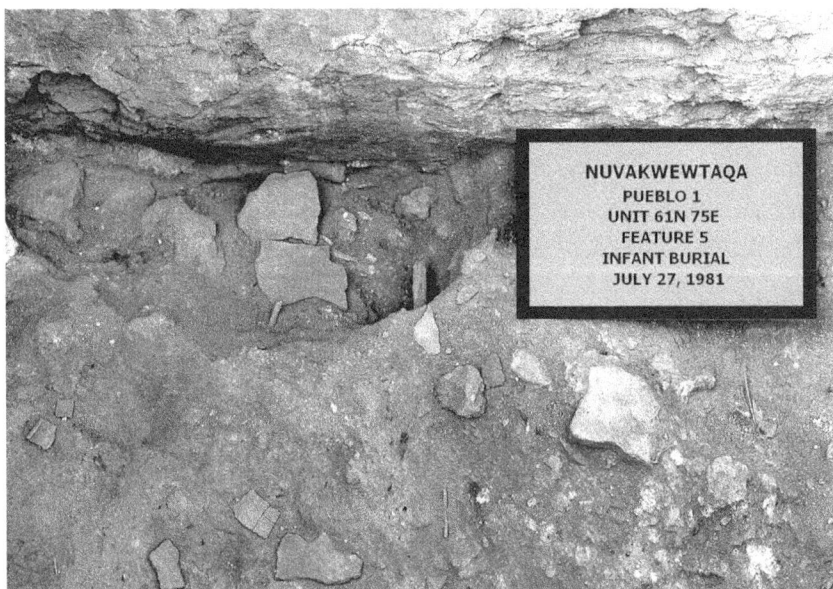

Figure 15.3. Subfloor burial pit in room corner.

pots were aligned in a row parallel with the left side of this skeleton. Beneath this skeleton were the scattered bones of two other, much younger infants. This grave appears to represent a sequence of three separate burials. The first infant was buried, then, after some interval, the grave was opened to receive the body of a second infant, with the bones of the first infant being disturbed in the process. This second infant showed evidence of severe pathology, which resulted in its bones being very light and deformed. After another interval, the process was repeated when a third infant was added. This third burial disturbed the bones of the second infant.

The other grave dug into the original floor contained the skeleton of a middle-age adult woman fully extended on her back. Four ceramic pots and an unusual polychrome lacquered basket were buried with her. The pelvis of this woman displays extremely well marked parturition scars, which suggest difficult birth. The scars are deep and run nearly the entire vertical length of the pubic elements. The center areas of both auricular surfaces of the pelvis are unusually rough, another condition that may be related to difficult birth.

The Infant Skeleton

The infant skeleton was relatively complete, but with some parts broken, probably long after death. Several missing parts, all very small in size, had probably been removed by rodents, likely when the living floor and grave were much closer to the surface. Of special interest is the thorax of this individual, particularly the ribs. Recovered complete ribs from the left side included numbers 1, 4, 5, 7, 8, and 11, and an extra rib (13). Partial left ribs included 2, 3, 6, 10, and 12. Recovered complete ribs from the right side included 1–3 and 5–12. A partial right rib 4 was also recovered.

The ribs bear evidence of five fractures. Healing complete fractures extending straight across the shaft were observed in ribs 6–8 on the left side and rib 7 on the right side (figure 15.4). (The rib shaft anterior to the fracture of the sixth rib was not recovered.) In each case the fracture site displays considerable bony callus, but the fracture line is clearly visible on a radiograph (figure 15.5). The fifth fracture also involves the right seventh rib, the fracture occurring near the rib's articulation with the body of the vertebra. A small portion of the vertebral end of the rib was fractured and not recovered. The presence of cortex on the surface suggests a fracture that underwent some healing but failed to unite. The same degree of healing suggests that all five fractures occurred during the same traumatic event.

Pueblo Infant Mortality

The ancestral Puebloans who lived in the American Southwest prior to European contact were sedentary agriculturalists who augmented their diet with hunted and gathered resources. They appear to have suffered a high rate of infant mortality. This can be seen at Arroyo Hondo, an ancestral Puebloan site near Santa Fe, New Mexico. Excavated from 1970 through 1974 by the School of American Research, Arroyo Hondo was occupied between A.D. 1300 and 1425, having its largest population during its first three decades of existence

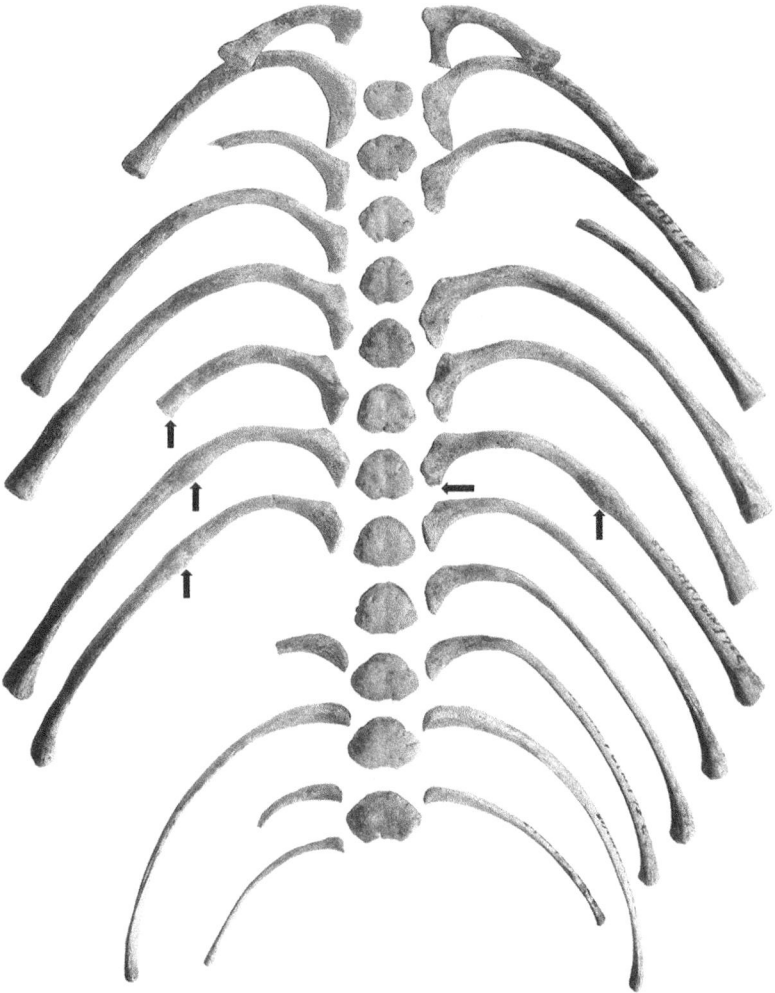

Figure 15.4. Ribs showing fracture locations.

(Palkovich 1980; and see Chapter 16 this volume). This makes it roughly contemporary with Nuvakwewtaqa. Nearly 27 percent of the 100-plus skeletons recovered at Arroyo Hondo were infants less than one year of age, and another 18 percent were between one and ten years of age.

Another example of high infant mortality is Grasshopper Ruin, a Mogollon pueblo site in east-central Arizona. Grasshopper was occupied from approximately A.D. 1275 to 1400, experiencing its maximum population between A.D. 1300 and 1350. Again, this makes it roughly contemporary with Nuvakwewtaqa. Of over 600 skeletons recovered from pueblo rooms and cemetery

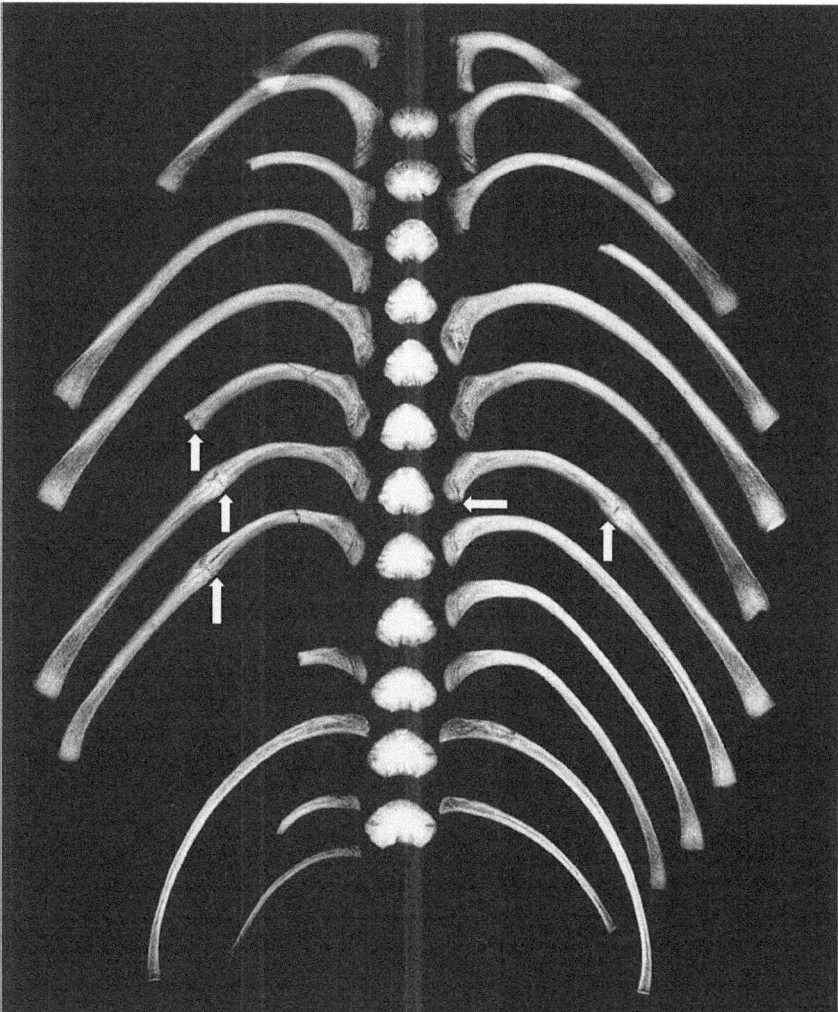

Figure 15.5. Radiograph of ribs showing fracture locations.

areas, approximately one-quarter were less than two years of age, and more than half were less than five years of age. It was only after age eight that the death rate dropped, and it did so dramatically, with those who survived living relatively long lives (Clark 1969; Hinkes 1983).

Arizona State University carried out excavations at Nuvakwewtaqa for five seasons, from 1978 to 1982 (Brown 1990). Efforts were concentrated on the main burial locations, the midden areas of the pueblos, which had been heavily plundered for over a century. These excavations produced a large number of individuals of all ages beyond infancy, but no infants. The only infant skeletons recovered at the site came from rooms, only a few of which were excavated as part of the general testing of the site. It seems likely that Nuvakwewtaqa follows the burial pattern observed in other prehistoric communities in the region, a pattern in which very young individuals were buried in the floors of rooms while most older individuals were buried in extramural midden areas.

Rib Fractures in Infants

In clinical practice today, rib fractures in older children and adults are usually associated with trauma, such as falls and motor vehicle accidents. They are not commonly seen in infants because the plasticity of the infant rib cage allows the skeletal structures to deform rather than break. It is only after a high threshold is met that fracturing occurs in infants (Lonergan et al. 2003; Oppenheim et al. 1990; Thomas 1977).

When identified in infants, rib fractures are usually attributed to one of three causes: child abuse, accident trauma, or birth trauma. With improved childbirth practices in modern times, fractures of the first rib are considered virtually diagnostic of child abuse because of the considerable force required to produce them (Strouse and Owings 1995). In a study carried out in Cincinnati and Winnipeg hospitals from 1994 through 1997, 32 of 39 cases of fractured ribs (usually located posterior or laterally on the thorax) identified in infants less than 12 months of age were attributed to child abuse (Bulloch et al. 2000). Three cases were associated with accidental trauma: a motor vehicle collision, a forceful direct blow, and a fall from a height. In three other cases the fractures were secondary to bone fragility resulting from osteogenesis imperfecta in one case, rickets in another, and fragile bones due to prematurity (born at 23 weeks gestation) in the third (Bulloch et al. 2000).

Only one of the 39 cases of fractured ribs in this study was attributed to trauma associated with birth. This was an infant of 40 weeks gestation born by vacuum pump extraction. The birth was complicated because the right side of the infant's chest and right shoulder were flexed up under the pubic symphysis of the mother's pelvis. The newborn infant suffered from respiratory problems and was immediately admitted to an intermediate care nursery. It was only on the fourth day after birth that fractures of the posterior arcs of the fourth, fifth, and sixth right ribs, plus a fractured right clavicle, were identified. The infant survived, probably thanks to the immediate hospital care it received (Bulloch et al. 2000), but this case also illustrates that significant trauma during childbirth can result in rib fractures that are not immediately detected.

Reports of rib fractures at childbirth are rare in the modern clinical literature (Rizzolo and Coleman 1989; Hartmann 1997), and when they do occur they are usually associated with large babies or difficult deliveries (Lonergan et al. 2003). Infant rib fractures may be caused by direct trauma of sufficient force to the thorax, with the fracture occurring at the site of impact (Bulloch et al. 2000). They may also occur when anterior-posterior compression is applied to the thorax. If the pressure is sufficient, the stress over the anterior cortex of the posterior part of the rib, where the rib tubercle articulates with the transverse process, may produce a fracture (Kleinman and Schlesinger 1997). This anterior-posterior compression also stresses the lateral aspects of the ribs that can result in lateral rib fractures (Kleinman and Schlesinger 1997). Because the forces are distributed in an area similar to the size of the fingers or hands of the person applying the pressure, fractures are typically seen in similar locations in multiple adjacent ribs and are often bilateral (Lonergan et al. 2003).

The healing of rib fractures in infants takes place in three stages. In three to seven days, the fracture site is characterized by inflammation, soft tissue swelling, and pain. Soft callus formation may be observed from seven to ten days. This is followed by bony callus formation, which may be completed in infants in three to six weeks. The last stage is that of remodeling, which may take from three months to one year (O'Connor and Cohen 1987). Fractures involving the lateral or anterior parts of the thorax tended to impact along the inner cortex of the rib rather than the entire shaft. The rib fractures in abused infants observed by Kleinman and colleagues (1996) ranged from unhealed through various stages of healing. Evidence of healing enhanced the ability to detect a fracture.

It is important to note that all of the clinical data referred to here deal with a birth situation very different from that faced by the Sinagua people of Nuvakwewtaqa. In modern cases, anticipation of a difficult birth usually results in a decision to perform a caesarean, an option not thought to be available to the ancient Puebloan people of the Southwest. Although there are still some questions as to how frequently rib fracturing occurs during birth today, the more important question is how frequently might it occur if caesarean were not an option. It would likely be a much more common event.

Of the two usual causes of rib fracturing in infants, child abuse and birth trauma, the first seems highly unlikely for the Nuvakwewtaqa infant. It does not fit with what we know ethnographically of Puebloan people today regarding their behavior toward infants. Also, the pattern of fracturing does not match a pattern of child abuse. The pressure on the thorax of the Nuvakwewtaqa infant appears to have been applied to the back of the chest, not the front as is usually the case in child abuse. The bilateral chest trauma of the Nuvakwewtaqa infant appears to have resulted from anterior-posterior compression, not from pressure applied from one direction and from the back or side as is usually the case in child abuse. In addition, all the fractures in the child appear to date from the same event rather than multiple events as might be the case in child abuse.

The Death of an Infant at Nuvakwewtaqa

What happened around A.D. 1350 in a room located near the northeast corner of Pueblo I at Nuvakwewtaqa that produced three graves containing five skeletons? In particular, what is the story behind the most recent of the burials, the one containing an infant who died several weeks after birth? The following is a plausible explanation that fits the available data.

The family living in this room experienced the death of a very young infant. In keeping with Puebloan beliefs (Parsons 1939; White 1942; Eggan 1950; Ellis 1968), there was assurance that although the body was dead, the infant's soul would continue to enter the body of another infant born in this room. To facilitate the transference of the soul to the newborn, the dead body in which it resided was buried in the floor of the room, in close proximity to where the new child would be born.

Another child was indeed born in this room, and the soul of the previous child established residence in this new body. Sadly, in time, this second child also died in early infancy, and the process was repeated. The grave in the floor of the room was reopened to receive the body of the second child, with the remains of the first child moved aside to make room for the new body. The soul waited in this grave until yet another infant was born, entering the body of the new infant at birth. Again this was accomplished smoothly, thanks to the proximity of the soul and the birth in the room.

Infant mortality among these people was common, however, so it probably came as no great surprise that the same sad event was to repeat itself yet again. The third child lived longer than the first two, more than a year, but the grave in the floor of the room had to be opened once again. The skeletal remains of the second child were now moved aside, and the third body was interred. The grave also contained three clay pots. Whether one was added at each burial event or all three date from the third event is unknown.

The next chapter in this story appears to have been the death of the mother. She was also interred in the floor of the room, next to her children. Why she was buried here and not in the regular adult burying area outside the pueblo is unknown. It may be that it was because she died giving birth to the infant with the broken ribs. Her grave, like the pit of the earlier infant deaths, was dug into the first floor surface. Debris-laden soil was added to the room to create a new floor above the one into which the two graves had been dug, allowing the room to continue being used. Several weeks later the infant injured in birth also died, and its tiny grave was dug into the new floor, just above where its three siblings lay buried. This infant appears to show evidence in the form of rib fractures of a very traumatic birth. Perhaps the infant was in breach position or some other complication presented itself, or perhaps the mother was assisted by an inexperienced midwife. Regardless of the cause, it appears as though the midwife was forced to exert considerable force on the thorax of the infant during birth, the fractures corresponding to where she would have placed her thumbs.

The death of infants was a sad fact of life during the fourteenth century in the Sinagua region of Arizona. Did a difficult birth result in the death of the mother, thus accounting for the grave of the adult woman in the floor of the room? What is clear is that the infant survived for some weeks after the birth trauma. Four of the fractures had been united by bony callus when the infant died, and the fifth showed healing with non-union. The fractures were probably caused by the thumbs of the midwife as she tried to force the infant through the birth canal. Partial healing of the fractures indicates that the infant survived birth but died several weeks later. Was the death of the infant within weeks of its birth related to its traumatic birth, causing lung damage or other complications? The bones are silent on this subject.

At the very least, the infant skeleton does speak eloquently to the difficulties of birth and infant survival in this ancient community. It certainly highlights the hazards facing the newborn, but it also speaks to the hazards facing women in childbirth. As difficult as birth is today, it was far more difficult in the past.

Acknowledgments

I want to thank Ursula Iwaniec, who analyzed Nuvakwewtaqa skeletal material for her master's thesis and first brought the rib pathology in the infant to my attention; my wife, Barbara, who first suggested that it might represent birth trauma; and to several midwives in the Phoenix area, who were willing to add their expertise to the case, indicating that, based on their experience, the scenario presented here was credible.

References Cited

Brown, Gary M.
1990   Nuvakwewtaqa and the Chavez Pass Region: An Overview. In *Technological Change in the Chavez Pass Region, North-Central Arizona*, edited by Gary M. Brown, pp. 5–19. Arizona State University Anthropological Research Papers No. 41. Arizona State University Press, Tempe.

Bulloch, Blake, Charles J. Schubert, Patrick D. Brophy, Neil Johnson, Martin H. Reed, and Robert A. Shapiro
2000   Cause and Clinical Characteristics of Rib Fractures in Infants. *Pediatrics* 105(4): e48.

Clark, Geoffrey A.
1969   A Preliminary Analysis of Burial Clusters in the Grasshopper Site, East Central Arizona. *Kiva* 35: 57–86.

Coinman, Nancy R.
1990   Ceramics from the North Pueblo at Nuvakwewtaqa. In *Technological Change in the Chavez Pass Region, North-Central Arizona*, edited by Gary M. Brown, pp. 21–72. Arizona State University Anthropological Research Papers No. 41. Arizona State University Press, Tempe.

Eggan, Fred
1950   *Social Organization of the Western Pueblos.* University of Chicago Press, Chicago.

Ellis, Florence Hawley
1968   An Interpretation of Prehistoric Death Customs in Terms of Modern Southwestern Parallels. In *Collected Papers in Honor of Lyndon Lane Hargrave*, edited by A. H. Schroeder, pp. 57–76. Papers of the Anthropological Society of New Mexico No. 1. Anthropological Society of New Mexico, Santa Fe.

Fewkes, Jesse W.
1904   Two Summers' Work in Pueblo Ruins. Twenty-second Report of the Bureau of American Ethnology, part 1, pp. 3–195. U.S. Government Printing Office, Washington, D.C.

Hartmann, R. W., Jr.
1997   Radiological Case of the Month: Rib Fractures Produced by Birth Trauma. *Archives of Pediatrics and Adolescent Medicine* 151: 947–48.

Hinkes, Madeleine J.
1983   Skeletal Evidence of Stress in Subadults: Trying to Come of Age at Grasshopper Pueblo. Ph.D. dissertation, Department of Anthropology, University of Arizona, Tucson.

Kleinman, Paul K., and Alan E. Schlesinger
1997   Mechanical Factors Associated with Posterior Rib Fractures: Laboratory and Case Studies. *Pediatric Radiology* 27(1): 87–91.

Kleinman, Paul K., Sandy C. Marks Jr., Katherine Nimkin, Shawn M. Rayder, and Stanton C. Kessler

1996   Rib Fractures in 31 Abused Infants: Postmortem Radiologic-Histopathologic Study. *Radiology* 200: 807–10.

Lonergan, Gael J., Andrew M. Baker, Mitchel K. Morey, and Steven C. Boos

2003   Child Abuse: Radiologic-Pathologic Correlation. *Radiographics* 23: 811–45.

O'Connor, John F., and Jonathan Cohen

1987   Dating Fractures. In *Diagnostic Imaging in Child Abuse*, edited by Paul K. Kleinman, pp. 101–13. William and Wilkins, Baltimore.

Oppenheim, William L., Alexander Davis, William A. Growdon, Frederick J. Dorey, and Lance B. Davlin

1990   Clavicle Fractures in the Newborn. *Clinical Orthopaedics and Related Research* 250: 176–80.

Palkovich, Ann M.

1980   *Pueblo Population and Society: The Arroyo Hondo Skeletal and Mortuary Remains.* Arroyo Hondo Archaeological Series, Vol. 3. School of American Research Press, Santa Fe, N.Mex.

Parsons, Elsie Clews

1939   *Pueblo Indian Religion.* University of Chicago Press, Chicago.

Rizzolo, Peter J., and Peter R. Coleman

1989   Neonatal Rib Fracture: Birth Trauma or Child Abuse? *Journal of Family Practice* 29(5): 561–63.

Strouse, Peter J., and Clyde L. Owings

1995   Fractures of the First Rib in Child Abuse. *Radiology* 197: 763–65.

Thomas, Paul S.

1977   Rib Fractures in Infancy. *Annals of Radiology* 20: 115–22.

White, Leslie A.

1942   *The Pueblo of Santa Ana, New Mexico.* American Anthropological Association Memoir No. 60. American Anthropological Association, Menasha, Wis.

16 ◈ Reading a Life

A FOURTEENTH-CENTURY ANCESTRAL
PUEBLOAN WOMAN

Ann M. Palkovich

Individual Profile

Site: Arroyo Hondo (LA 12)
Location: 4.5 miles south of Santa Fe, New Mexico
Cultural Affiliation: Ancestral Puebloan, Pueblo IV, Late Prehistoric
Date: A.D. 1310–1330, based on tree-ring dating of Plaza area
Feature: 12-G-2-3-35
Location of Grave: Southeast corner, Plaza G, Component I occupation
Burial and Grave Type: Single primary inhumation, semiflexed on left side, head to west; oval straight-walled pit dug into uppermost plaza surface, filled with trash-laden dirt, and sealed with adobe plaster at plaza surface
Associated Materials: Woven yucca mat covering body
Preservation and Completeness: Fair preservation, some skeletal elements highly fragmentary and incomplete; cranium highly fragmentary, long bones partly reconstructed
Age at Death and Basis of Estimate: 35–40 years, based on auricular surface and dental wear
Sex and Basis of Determination: Female, based on pelvic morphology and femoral head diameters
Conditions Observed: Severe bowing of humeri, radii, ulnas, femurs, tibias, and fibulas attributed to rickets
Specialized Analysis: None
Excavated: June 1974, Arroyo Hondo Archaeological Project directed by Douglas W. Schwartz, School of American Research, Santa Fe, New Mexico
Archaeological Report: Palkovich 1980
Current Disposition: Reburied in March 2006; no photographs of remains are included here in accord with the wishes of the descendant population

This study focuses on an adult female who lived at the fourteenth-century Puebloan village of Arroyo Hondo, New Mexico (figure 16.1). Sedentary dry farming as a way of life dates to A.D. 700. in the Galisteo Basin of northern New Mexico. Population in this basin increased notably during the mid-1200s, leading to large farm settlements in the Galisteo by 1300, of which Arroyo Hondo is a part. These communities were formed when smaller groups—perhaps extended families—moved from isolated hamlets to build complex, extended multistoried roomblocks arranged to form distinct plazas (figure 16.2). Subsistence diets of corn, beans, and squash were supplemented by domesticated turkeys and various wild game, including deer, rabbits, and rodents. Like most ancestral Pueblo settlements, Arroyo Hondo was occupied for only a few generations as farming populations built and then abandoned settlements in response to unpredictable rainfall in marginal environments (Wetterstrom 1986; Stuart 2000; Plog 2008; Cordell 2009).

Arroyo Hondo village life appears to have been unusually harsh, even when compared to other ancestral Pueblos. Severe, chronic health problems suffered by these villagers are indicated by the high incidence of skeletal pathologies and low life expectancy (Palkovich 1980; Martin 1994; Nelson et al. 1994; Stodder 2007). Ubiquitous porotic lesions associated with nutritional inadequacies and infections and the accompanying impact poor health had on fertility and mortality are well documented throughout prehistoric southwestern populations. However, the significance of varying dietary and health problems from village to village is less well understood. Settlement patterns clearly suggest that groups continually moved, reorganized, and resettled in response to environmental limitations such as local carrying capacity and shifting annual rainfall. The aggregation into larger villages such as Arroyo Hondo certainly impacted farming and food-gathering strategies. Families once accustomed to living in small hamlets now cooped with village neighbors making a living from the same limited resources likely created new, complex sociopolitical issues (Swedlund 1994). Villagers may have also been subject to the emergence of new health and hygiene problems, the result of denser concentrations of people.

A Woman of Plaza G

Among the villagers buried at Arroyo Hondo is this Plaza G woman (12-G-2-3-35). Her life history was shaped by the larger social and environmental dynamics of fourteenth-century Puebloan village life in New Mexico. This woman's life experiences provide us with a window on the intimate links between ancestral Puebloan health and social life.

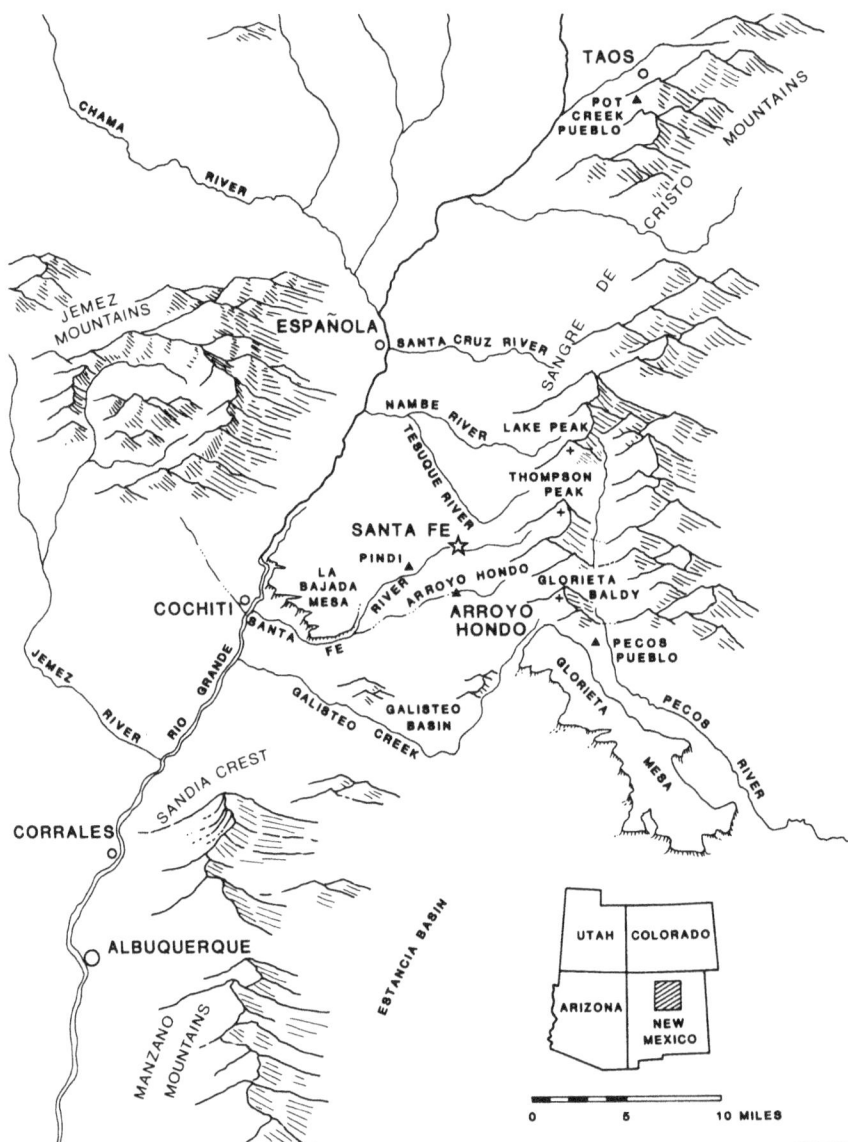

Figure 16.1. Location of Arroyo Hondo Pueblo. (Reprinted by permission from *Food, Diet and Population at Prehistoric Arroyo Hondo Pueblo, New Mexico*, ©1986 by the School of Advanced Research, Santa Fe, New Mexico.)

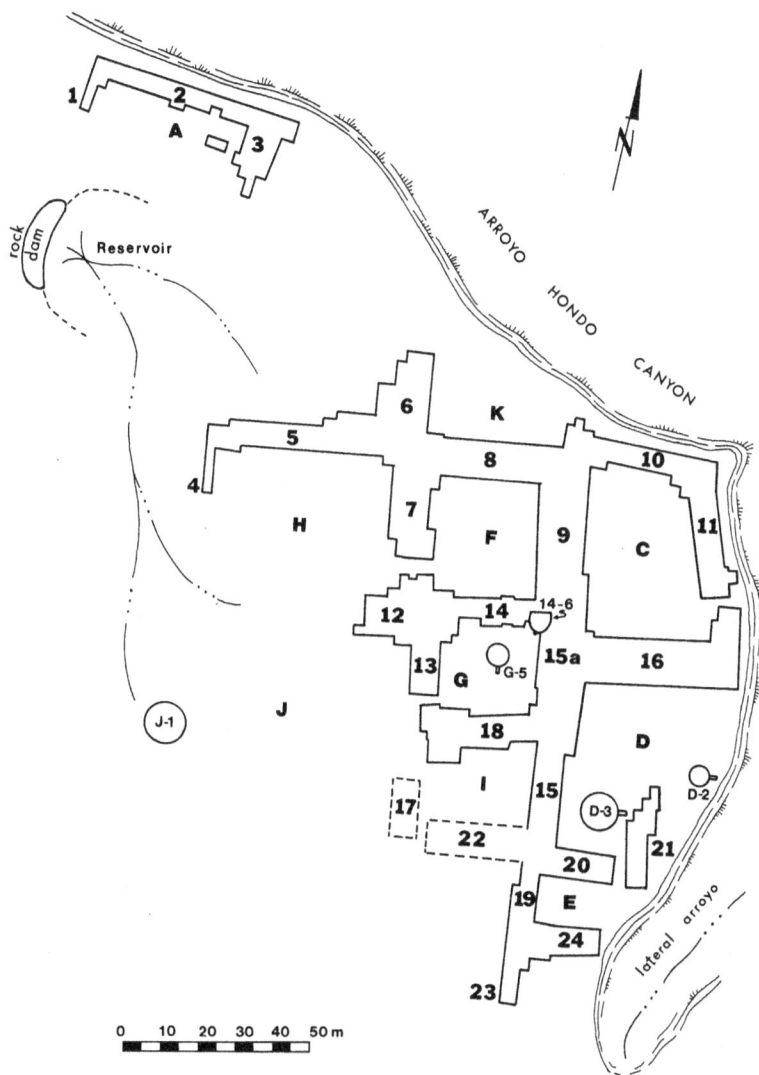

Figure 16.2. Organization of Arroyo Hondo Pueblo. Plazas labeled. (Reprinted by permission from *The Arroyo Hondo Skeletal and Mortuary Remains*, ©1980 by the School of Advanced Research, Santa Fe, New Mexico.)

Childhood

Infancy and childhood were times of great health perils among ancestral Puebloans. The prevalence of porotic skeletal lesions among the very young suggests the Arroyo Hondoan community suffered high infant and childhood mortality rates as is commonly experienced in undeveloped populations. Various studies (Kunitz and Euler 1972; Martin 1994; Stodder 2007) link these mortality/morbidity patterns to the combined effects of childhood diseases such as diarrhea and parasitic infections, acting in concert with dietary protein and micronutrient deficiencies. Many infants and children sickened, some from birth, with both acute and chronic illness leading to the early deaths of many.

Most striking in Plaza G woman is the bowing of all her limbs. Bones respond to increasing muscle size and strength during normal childhood growth. This growth dynamic can be affected by nutritional deficiencies, sometimes leading to lifelong changes in bone size, shape, and overall morphology.

Plaza G woman's right femur shows unusual medial bowing and very poor development of the areas of muscle attachment (such as the linea aspera that runs the posterior length of the bone) as well as fine porous lesions just above the knee (posterior aspect of diaphysis adjacent to condyles). Her left femur shows no natural anterior curve, but instead is unusually straight and thickened at its distal end, and also shows poorly developed areas where muscles attach. Her right tibia is unusually bowed medially and flattened in cross section, while her left tibia exhibits unusual lateral bowing, pronounced counterclockwise twisting, and cortical thickening. Her right fibula has an unusual, oval cross section and matches the bowing of her right tibia (the left tibia was missing). Her lower legs also show poor muscle attachment development.

This woman's arms exhibit similar deformities. Both her right and left humerus of her upper arms are slightly bowed and show unusual curvature. Her forearms are similarly bowed and show unusual flaring of bony crests. As with her legs, her arms exhibit poor muscle development, such as unusually shallow bicipital grooves, which are normally pronounced areas of muscle attachment. All of these long bones were poorly calcified and retained abnormally thin cortical bone throughout her life. Her ribs also exhibit similar cortical thinning. Despite the variable preservation of her skeleton, these abnormal skeletal features clearly indicate she was severely impaired by rickets, a disease of childhood.

Rickets is a metabolic disturbance resulting from vitamin D deficiency. Sunshine exposure is the single most important source of vitamin D in humans (Mankin 1974). Infants concealed from direct exposure to ultraviolet rays must depend solely on dietary sources of vitamin D, either from maternal supplies via breast-feeding or from other dietary sources such as green vegetables. However, exclusive or prolonged breast-feeding can result in vitamin D deficiency early in infancy and is exacerbated in premature infants (Hess 1922; Mughal et al. 1999; Hatun et al. 2005). As little as 15 minutes of exposure of one's face to the sun is sufficient to synthesize adequate vitamin D in healthy individuals. In contemporary populations, continuously cloistering children indoors for prolonged periods can result in rickets. Rickets also can develop from or be compounded by other micronutrient deficiencies, in particular phosphorous, which inhibits normal bone synthesis even when calcium is readily available from food intake and in the blood (Hess 1922).

Plaza G woman first experienced vitamin D deficiency between one and three years of age. Crawling in infancy meant weight bearing on her arms as well as her legs painlessly deformed her poorly mineralized limb bones. Ironically, even though residing in the sunny climate of the American Southwest, this woman developed childhood rickets. It is likely Plaza G woman was cloistered as an infant but was allowed to move about in a windowless adobe room for weeks or months. Once deformed, the abnormal bone morphology resulting from rickets is retained for life, even if normal amounts of vitamin D are restored.

The role of protein calorie malnutrition is also significant in this woman's life. Unlike many other inhabitants of her village and other ancestral Pueblos, this woman does not exhibit any skeletal indicators of cribra orbitalia, porotic hyperostosis, or skeletal porosities related to specific dietary deficiencies. Protein malnutrition plays an ironic role among those who develop rickets, specifically because rickets is a disease of "growth" (Mankin 1974: 116). Children who are severely malnourished or who grow sicker systemically as they develop rickets (tracked clinically in living individuals by increasingly abnormal blood chemistry) tend to exhibit milder rachitic symptoms as growth ceases. Moderately malnourished children (based on protein nutritional status) will exhibit rickets while severely malnourished individuals from the same population showed no symptoms (Walter et al. 1997). Children who develop dietary absorption problems associated with infections or diarrheal diseases often also develop vitamin D, calcium, and phosphorous deficiencies that result in undermineralized bones and rachitic deformities (Mankin 1974).

Like other children born at Arroyo Hondo, Plaza G woman may have suffered from malnutrition, diarrhea, and other infections as an infant. However, she developed rickets precisely because these other metabolic disturbances were not severe enough to significantly inhibit or halt her growth as an infant.

Though bone deformities resulting from vitamin D deficiency, termed osteo-malacia, can occur in adulthood, these deformities are generally limited to the pelvis and vertebral column. Limbs deformed from rickets develop only in young children. For this woman, it appears rickets resulted from child-care practices certainly intended to keep her alive and dietary deficiencies faced by many at Arroyo Hondo.

Early in her life, this ancestral Puebloan woman likely was kept inside her family's adobe room, away from sunlight for prolonged periods. Breast-fed by her mother or fed food deficient in protein as well as calcium and/or phospho-rous, she likely became malnourished, thus also increasing her susceptibility to typical childhood infections such as diarrhea and pneumonia. Severe seasonal weather or chronic illness may have prompted her mother to keep her young daughter cloistered indoors or completely bundled in clothing, thus severely curtailing the child's natural vitamin D synthesis from sunlight. Her undermin-eralized bones painlessly bent under her weight as she crawled and then walked during her first few years. Sometimes referred to as residual rickets (Haduch et al. 2009; Brickley et al. 2010), rachitic bowing that occurs early in childhood results in uncorrected, permanent bone deformation evident throughout life. Her early care and available diet were sufficient to keep her alive as an infant but became the underlying cause of this woman's lifelong impairment.

Adulthood

Residual rickets clearly limited Plaza G woman's everyday life as an adult. Poor muscle development as she grew provided little strength to her deformed legs and arms, and limited her ability to carry out the physically demanding every-day chores of ancestral Puebloan life such as grinding corn, climbing in and out of multistoried structures, and maintaining her family's adobe residence. Getting water at Arroyo Hondo required a steep, tiring, and difficult 100-foot descent to the spring in the arroyo at the base of the plateau. She has no signs of osteomalacia, rachitic changes in adults typified by pelvic and sometimes vertebral and rib deformities, so apparently did not suffer from vitamin D de-ficiency as an adult. Ethnographic accounts suggest that ancestral Puebloan women likely married and had children. Plaza G woman's physical impairments would not have necessarily precluded her from bearing children.

Importantly, she was not alone. Others—both adults and children—interred in and near Plaza G at Arroyo Hondo were similarly affected. Seven of the nine rachitic adults among the burials from Arroyo Hondo were interred in Plaza G, and one similarly affected adult female was interred in adjacent Roomblock 18.

Fifteen juveniles associated with this first occupation phase of the site were diagnosed with rickets. Nearly half of these children (7 of 15) were buried nearby—four of these children were interred in Plaza G, with an additional three children interred in adjoining Roomblock 18.

We have no way of assessing if individuals with physical impairments like rickets at Arroyo Hondo were provided with special care or assistance. Skeletally, none of the rachitic individuals appear to have been immobile or would have required extraordinary assistance to move about. However, the usual number of rachitic cases at Arroyo Hondo, with most clustered in one area, suggests that dietary problems compounded by child-care practices leading to physical impairment were experienced by some families in this village and not by others.

Death and Burial

Plaza G woman is estimated to have been in her mid-to-late thirties at the time of death; her cause of death could not be determined, though it is certainly possible her poor health early in life and physical impairments could also have contributed to a shortened lifespan. Life expectancy at Arroyo Hondo, as in most prehistoric populations, was short, with most adults dying in their thirties and forties, so her early death was not atypical among these villagers.

The location and construction of her grave suggest Plaza G woman was buried in the traditional manner of the village despite her physical impairment, which would have been obvious in life. She was interred during the height of the Component I occupation at Arroyo Hondo, buried along the east wall of Plaza G. Ancestral Puebloans did not maintain separate cemetery areas; rather, the dead return to the underworld in Puebloan cosmology (Ortiz 1969) through interment within the pueblo's living spaces, including the village trash middens. Plaza G was established during the third building phase at the site, so this woman's death and interment likely date between A.D. 1320 and 1330. Eventually, 23 children, six men, eight women, and one other adult were interred within this defined plaza space, just predating the drastic decline in the village's population during the 1350s. Those interred in and around Plaza G represent one or two generations of villagers.

Her grave was an oval-shaped pit dug into the subsoil, with straight walls and a flat base that accommodated her body in a tightly flexed position. Though preservation at the site is not good, fragments remained of the woven yucca mat that covered her body. No other perishable items were found. Personal items (for example, pots, projectile points, necklaces) were occasionally buried with the deceased at Arroyo Hondo; however, no other items were found with this woman. Her grave was filled with trash-laden soil, then sealed with a plaster layer at the plaza surface. Plaza G continued to be used by the living after her interment.

Physical Impairments and Disabilities

Bioarchaeologists and others have often speculated that observed skeletal physical impairment (such as seen in Plaza G woman) or unusual morphology among individuals from the prehistoric past is evidence of a physical disability suffered during life. And there are instances where one can offer a compelling argument that an individual's physical impairment was severe enough to require the help and support of others for simple survival. For example, an adult male from Gran Quivira suffered a progressive, debilitating musculoskeletal disease rendering him largely unable to care for himself for many years prior to his death (Hawkey 1998). However, that all skeletal evidence of physical impairment indicates a "disability" in both physical and social terms is an assumption we make about prehistoric peoples. Our ideas about "disability" as well as the care of people with disabilities as moral acts of "compassion" are defined within culturally bounded norms (Dettwyler 1991). What we as bioarchaeologists assess as "physical impairment" and interpret as a "disability" may or may not have been understood, experienced, or acknowledged as a handicap by those affected individuals in the past. Careful assessment of the archaeological context for these unusual individuals as well as ethnographic analogies and comparisons where appropriate provide our only well-grounded clues to understanding the lives of such individuals.

Both ethnographic and archaeological evidence in the American Southwest indicate that Puebloans noted and responded to unusual body forms. For example, ethnographic reports for the Hopi note that infanticide was practiced in cases of malformed newborns (Hrdlicka 1908; Beaglehole and Beaglehole 1935; Brandt 1954), and historically Puebloan villagers clearly understood and responded to the presence of illnesses, infant/childhood deaths, and various other maladies. However, ethnographic accounts suggest that some physical differences such as albinism (Woolf 2005) or cranial deformation (Stodder 2009) were noticed but did not necessarily affect the status or treatment of a person. In addition, rock art depictions of polydactyly and the varying treatment of adults and children with extra fingers or toes again suggests that this condition was noted, but may have only occasionally warranted special treatment of the individual at death (Barnes 1994; Case et al. 2006).

At Arroyo Hondo, there is no evidence to suggest that physically impaired adults or children were treated any differently than other villagers at death. They were afforded the same kinds of burial treatment and interred in the same kinds of locations, and their graves were not markedly devoid of accoutrements, nor did they contain anything usual. The clustering of these individuals in and around Plaza G suggests those residing in that part of the village were unduly affected by vitamin D and accompanying dietary deficiencies. This clustering of rachitic individuals at Arroyo Hondo also may reflect internal social dynamics of the village. Perhaps kinship or other group tensions may have resulted in differential access to food resources for the residents of Plaza G. Differences in dietary and feeding practices among different social groups also could have severely impacted Plaza G inhabitants more than others. The physical impairments of rickets would have likely been noticed. However, it does not appear that Plaza G woman or the others affected by residual rickets were treated different socially. The interment cluster of physically impaired and severely ill individuals in and around Plaza G does, however, suggest that some social groups within the community suffered more severe health issues than others.

Was Plaza G woman "disabled"? Certainly her physical impairment presented her with challenges of mobility and limited strength. However, it is not clear that she or others considered her "disabled," unable to carry out the necessary tasks of everyday life or unable to fulfill particular social roles. The archaeological record provides no evidence she was treated differently at the time of her death, and ethnographic comparisons are silent about whether she and others with similar physical challenges at Arroyo Hondo may have been seen as different or treated differently than others during life. For Plaza G woman, we can draw no definitive conclusions about what impact her physical limitations placed on her social life.

Conclusion

Starting in infancy, the woman in Plaza G suffered from rickets, possibly complicated by moderate malnutrition. Her limb deformities persisted into adulthood, affecting her daily life. It appears from the archaeological context that child-care practices shared by Plaza G families resulted in a clustering of those afflicted with rickets in this fourteenth-century village. Rickets seems an odd malady to suffer in the sun-rich American Southwest, though studies have occasionally noted rachitic cases among other ancestral Puebloan groups (e.g., Brues 1946; Ortner 2003; Schultz et al. 2007; Schultz et al. 2008). At Arroyo Hondo, the number of individuals surviving to adulthood with rickets as well the number of children who died with this health complication is striking. Social dynamics among the families who lived in and around Plaza G clearly played a significant role in the shaping the health of these women, men, and children.

Metabolic disturbances had a severe impact on the health and longevity of people living in and around Plaza G during the height of occupation at Arroyo Hondo. Sick children were cloistered indoors, and the resulting lifelong effects of childhood illness and rickets persisting into adulthood would likely have been evident to everyone in the village. The burial evidence, however, suggests those impaired by rickets were afforded the same social customs at death. In addition, affected individuals were clustered in Plaza G and surrounding room-blocks, suggesting these health issues impacted some families or extended kin groups more than others. These misfortunes may possibly reflect social inequalities, such as differential access to adequate food resources or productive land for dry farming. However, it is not possible to know whether the misfortune of physical impairments also impacted aspects of Plaza G woman's social life (for example, social shunning or exclusion from certain social status).

This fourteenth-century woman at Arroyo Hondo was among a number of villagers who experienced the impairment of rickets throughout their lives. She was interred in the same manner as other adult women of her time. However, the physical challenges shared by other adults and an unusual prevalence of severe illness among some children around Plaza G at Arroyo Hondo set this segment of the village apart, and may have created real or perceived hardships that resonated in other social, political, economic, and religious arenas.

References Cited

Barnes, Ethne
1994   Polydactyly in the Southwest. *Kiva* 59: 419–31.
Beaglehole, E., and P. Beaglehole
1935   *Hopi of the Second Mesa*. Memoirs of the American Anthropological Association No. 44. American Anthropological Association, Menasha, Wis.
Brandt, R. B.
1954   *Hopi Ethics: A Theoretical Analysis*. University of Chicago Press, Chicago.
Brickley, Megan, Simon Mays, and Rebecca Ives
2010   Evaluation and Interpretation of Residual Rickets Deformities in Adults. *International Journal of Osteoarchaeology* 20(1): 54–66.
Brues, Alice M.
1946   Alkalai Ridge Skeletons, Pathology and Anomaly. In *Archaeology of Alkalai Ridge, Southeastern Utah*, edited by J. O. Brew, pp. 327–29. Papers of the Peabody Museum No. 21. Peabody Museum, New Haven, Conn.

Case, D. Troy, Rebecca J. Hill, Charles F. Merbs, and M. Fong

2006   Polydactyly in the Prehistoric American Southwest. *International Journal of Osteo-archaeology* 16: 221–35.

Cordell, Linda

2009   *Archaeology of the Prehistoric Southwest*. 2nd ed. Left Coast Press, Walnut Creek, Calif.

Dettwyler, Katherine A.

1991   Can Paleopathology Provide Evidence for "Compassion"? *American Journal of Physical Anthropology* 84: 375–84.

Haduch, E., A. Szczepanak, J. Skrzat, R. Srodek, and P. Brzegowy

2009   Residual Rickets or Osteomalacia: A Case Dating from the 16–18th Centuries from Krosno Odrzanskie, Poland. *International Journal of Osteoarchaeology* 19: 593–612.

Hatun, Sukru, Behzat Ozkan, Zerrin Orbak, Hakan Doneray, Filiz Cizmecioglu, Demet Toprak, and Ali Calikoglu

2005   Vitamin D Deficiency in Early Infancy. *Journal of Nutrition* 135: 279–82.

Hawkey, Diane

1998   Disability, Compassion and the Skeletal Record: Using Musculoskeletal Stress Markers (MSM) to Construct an Osteobiography from Early New Mexico. *International Journal of Osteoarchaeology* 8: 326–40.

Hess, Julius

1922   Diseases Peculiar to Premature Infants. In *Premature and Congenitally Diseased Infants*, by Julius Hess. Lea and Febiger, Philadelphia. See www.neonatology.org/classics/hess1922/hess.18.html.

Hrdlicka, Alês

1908   *Physiological and Medical Observations among the Indians of the Southwestern United States and Northern Mexico*. Bureau of Ethnology Bulletin 34. Government Printing Office, Washington, D.C.

Kunitz, Stephen, and Robert Euler

1972   Aspects of Southwestern Paleoepidemiology. Anthropological Reports No. 2. Prescott College Press, Prescott, Ariz.

Mankin, Henry

1974   Rickets, Osteomalacia and Renal Osteodystrophy. *Journal of Bone and Joint Surgery* 56: 101–28.

Martin, Debra L.

1994   Patterns of Diet and Disease: Stress Profiles for the Prehistoric Southwest. In *Themes in Southwest Prehistory*, edited by George J. Gumerman, pp. 87–108. School of American Research Press, Santa Fe, N.Mex.

Mughal, M. Z., H. Salama, T. Greenway, I. Laing, and E. B. Mawer

1999   Florid Rickets Associated with Prolonged Breast Feeding without Vitamin D Supplementation. *British Medical Journal* 318: 39–40.

Nelson, Ben, Timothy Kohler, and Keith Kintigh

1994   Studies in Disruption: Demography and Health in the Prehistoric Southwest. In *Understanding Complexity in the Prehistoric Southwest*, edited by George Gumerman and Murray Gell-Mann, pp. 59–112. Proceedings Vol. 16, Santa Fe Institute Studies in the Sciences of Complexity. Addison-Wesley, Reading, Mass.

Ortiz, Alfonso
1969   *The Tewa World: Space, Time, Being and Becoming in a Pueblo Society*. University of Chicago Press, Chicago.
Ortner, Donald
2003   *Identification of Pathological Conditions in Human Skeletal Remains*. 2nd ed. Academic Press, New York.
Palkovich, Ann M.
1980   *Pueblo Population and Society: The Arroyo Hondo Skeletal and Mortuary Remains*. Arroyo Hondo Archaeological Series, Vol. 3. School of American Research Press, Santa Fe, N.Mex.
Plog, Stephen
2008   *Ancient Peoples of the American Southwest*. 2nd ed. Thames and Hudson, London.
Schultz, Michael, Ulrich Timme, and Tyede H. Schmidt-Schultz
2007   Infancy and Childhood in the Pre-Columbian North American Southwest—First Results of the Paleopathological Investigation of the Skeletons from the Grasshopper Pueblo, Arizona. *International Journal of Osteoarchaeology* 17: 369–79.
Schultz, Michael, Ulrich Timme, Reinhard Hilgers, and Tyede H. Schmidt-Schultz
2008   Preliminary Results of the Bioarchaeological and Sociobiological Investigation of the Infants and Children of Grasshopper Pueblo. In *Reanalysis and Reinterpretation in Southwestern Bioarchaeology*, edited by Ann L. W. Stodder, pp. 127–39. Arizona State University Anthropological Research Papers No. 59. Arizona State University Press, Tempe.
Stodder, Ann L. W.
2007   Skeletal Biology: Southwest. In *Handbook of North American Indians*, Vol. 3, *Environment, Origins and Population*, edited by Douglas Ubelaker, pp. 557–80. Smithsonian Institution Press, Washington, D.C.
2009   Variation, Group Identity and the Visible "Other" in the Prehistoric Southwest. Paper presented at the 74th Annual Meeting, Society for American Archaeology, Atlanta.
Stuart, David
2000   *Anazasi America: Seventeen Centuries on the Road from Center Place*. University of New Mexico Press, Albuquerque.
Swedlund, Alan
1994   Issues in Demography and Health. In *Understanding Complexity in the Prehistoric Southwest*, edited by George Gumerman and Murray Gell-Mann, pp. 39–58. Proceedings Vol. 16, Santa Fe Institute, Studies in the Sciences of Complexity. Addison-Wesley, Reading, Mass.
Walter, E. A., J. K. Scariano, C. R. Easington, A. M. Polaco, B. W. Hollis, A. Daspuota, S. Pam, and R. H. Glew
1997   Rickets and Protein Malnutrition in Northern Nigeria. *Journal of Tropical Pediatrics* 43(2): 98–102.
Wetterstrom, Wilma
1986   *Food, Diet and Population at Prehistoric Arroyo Hondo Pueblo, New Mexico*. Arroyo Hondo Archaeological Series, Vol. 6. School of American Research Press, Santa Fe, N.Mex.
Woolf, Charles
2005   Albinism (OCA2) in Amerindians. *Yearbook of Physical Anthropology* 48: 118–40.

17 ◆ From Cradle to Grave and Beyond

A Maya Life and Death

Pamela L. Geller

Individual Profile

Site: Bajo Hill (RB 25)
Location: 3 km west-northwest of La Milpa, Río Bravo Conservation and Management Area, northwestern Belize, C.A.
Cultural Affiliation: Pre-Columbian Maya
Date: Late/Terminal Classic period, Tepeu 2–3 phase, ca. A.D. 700–900; based on ceramic analysis
Feature: V42-B-13
Location of Grave: Under house floor, Structure 2, Group B
Burial and Grave Type: Single primary inhumation tightly flexed on left side, north–south orientation; circular pit cut into floor with modification of underlying bedrock, filled with subfloor fill, sealed with plaster floor, and topped by an architectural feature—a masonry bench with construction fill comprised of red plaster chunks, lithics, sherds, marl, and cobble
Associated Materials: Miniature ceramic jar, three hematite disks, obsidian blade, vertical headstone
Preservation and Completeness: Poor preservation, skeletal elements highly fragmentary and incomplete; 12 teeth; eroded cranial fragments primarily from occiput; very eroded shafts of right and left femora, tibiae, humeri, and radius or ulna; very eroded fragments of right and left scapulae
Age at Death and Basis of Estimate: 20–34 years, based on dental wear
Sex and Basis of Determination: Probable male, based on robusticity of occipital and long bones
Conditions Observed: Peg incisor (RI^2), LEH on canines (one episode at 3–5 years)
Specialized Analysis: None
Excavated: June 1999, Programme for Belize Archaeological Project directed by Fred Valdez Jr., University of Texas–Austin
Archaeological Report: Geller 1999, 2004; Saul and Saul 2004
Current Disposition: PfBAP field laboratory, Río Bravo Conservation and Management Area, northwestern Belize, C.A.

Feminist archaeology means writing the prehistory of people. This means social actors who have gender, personalities, biographies.

—Ruth Tringham, "Engendered Places in Prehistory," 183.

Bioarchaeologists, those whose studies take the remains of people as their terminus a quo, are neither unfamiliar with nor hostile to the notion of peopling the past. On the contrary, Buikstra (2006: xix) reminds us that bioarchaeology as an outgrowth of American anthropology emphasizes "peopling the past." Yet many bioarchaeologists' efforts at peopling call to my mind Tringham's statements about pasts comprised of "faceless blobs" (1991: 94). After reflecting upon her own archaeological work, Tringham realized that the material data she examined "had a richer role to play in archaeology than a passive reflection on human behavior" (1991: 98). That is, to truly and effectively people the past required critical evaluation of knowledge production and expansion of research concerns, which Tringham and her fellow feminist archaeologists proceeded to do.

Since its fomentation, feminist archaeology has endeavored to people the past in three ways. First, in reaction to processualists' limited focus on macroscale phenomena, feminist archaeologists take a multiscalar approach in their studies—from the quotidian and interpersonal to the long term and large scale (Conkey 2003: 870–71). Second, feminist archaeologists think about difference beyond dichotomy, exploring individuals' identities as intersected by multiple, materially recoverable attributes. While sex and gender remain prominent concerns, practitioners also think about the ways in which these facets of identity intersect with age, race, ethnicity, class, and sexuality (e.g., Gilchrist 1999; Meskell 1999; Dowson 2000; Schmidt and Voss 2000). Conceptualizing identities as the complex outcome of varied characteristics allows for a more nuanced construction of past categories of personhood. The past is no longer comprised of "faceless blobs," but encompasses diverse peoples whose identities were contextually contingent and mutable throughout their lives. Third, feminist archaeologists advocate alternative and creative ways to write the past, such as first-person anecdote, hypertext, and informed fiction (e.g., Spector 1993; Joyce et al. 2000; Dowson 2006). To do so, Conkey and Gero (1991: 22) remarked, undermines "cults of authority: the authority of statistics, of the passive voice, the exaggeratedly objective eye, the single line of evidence, the single cause, the only perspective." Accordingly, a more vibrant and holistic prehistory materializes.

With these lessons learned from feminist archaeology, critical evaluation of bioarchaeology's peopling project reveals a shortcoming. Many researchers retain a preference for population research; they eschew the individual, an oversight that this volume seeks to remedy. This is not to say that population perspectives have failed to advance our understanding of the human condition. Posing population-based questions, bioarchaeologists have, for example, fruitfully explored the immediate and future effects of agricultural intensification on health status (Cohen and Armelagos 1984; Armelagos 2003; Cohen and Crane-Kramer 2007). However, strictly focusing on populational patterns elides exploration of individuals' idiosyncrasies and identities. And, as feminist archaeologists note, confining analysis to the macroscale lends itself to presentations of past peoples as homogeneous and indistinguishable.

Previous studies of burials informed by feminist perspectives have shed much light on the life histories of past peoples (e.g., Meskell 1996; Hollimon 1997; Joyce 1999; Arnold and Wicker 2001; Sofaer 2006). In this chapter, my use of a bioarchaeological approach furthers these efforts by scaling down, reflecting upon the materiality of identity, and writing in an explicitly humanistic manner. I begin by considering the unassuming burial of a pre-Columbian Maya villager who lived some 1,200 years ago in what today is the modern nation-state of Belize. The decedent was venerated as an ancestor after death, and there is evidence that in life the individual performed medico-religious practices associated with the specialized and communally significant profession of healer.

Were we to assess only his highly fragmented skeletal remains, we would learn little about this person's life. Hence, to flesh out this story, I also examine additional salient information gleaned from architectural context, associated artifacts, and critically utilized ethnohistory, ethnography, and artistic imagery. I recognize that not all investigators have access to such resources. Yet a multivariate approach inevitably enriches the study of mortuary features and the bodies therein. This perspective emphasizes that we consider bodies not just as spaces unto themselves but also as situated within space. And, accordingly, it can reveal much about an individual and his or her society from cradle to grave and beyond. Of course, bioarchaeologists reverse this sequence, as we first encounter graves and not cradles.

Case Study: Late Classic Maya of the Lowlands

Late Classic peoples of the Maya Lowlands intentionally buried select decedents beneath structures that mourners continued to use. Spatial proximity indicates that the living granted social viability to the biologically dead, thereby ensuring an ongoing dialogue with powerful ancestors (McAnany 1995; Gillespie 2001).

Interactions between living and dead members of Maya society were pervasive and complex, shaped by religious tenets, cosmological beliefs, and social norms but also by mourners' personal memories and decedents' life histories. The patterning in Maya burial assemblages indicates shared cultural practices and beliefs, which population-based questions bring to light. Yet analysts' search for patterns often yields information about particulars, which complicate interpretations and hence require explanation.

In Maya studies, Frank Saul's osteobiographic approach set an important precedent for identifying patterns and particulars (1972). Accounts of royal individuals' life histories—from Altar de Sacrificios (Saul and Saul 1989: 291–92), Copán (Bell 2002; Buikstra et al. 2004), and Palenque (Tiesler et al. 2004; Tiesler and Cucina 2006)—have revealed their large-scale sociopolitical impacts and personal pains. Mourners celebrated these charismatic movers and shakers, as evidenced by grand tombs, rich funerary accoutrements, historic narration carved onto stone stelae, and artistically rendered portraiture on vessels or murals. For these reasons, such individuals' life histories are likely to come to light. But what of the individuals whose lives resonated on a local scale? And what can these individuals' life histories relate about broader cultural practices and beliefs or particular circumstances?

Background Information: Be It Ever So Humble . . .

Pre-Columbian peoples of the Maya lowlands resided in an exceedingly humid environment with continual wet-dry fluctuations. As a consequence, preservation in such tropical settings is generally poor. As a rule, excavators encounter bones that are highly fragmented and eroded. Such fragility guarantees that information will be lost as researchers move remains from field setting to laboratories. Careful attention to detail and context during the excavation process, therefore, is essential. Such is especially the case when excavating the burials of commoners, who lacked the material and historical riches of royalty.

Though not the only type of burial utilized by Classic commoners, house burial was ubiquitous. One intriguing example is the commoner burial of Individual 102 at the Bajo Hill site in northwestern Belize (figure 17.1). The Bajo Hill site is located on the western outskirts of La Milpa, a regional ceremonial center (Kunen 2001, 2004). According to the site's excavator, Julie Kunen, inhabitants of this farming community thrived in a seasonally inundated wetland environment for six centuries (2001, 2004). In its final form, the Bajo Hill site had 17 distinct clusters of structures. Group B was one such cluster, and its occupation extended from ca. A.D. 250 to 850. This group was comprised of two structures positioned to form a right angle (Kunen 2001, 2004). Throughout the site's occupation, the group's structures had been renovated at least three times. The death of a presumed kin member, Individual 102, was the impetus for one of these architectural renovations. Some time after the start of the Late/Terminal Classic period (A.D. 750), mourners interred this decedent beneath the northeastern section of Structure 2's platform.

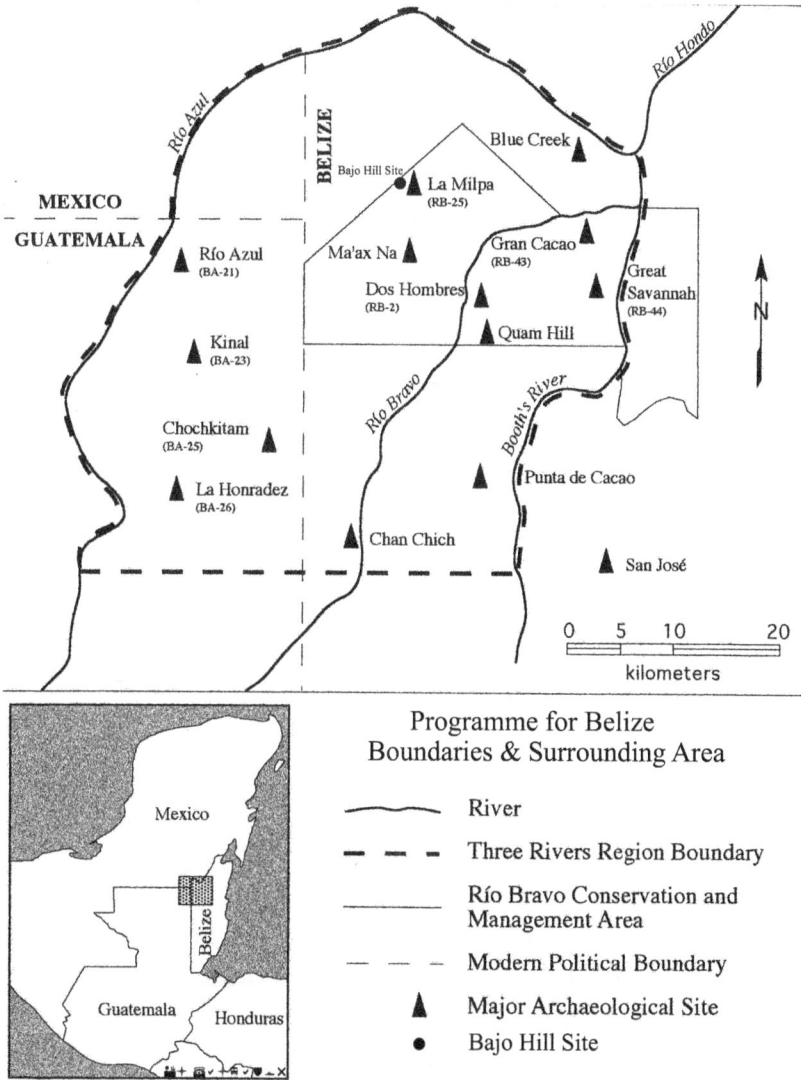

Figure 17.1. Map of sites in the Programme for Belize, northwestern Belize. A black dot indicates the Bajo Hill site.

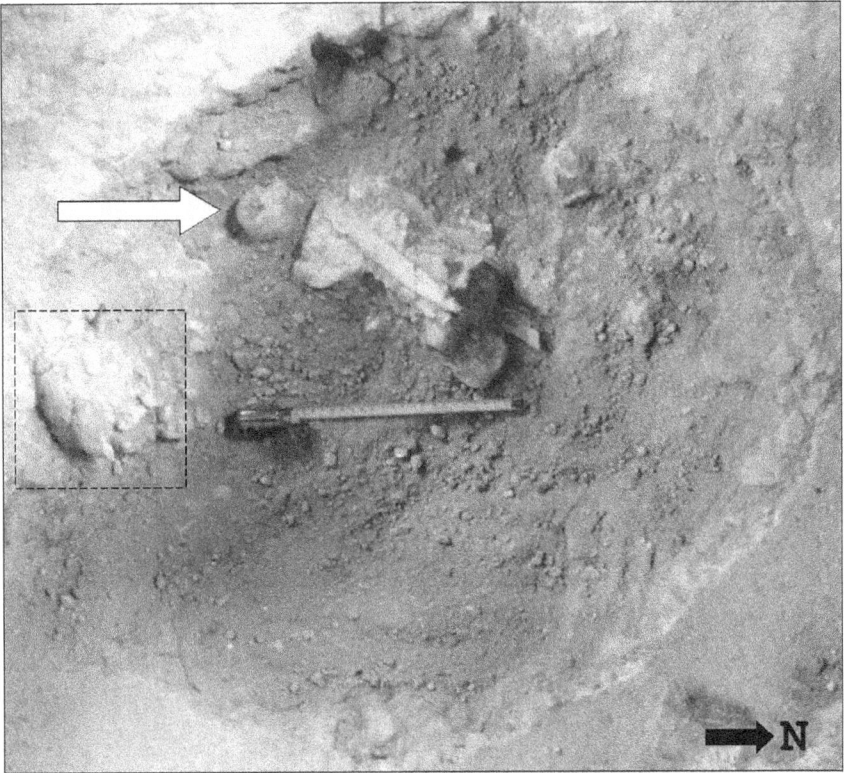

Figure 17.2. Individual 102's pit grave. A white arrow indicates the jar's location. A dashed-lined box gives a rough estimate of where the headstone had been; it was removed before this photograph was taken in order to excavate the human remains.

The grave builders, who were presumably kin members, excavated a shallow pit approximately 60 cm wide and 10 cm deep. The pit, which was oriented on the north–south axis, extended down through Structure 2's plaster floor and into subfloor fill (figure 17.2). Bedrock, located just beneath this construction fill, had been modified in order to accommodate the decedent's body. Those who handled the corpse placed Individual 102 into a tightly flexed position, the body oriented north–south with the head to the south, facing west. The flexed position suggests that funerary attendants bundled the corpse with perishable materials prior to its interment, a practice that was widespread throughout the Maya world (Reese-Taylor et al. 2006). Tightly flexed burials were not rare in the Programme for Belize Archaeological Project (PfBAP) sample (n = 135); 15.2 percent of individuals had been positioned in such a manner. Yet Individual 102's assortment of grave goods was unique. Adjacent to the decedent's bent knees, mourners placed a miniature ceramic jar (figure 17.3). Three hematite disks ran parallel to Individual 102's thighs, an arrangement that suggests they were wedged between the decedent's flexed thighs and upper torso during corpse preparation (figure 17.4). The largest measures 20 mm in diameter, has a thickness of 4.5 mm, and weighs 4 g. The second disk's diameter, thickness, and weight are 19.4 mm, 3.85 mm, 5.5 g, respectively. And the smallest disk is 16 mm in diameter, is 4.2 mm thick, and weighs 2.8 g. The diameters of the raised circles in the center of all three disks are about 5.6 mm.

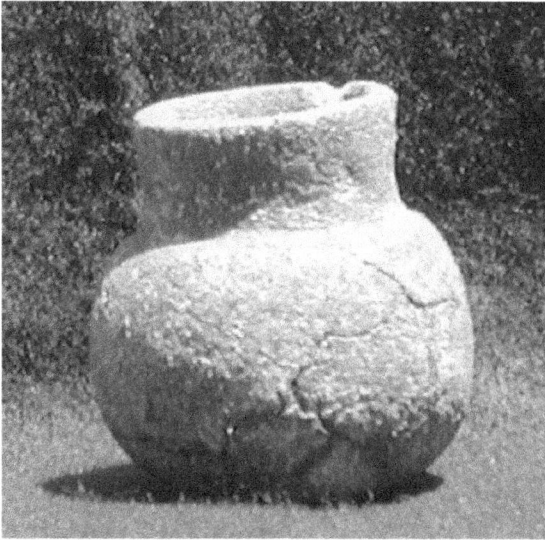

Figure 17.3. This Late/Terminal Classic jar has a body diameter of 5.5 cm and a rim diameter of 3.75 cm. The vessel is 5.8 cm high and weighs 55.3 g. The jar has no traces of red paint inside, and no residue analyses were conducted on its contents.

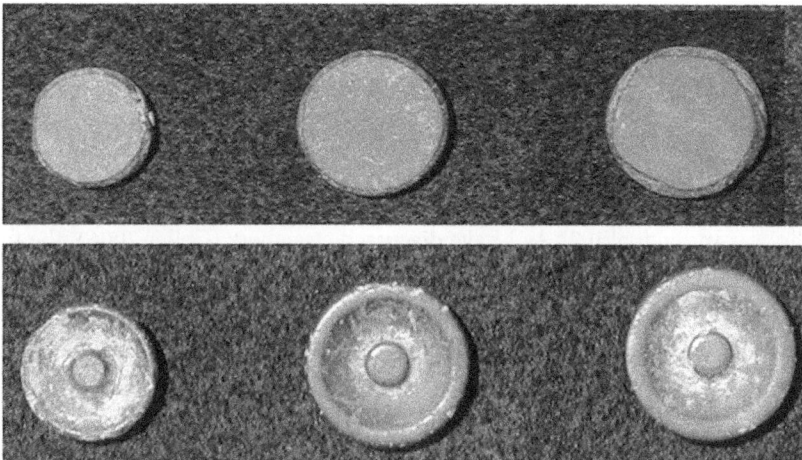

Figure 17.4. Carved sides (*below*) and polished sides (*above*) of three hematite disks. The disk to the far right measures 19.4 mm in diameter, is 3.85 mm thick, and weighs 5.5 g.

Mourners also included an obsidian blade in the grave. The exact placement of the blade is unknown; it was recovered while screening the fill removed from the grave. Then mourners placed a roughly hewn vertical headstone, which was 36 cm in height and about 30 cm at its widest points, above Individual 102's head and filled the grave with a cementlike subfloor fill. And finally, Individual 102's kin resurfaced the plaster floor to seal over the grave space.

Sometime after Individual 102's burial, mourners interred a second individual, Individual 101, just slightly east of Individual 102 and above the plaster floor. They entombed Individual 101 in a plaster bench measuring 2 m long and 40–60 cm high. In contrast to Individual 102, this second body was oriented in an east–west direction with the head to the west. This decedent was also flexed, but attendants placed the body on its back. No grave goods were recovered in association with Individual 101. However, as with Individual 102, mourners had intentionally placed a roughly hewn and vertical limestone slab adjacent to the decedent's head, though just to the west.

By the time I disturbed Individual 102 some 1,250 years later, this ancestor's remains were exceedingly fragmentary and incomplete. Without contextual information, they offer the meagerest of osteobiographic insights. Per Saul and Saul's initial analysis (in Kunen 2004: 147), slight dental attrition indicates that Individual 102 died between 20 and 34 years of age, while robusticity of the occipital and long bones intimate a probable male sex. However, intense physical activity characterized the lifestyle of all Maya commoners, and the extreme fragmentation of these remains makes robusticity an unreliable indicator of sex. The skeletal remains of Individual 101, on the other hand, have definite female features: an elevated auricular surface on the pelvis, a sharp upper orbital margin, and overall gracility (Saul and Saul in Kunen 2004: 147). Like Individual 102, she died between the ages of 20 and 34 years.

Discussion: Materializing Identity

Who was Individual 102? As I have discussed elsewhere (Geller 2006), the funerary treatment of Individuals 102 and 101 transformed their liminal corpses into venerated ancestors, as was the case for decedents throughout the Maya world. Their graves likely replicated caves, which the Maya considered to be conduits between the terrestrial realm and the supernatural underworld (Brady and Ashmore 1999). The bench functioned as an ancestral shrine where the living could continue to dialogue with the biologically dead though socially viable. But what did Individuals 102 and 101 do during life to warrant such a special identity after death?

To answer this query, I return to Individual 102's unique assortment of funerary goods. Chronicling by sixteenth-century missionary Diego de Landa illumines the significance of such an assemblage. He writes of a festival celebrated annually in the month *Zip*:

> The physicians and the sorcerers assembled in one of their houses with their wives. . . . They opened the bundles of their medicine, in which they kept many trifles and, each having his own, little idols of the goddess of medicine, whom they called Ix Chel . . . as well as some small stones, called *am*, of the kind which they used for casting lots. (in Tozzer 1941: 154)

Landa also relates that medico-ritual specialists were interred beneath their houses with toolkits in hand (in Tozzer 1941: 130). Despite the corrosive effect of Spanish colonialism on indigenous cultures, medico-religious specialists continued administering to body and soul, and healers remain esteemed figures in modern Maya communities, notwithstanding Western biomedicine's delegitimization of their practices and knowledge. Ethnographies proffer a wealth of details about bonesetters, midwives, herbalists, and shamans (e.g., Wisdom 1940; Woods 1968; Fabrega and Silver 1973; Paul and Paul 1975; Paul 1976; Hinojosa 2002). And contra to Landa's comments, women functioned as wives *and* medico-religious specialists.

From this corpus, we see that individuals become medico-religious specialists during "a series of personal experiential events that eventually are resolved through self identification with a new social status" (Brown 2000: 328). They are divinely elected in their dreams and via the discovery of sacred objects, or *sacra*. *Sacra* have a connection to the supernatural, and in medico-ritual practices they vary in form and function (Brown 2000). Practitioners may use items to divine an illness's etiology. Bonesetters, for instance, utilize a special little bone to locate where a patient's bone is broken (Paul 1976: 77; Hinojosa 2002: 31). Other items simultaneously possess symbolic and utilitarian value. A midwife from the Zutuhil-Maya community of San Pedro la Laguna, for example, recounted to Paul and Paul (1975: 711) her discovery of a conch shell and penknife while out walking. During dreams, her predecessors instructed the midwife to collect these items, for the shell symbolically represented her power while the knife would aid in cutting infants' umbilical cords.

The endurance and materiality of medico-religious practices and beliefs invite consideration of ancient phenomena. In her analysis of artifacts' types and spatial locations, Brown (2000) makes a convincing case that Structure 12 at Joya de Cerén, the Classic period site in El Salvador, contained diverse portable objects that served as *sacra* and divination tools: obsidian blades, crystals, a greenstone disk, a miniature frog effigy pot, and more. The objects interred with Individual 102 likely functioned as *sacra* as well.

There is substantial evidence to support the notion that Individual 102's obsidian blade doubled as a symbolic and utilitarian object. Numerous images depict pre-Columbian Maya peoples' use of obsidian blades for bloodletting during ritual events (Schele and Miller 1986). Ancient practices persisted after conquest and into modern times; Maya healers bleed the ailing with exceedingly sharp obsidian blades (Roys 1931; Ximénez 1967; Orellana 1987: 71–74), and these practitioners are described as possessing surgical skill and specialized knowledge of the body.

To convincingly argue that Individual 102's hematite disks served as divination stones, I similarly draw on ethnohistory and ethnography. The Maya used crystals for divinatory purposes (e.g., Redfield and Villa Rojas 1934; Kunow 1996: 72–73), and curers also utilized special items. In the case of the Chorti Maya, medico-religious practitioners utilized sanctified stone celts and chipped stone (Wisdom 1940: 382). Woods (1968: 129) described a Cakchiquel curer's assemblage that included oblong pieces of obsidian and small rocks of various sizes and shapes. The resemblance between these sacred items and Individual 102's hematite disks, which were also small and fashioned from a dark-colored stone, is striking.

In her study of the Lacandon Maya, Davis (1978) identifies an intriguing link between sacred stones and ceramic vessels. Stones were put into god pots, which were "clay bowls approximately six to eight inches in diameter . . . [with] a small anthropomorphous head jutting above the rim on one side that represents the god to whom the pot is dedicated" (Davis 1978: 73). Placing stones in god pots allowed the vessels' owners to commune with the supernatural. The Lacandon also made a smaller version of the god pot called a *sihir*. Mainly produced during god pot renewal ceremonies, the *sihirs* were deposited in caves as offerings to the gods. It was in these sacred spaces that the soul (*pishan*) of each pot ascended to heaven and transformed into a man (Davis 1978: 76).

Sihirs appear to have ancient antecedents; miniature vessels like Individual 102's jar are found at Classic period sites throughout the Maya lowland. Colloquially, these jars are referred to as "poison" or "perfume" bottles, though there is no archaeological support for such designations. Archaeologists have argued that these vessels were children's toys (Satterthwaite et al. 2006: 105) or scribes' pigment jars (Smith 1955: 103, 138). An alternative explanation for these vessels' function is indicated by iconography on painted and molded examples. Poor preservation may account for the blank surfaces of some vessels like Individual 102's, but many jars have painted glyphs or mold-made images of animals and deities. Often featured on these vessels is God L, a principal underworld deity (Reents-Budet 1994: 215). Many small jars depict God L with tobacco leaves

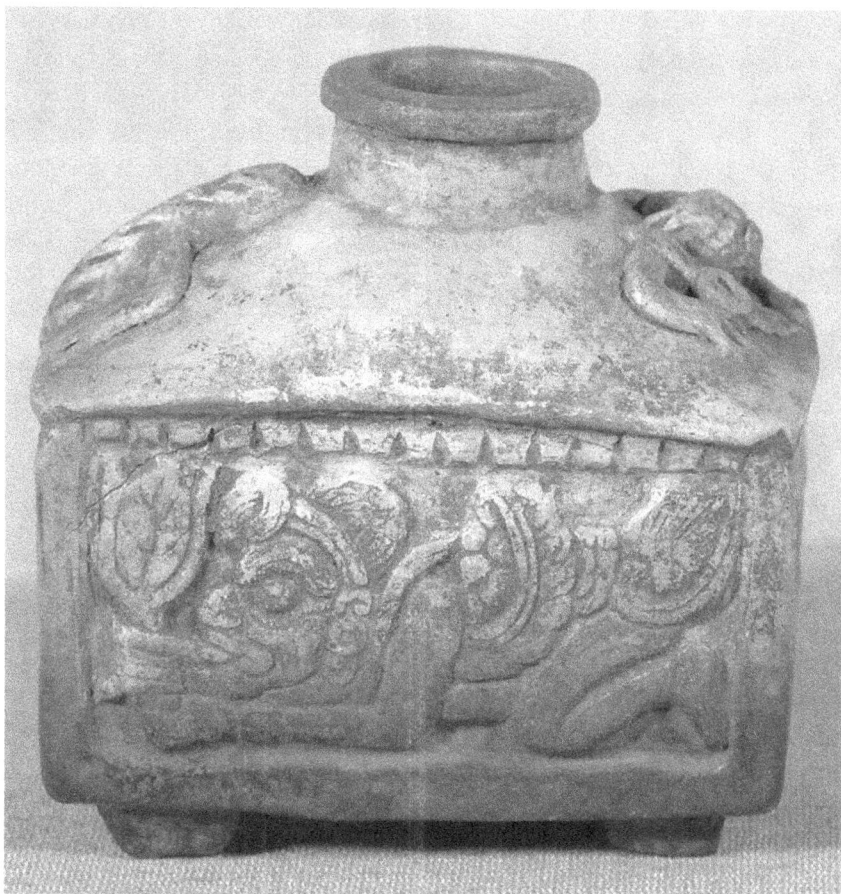

Figure 17.5. Miniature jar with God L holding tobacco leaf. Dates to ca. A.D. 600–900; measures 8.9 cm high and 9.1 cm wide. Part of the Jay I. Kislak Collection, Rare Books and Special Collections Division, Library of Congress, Washington, D.C. (96.070.00.003). (Photograph courtesy of Arthur Dunkelman.)

(Kerr and Kerr 2006: 75–76) (figure 17.5). They are believed to have contained tobacco snuff used for medico-ritual purposes (John Carlson, personal communication 2006). From pre-Columbian times onward, tobacco snuff has figured prominently in the ritual and medicinal practices of the Maya (Orellana 1987: 81–82). Roys (1931: 259) documented the widespread use of green tobacco to remedy ailments such as asthma, fevers, convulsions, insect bites, skin diseases, sore eyes, and bowel complaints (see also Osado 1979: 114, 205; Orellana 1987: 31, 221–23). The Maya also used tobacco during rituals to conjure visions and to dialogue with the gods (Sharer 1994: 542).

With this in mind, I suggest that Individual 102's small pot held substances used by the decedent during curing practices. Or mourners could have expressly created the jar as an offering in the wake of Individual 102's death. Interment of the vessel in Individual 102's cavelike grave would have instigated transformation of the pot's soul. Regardless of the jar's exact function, the complete funerary assemblage of pot, disks, and blade is suggestive of a medico-religious specialist's toolkit. Hence, there is support for the notion that Individual 102 carried out practices and retained the knowledge related to this communally significant position. Given the spatial association, perhaps Individual 101 fulfilled a similar role, but the absence of material signatures makes it difficult to speculate further.

Conclusion: Living la Vida Local

From pre-Columbian times onward, medico-religious specialists have played central roles in Maya communities, and as with Individual 102, their lives were commemorated after death. A bioarchaeological approach to burials and the bodies therein provides important clues about the formation of these individuals' identities, as they first became specialized practitioners and later venerated ancestors. In scaling down to the level of the individual, we may begin to repopulate the past with the varied people who comprised it—the celebrated, the downtrodden, and everybody in between. The identification of these individuals in burials is not just an exercise in the idiosyncratic; this study of Individual 102 demonstrates that the single burial has much to communicate about larger-scale social phenomena, and for the Maya, in particular, this multiscalar approach allows us to recognize the ways in which their practices and beliefs intimately intertwined the mundane and sacred, the practical and religious, the ordinary and extraordinary.

Acknowledgments

For the opportunity to participate in the Programme for Belize Archaeological Project (PfBAP) and permission to draw on its data, I thank Fred Valdez Jr. I also thank Frank and Julie Saul, who have directed skeletal analyses for the PfBAP since its inception and who trained me in the excavation and analysis of burials during my time in Belize. I am grateful to Julie Kunen for her work in La Milpa's Far West Bajo. Additional research was conducted at the Library of Congress during my 2006–2007 tenure as the Kislak Fellow in American Studies, and I would like to thank Arthur Dunkelman, who was the collection's curator during this time. This essay was originally presented in poster form for the seventy-sixth annual American Association of Physical Anthropologists meeting in Philadelphia (March 27–April 1, 2007). I would like to thank Ann Stodder and Ann Palkovich for organizing and inviting me to participate in the session and the volume.

References Cited

Armelagos, George J.
2003   Bioarchaeology as Anthropology. In *Archaeology Is Anthropology*, edited by S. D. Gillespie and D. L. Nichols, pp. 27–40. American Anthropological Association, Arlington, Va.

Arnold, Bettina, and Nancy L. Wicker (editors)
2001   *Gender and the Archaeology of Death.* AltaMira Press, Walnut Creek, Calif.

Bell, Ellen E.
2002   Engendering a Dynasty: A Royal Woman in the Margarita Tomb, Copan. In *Ancient Maya Women*, edited by T. Ardren, pp. 89–104. AltaMira Press, Walnut Creek, Calif.

Brady, James E., and Wendy Ashmore
1999   Mountains, Caves, Water: Ideational Landscapes of the Ancient Maya. In *Archaeologies of Landscape*, edited by W. Ashmore and A. B. Knapp, pp. 124–45. Blackwell, Malden, Mass.

Brown, Linda A.
2000   From Discard to Divination: Demarcating the Sacred through the Collection and Curation of Discarded Objects. *Latin American Antiquity* 11(4): 319–33.

Buikstra, Jane E.
2006   Preface. In *Bioarchaeology: The Contextual Analysis of Human Remains*, edited by J. E. Buikstra and L. A. Beck, pp. xvii–xx. Academic Press, Burlington, Mass.

Buikstra, Jane E., T. Douglas Price, James Burton, and Lori Wright
2004   Tombs from Copan's Acropolis: A Life History Approach. In *Understanding Early Classic Copan*, edited by E. Bell, M. Canuto, and R. Sharer, pp. 185–206. University of Pennsylvania Museum of Archaeology and Anthropology, Philadelphia.

Cohen, Mark N., and George J. Armelagos (editors)
1984   *Paleopathology at the Origins of Agriculture.* Academic Press, New York.

Cohen, Mark N., and Gillian M. M. Crane-Kramer (editors)
2007   *Ancient Health: Skeletal Indicators of Agricultural and Economic Intensification.* University Press of Florida, Gainesville.

Conkey, Margaret W.
2003   Has Feminism Changed Archaeology? *Signs* 28(3): 867–80.

Conkey, Margaret W., and Joan M. Gero
1991   Tensions, Pluralities and Engendering Archaeology: An Introduction to Women and Prehistory. In *Engendering Archaeology*, edited by J. M. Gero and M. W. Conkey, pp. 3–30. Blackwell, Malden, Mass.

Davis, Virginia Dale
1978   Ritual of the Northern Lacandon Maya. Ph.D. dissertation, Department of Anthropology, Tulane University.

Dowson, Thomas (editor)

2000   Queer Archaeology. *World Archaeology* 32(2).

Dowson, Thomas

2006   Archaeologists, Feminists, and Queers: Sexual Politics in the Construction of the Past. In *Feminist Anthropology: Past, Present, and Future*, edited by P. L. Geller and M. K. Stockett, pp. 89–102. University of Pennsylvania Press, Philadelphia.

Fabrega, Horacio, Jr., and Daniel B. Silver

1973   *Illness and Shamanistic Curing in Zinacantan: An Ethnomedical Analysis.* Stanford University Press, Stanford, Calif.

Geller, Pamela

1999   Field notes. On file with author.

2004   Transforming Bodies, Transforming Identities: A Consideration of Pre-Columbian Maya Corporeal Beliefs and Practices. Ph.D. dissertation, Department of Anthropology, University of Pennsylvania.

2006   Maya Mortuary Spaces as Cosmological Metaphors. In *Space and Spatial Analysis in Archaeology*, edited by E. Robertson, J. Seibert, D. Fernandez, and M. Zender, pp. 37–48. University of Calgary Press, Calgary.

Gilchrist, Roberta

1999   *Gender and Archaeology.* Routledge, London.

Gillespie, Susan

2001   Personhood, Agency, and Mortuary Ritual: A Case Study from the Ancient Maya. *Journal of Anthropological Archaeology* 20: 73–112.

Hinojosa, Servando Z.

2002   "The Hands Know": Bodily Engagement and Medical Impasse in Highland Maya Bonesetting. *Medical Anthropology Quarterly* 16(1): 22–40.

Hollimon Sandra E.

1997   The Third Gender in Native California: Two-Spirit Undertakers among the Chumash and Their Neighbors. In *Women in Prehistory*, edited by C. Claassen and R. Joyce, pp. 173–88. University of Pennsylvania Press, Philadelphia.

Joyce, Rosemary A.

1999   Social Dimensions of Pre-Classic Burials. In *Social Patterns in Pre-Classic Meso-america*, edited by D. Grove and R. Joyce, pp. 15–47. Dumbarton Oaks, Washington, D.C.

Joyce, Rosemary A., Carolyn Guyer, and Michael Joyce

2000   *Sister Stories.* New York University Press, New York.

Kerr, Barbara, and Justin Kerr

2006   The Way of God L: The Princeton Vase Revisited. *Record of the Art Museum, Princeton University* 64: 71–79.

Kunen, Julie L.

2001   Study of an Ancient Maya Bajo Landscape in Northwestern Belize. Ph.D. dissertation, Department of Anthropology, University of Arizona.

2004   *Ancient Maya Life in the Far West Bajo: Social and Environmental Change in the Wetlands of Belize.* University of Arizona Press, Tucson.

Kunow, Marianna A.

1996   Curing and Curers in Pisté, Yucatán, Mexico. Ph.D. dissertation, Department of Anthropology, Tulane University.

McAnany, Patricia A.

1995   *Living with the Ancestors: Kinship and Kingship in Ancient Maya Society.* University of Texas Press, Austin.

Meskell, Lynn M.

1996   The Somatization of Archaeology: Institutions, Discourses, Corporality. *Norwegian Archaeological Review* 29: 1–16.

1999   *Archaeologies of Social Life: Age, Sex, Class et cetera in Ancient Egypt.* Blackwell, Malden, Mass.

Orellana, Sandra L.

1987   *Indian Medicine in Highland Guatemala.* University of New Mexico Press, Albuquerque.

Osado, Ricardo

1979   *El Libro Judio o Medicina Domestica: Descripción de los nombres de las Yerbas de Yucatán y las Enfermedades a que se Aplican.* Siglo XVII. Apartado 1456, Merida, Mexico.

Paul, Benjamin D.

1976   The Maya Bonesetter as Sacred Specialist. *Ethnology* 15(1): 77–81.

Paul, Lois, and Benjamin D. Paul

1975   The Maya Midwife as Sacred Specialist: A Guatemalan Case. *American Ethnologist* 2(4): 707–26.

Redfield, Robert, and Alfonso Villa Rojas

1934   *Chan Kom: A Maya Village.* Carnegie Institution of Washington, Washington, D.C.

Reents-Budet, Dorie

1994   *Painting the Maya Universe: Royal Ceramics of the Classic Period.* Duke University Press, Durham, N.C.

Reese-Taylor, Kathryn, Marc Zender, and Pamela L. Geller

2006   Fit to Be Tied: Funerary Practices among the Prehispanic Maya. In *Sacred Bundles: Ritual Acts of Wrapping and Binding in Mesoamerica*, edited by J. Guernsey and F. K. Reilly, pp. 40–58. Boundary End Archaeology Research Center, Barnardsville, N.C.

Roys, Ralph L.

1931   *The Ethno-Botany of the Maya.* Institute for the Study of Human Issues, Philadelphia.

Satterthwaite, Linton, Mary Butler, and J. Alden Mason

2006 [1935] Piedras Negras Archaeology, 1931–39. Piedras Negras Preliminary Papers. *Piedras Negras Archaeology: Architecture*, edited by J. M. Weeks, J. Hill, and C. Golden. University of Pennsylvania Museum of Archaeology and Anthropology, Philadelphia.

Saul, Frank P.

1972   *The Human Skeletal Remains of Altar de Sacrificios: An Osteobiographic Analysis.* Papers of the Peabody Museum of American Archaeology and Ethnology, Vol. 63. Harvard University, Cambridge, Mass.

Saul, Frank P., and Julie M. Saul

1989   Osteobiography: A Maya Example. In *Reconstruction of Life from the Skeleton*, edited by M. Y. Iscan and K. A. R. Kennedy, pp. 287–302. Alan R. Liss, New York.

Saul, Julie M., and Frank P. Saul

2004   Appendix G: Prehistoric Burials in the Far West Bajo, Belize. In *Ancient Maya Life in the Far West Bajo: Social and Environmental Change in the Wetlands of Belize*, by

J. Kunen, pp. 147–55. Anthropological Papers of the University of Arizona No. 69. University of Arizona Press, Tucson.

Schele, Linda, and Mary Ellen Miller
1986   *Blood of Kings: Dynasty and Ritual in Maya Art.* George Braziller, New York.

Schmidt, Robert A., and Barbara L. Voss (editors)
2000   *Archaeologies of Sexuality.* Routledge, London.

Sharer, Robert
1994   *The Ancient Maya.* Stanford University Press, Stanford, Calif.

Smith, Robert E.
1955   *Ceramic Sequence at Uaxactun, Guatemala.* Middle American Research Institute, Tulane University, New Orleans.

Sofaer, Joanna R.
2006   *The Body as Material Culture: A Theoretical Osteoarchaeology.* Cambridge University Press, Cambridge.

Spector, Janet D.
1993   *What This Awl Means: Feminist Archaeology at a Wahpeton Dakota Village.* Minnesota Historical Society Press, St. Paul.

Tiesler, Vera, and Andrea Cucina (editors)
2006   *Janaab' Pakal of Palenque: Reconstructing the Life and Death of a Maya Ruler.* University of Arizona Press, Tucson.

Tiesler, Vera, Andrea Cucina, and A. Romano Pacheco
2004   Who Was the Red Queen? Identity of the Female Maya Dignitary from the Sarcophagus Tomb of Temple XIII, Palenque, Mexico. *Homo* 55(1–2): 65–76.

Tozzer, Alfred M.
1941   *Landa's Relación de las Cosas de Yucatan: A Translation Edited with Notes.* Papers of the Peabody Museum of American Archaeology and Ethnology, Vol. 18. Harvard University, Cambridge, Mass.

Tringham, Ruth E.
1991   Household with Faces: The Challenge of Gender in Prehistoric Architectural Remains. In *Engendering Archaeology*, edited by J. M. Gero and M. W. Conkey, pp. 93–131. Blackwell, Malden, Mass.
1994   Engendered Places in Prehistory. *Gender, Place & Culture* 1(2): 169–203

Widsom, Charles
1940   *The Chorti Indian of Guatemala.* University of Chicago Press, Chicago.

Woods, Clyde M.
1968   Medicine and Culture Change in San Lucas Toliman: A Highland Guatemalan Community. Ph.D. dissertation, Department of Anthropology, Stanford University.

Ximénez, Francisco
1967 [1666–ca.1772] *Historia Natural del Reino de Guatemala.* Editorial "José de Pineda Ibarra," Guatemala.

Contributors

Brenda J. Baker is associate professor of anthropology at the Center for Bioarchaeological Research in Arizona State University's School of Human Evolution and Social Change. Her research concerns bioarchaeology, paleopathology, subadult osteology, and culture contact in the Nile Valley, Cyprus, and North America.

Alexis T. Boutin is assistant professor of anthropology at Sonoma State University. Her research and publications focus on the bioarchaeology of personhood in the ancient Near East, Arabian Gulf, and eastern Mediterranean.

Jane E. Buikstra is Regents Professor of Bioarchaeology at Arizona State University and director of the Center for Amerian Archaeology in Kampsville, IL. She has conducted research on funerary archaeology, paleodemography, paleopathology, and biodistance in the Americas and portions of the Old World.

Jesse Byock is professor of archaeology and medieval Scandinavia in the Cotsen Institute of Archaeology and the Scandinavian Section at the University of California, Los Angeles. He is also an affiliate professor at the University of Iceland in the Department of History and the Program in Viking Studies. He is the director of the Mosfell Archaeological Project and has published numerous books and articles on Viking Archaeology, Viking Age Iceland, feud, and the Icelandic Sagas.

Della Collins Cook is professor of anthropology at Indiana University, Bloomington. Her research interests center on paleopathology, growth and development, and mortuary practices in ancient peoples of North America, Belize, Brazil, and the Mediterranean.

Vincent P. Diego is a staff scientist in statistical genetics at the Texas Biomedical Research Institute, San Antonio, Texas, USA. His research interests include the genetics of complex disease and aging, gene-by-environment interaction, and the human biology of Pacific Island populations.

Michele Toomay Douglas is a consultant in bioarchaeology and affiliate graduate faculty at the University of Hawai'i at Manoa. Her research interests include paleopathology and skeletal biology in archaeological populations from the Pacific and Southeast Asia.

Jacqueline T. Eng is assistant professor of anthropology at Western Michigan University. She has conducted bioarchaeological and paleopathological research on archaeological human skeletal remains in China, Mongolia, Nepal, Iceland, Romania, and the United States.

Jon M. Erlandson is an archaeologist, professor of anthropology, and executive director of the Museum of Natural and Cultural History at the University of Oregon. He has written or edited nineteen books and published over 250 scholarly articles, most of them focused on the deep history of maritime peoples around the world.

Pamela L. Geller is an assistant professor of anthropology at the University of Miami. Her research interests include anthropological bioarchaeology, feminist and queer studies, the materiality of identity, and the sociopolitics of archaeology. She has conducted fieldwork in Israel, Hawai'i, Belize, Honduras, and Peru.

Rex C. Haydon is associate professor of surgery at the University of Chicago with an interest in orthopedic paleopathology.

Gary M. Heathcote is an adjunct professor of anthropology at St. Thomas University in Fredericton, New Brunswick, Canada. His research interests include human osteology and biomedical anthrpology, with areal focus on the Arctic and Western Pacific.

Per Holck is professor emeritus of anatomy at the Institute of Basic Medical Science, University of Oslo, Norway. His specialties are biological anthropology, forensic anthropology, and paleopathology.

Hajime Ishida is professor of human biology and anatomy at University of the Ryukyus, Okinawa, Japan. He has conducted research on skeletal biology and paleopathology in prehistoric skeletal series from northeastern and western Asia, and research on human genetics of East Asians.

Frederika Kaestle is associate professor of anthropology and fellow of the Institute of Molecular Biology at Indiana University, Bloomington. She has conducted research on population movement and contact, mortuary practices, and molecular evolution using ancient and modern DNA techniques on populations from around the world, with a particular focus on the Americas.

M. Anne Katzenberg is professor of physical anthropology in the Department of Archaeology, University of Calgary, Alberta, Canada. Her research interests focus on past dietary adaptations and health among prehistoric people from Canada, the United States, and Eurasia.

Kelly J. Knudson is associate professor at the Center for Bioarchaeological Research in the School of Human Evolution and Social Change at Arizona State University. She focuses on bioarchaeological and biogeochemical research in the Andes.

Maia M. Langley is a doctoral student at the University of Lisbon in Portugal and a researcher at Lisbon's National Museum of Archaeology. She focuses on spatial analysis of Iberian villas and on analysis of their material finds based on current excavations and archival records. She is currently editing three volumes dedicated to the archaeological site of Torre de Palma, the largest excavated villa in Iberia.

María Cecilia Lozada is a research associate in anthropology at the University of Chicago. She has conducted extensive multidisciplinary research in the Andes combining archaeology, ethnohistory, and human biological data.

Debra L. Martin is professor of bioarchaeology at the University of Nevada, Las Vegas. Her research addresses the origins and evolution of violence in prestate societies, with a focus on the relationship of violence to health, sex, age, and habitual activities.

Charles F. Merbs is professor emeritus at the School of Human Evolution and Social Change at Arizona State University, Tempe. His research interests and publications include work in paleopathology, forensic anthropology, and skeletal symbolism, with regional interests in the Arctic, American Southwest, and Peru.

Jill E. Neitzel is associate professor of anthropology at the University of Delaware. Her research interests include organizational complexity and regional interaction in the American Southwest.

Ann M. Palkovich is Krasnow Professor Emerita of anthropology at George Mason University. Her research interests include skeletal biology, archaeology of the American Southwest, paleopathology, and primate behavior.

Amy Papalexandrou is assistant professor at Richard Stockton College of New Jersey.

Michael Pietrusewsky is professor of anthropology at the University of Hawai'i at Manoa. His research interests and publications include multivariate methods, biological distance, skeletal biology, and bioarchaeology in Australia, the Pacific Islands, Southeast Asia, and East Asia.

Daniel T. Potts is Edwin Cuthbert Hall Professor of Middle Eastern Archaeology at the University of Sydney. He has excavated extensively in the United Arab

Emirates, Saudi Arabia, and Iran, where he currently codirects the Mamasani Archaeological Project in Fars Province.

Mary Lucas Powell is former editor of the *Paleopathology Newsletter*. She spent her first quarter century in bioarchaeology investigating health and disease in ancient Native American populations in the U.S. Midwest and Southeast, but since 1996 she has pursued her childhood dream of studying ancient lives in the Classical world, focusing on the site of Torre de Palma in eastern Portugal.

Jennifer Raff is a research fellow in the Department of Anthropology at the University of Texas in Austin. Her research focuses on the use of ancient and modern DNA to address questions of human population history, bioarchaeology, and pathogen evolution in American Midwestern and Arctic populations.

Shelley R. Saunders (1950–2008) was professor and Canada Research Chair in the Department of Anthropology at McMaster University, Ontario. She was a skeletal biologist with research interests in human growth and development, paleopathology, and skeletal studies of historic cemeteries.

Vincent J. Sava is a forensic anthropologist currently employed at the Joint POW/ MIA Accounting Command, Central Identification Laboratory in Hawai'i as a quality assurance manager. He has conducted research on paleopathology, health and disease, and occupational markers in archaeological skeletal series from the Pacific.

Henry P. Schwarcz is professor emeritus in earth sciences at McMaster University in Hamilton, Ontario. He has carried out research on the use of stable isotopes in determining the diet and migrational history of humans and animals from North America, Mesoamerica, Israel, and the Mediterranean.

Susan Dale Spencer is a Ph.D. candidate in anthropology at Indiana University, Bloomington. Her research interests include North American prehistory, paleopathology, taphonomy, and forensic anthropology.

Ann L. W. Stodder is an osteologist with the Office of Archaeological Studies, Museum of New Mexico, adjunct associate professor in the Department of Anthropology at the University of New Mexico, and research associate in Anthropology at the Field Museum. Her research addresses bioarchaeology, taphonomy, and mortuary archaeology in the US Southwest, Micronesia, and New Guinea.

Rebecca Storey is associate professor of anthropology at the University of Houston.

She specializes in the study of Prehispanic skeletons from Central Mexico and Maya in Central America, focusing on paleodemography and paleopathology.

Claire E. Terhune is an assistant professor in the Department of Anthropology at the University of Arkansas in Fayetteville, Arkansas. She has conducted research on morphological variation in the masticatory apparatus and cranium of living and fossil primates, and has interests in human evolution, skeletal biology, and functional morphology.

Jennifer L. Thompson is a paleoanthropologist. Her research addresses questions relating to the origin of modern humans, hominin growth and development, and childhood and adolescence in prehistory, and her interests include various aspects of skeletal biology and odontology.

Phillip L. Walker, who passed away in February 2009, was professor of anthropology at the University of California, Santa Barbara. His numerous publications and research interests encompassed the Mosfell Archaeological Project, Global History of Health Project, Western Hemisphere Project, Santa Barbara Channel Islands bioarchaeological history, as well as NAGPRA and forensic anthropology.

Randolph J. Widmer is associate professor of anthropology at the University of Houston. He has conducted archaeological research in Florida, Mexico, and Honduras and specializes in craft specialization, coastal adaptation, and prehistoric social structure and demography.

Gabriel D. Wrobel is associate professor of anthropology at Michigan State University, East Lansing. He is the director of the Central Belize Archaeological Survey project, focusing his research on Maya mortuary ritual in caves and rockshelters in west-central Belize.

Davide Zori received his Ph.D. from the Cotsen Institute of Archaeology at the University of California, Los Angeles (UCLA), and is currently a postdoctoral researcher at the Center for Medieval and Renaissance Studies at UCLA. His research focus is the archaeology of Viking Age and medieval Europe, and he is field director of the Mosfell Archaeological Project.

Index

Elliott, Orville, 132–33, 135, 135f

El-Najjar, Mahmoud, 17

El Yaral, 4, 85, 87, 88f, 89. See also *Curandero, of Yaral*

Enamel hypoplasia, 11, 17, 31, 33f, 39, 79–80, 174, 177, 185, 207

Endemic cretinism, 140

"Engendered Places in Prehistory" (Tringham), 256

Enthesopathies, 96, 119, 193, 199–200, 199f, 202

Epidemic disease: cholera, 219, 225; impact of, 5, 225; typhus, 225

Ermidas de São Domingos (Hermitage of Saint Dominic), 129, 142–43

Expedition to Alalakh, 193

Feminist archaeology, 256–57

Femora, asymmetry in, 122

Fictive narrative, osteobiography and, 203–6

Finnegan Mat Delta+XL mass spectrometer, 223

Fishing net, 202f

FORDISC 3.0, 136–37

Fractures: craniofacial, 85, 93f; foot, 225; long bone, 11, 17, 193, 200, 201f; Parry, 200, 201f; rib, 233–37, 234f–235f, 239; skull, 225; spiral, 118; vertebral, 55, 96, 104

Freydis, 36–37

Galt, 219

Gender, archaeology of, 2

George. *See* Neolithic Nomad, at Dakhleh Oasis

Giles, Eugene, 132–33, 135, 135f

God L, 264–65, 265f

God pot, 264–65, 265f

Goggles, Rain God, 171, 173–75

Gorman, Chester, 177–78

Gran Quivira, 250

Grasshopper Ruin, 235–36

Grave goods: of Burial 56, 168–70; of Burial 57, 165, 169–75, 170f, 172f; at Chau Hiix, 78–79; of *curandero* of Yaral, 89, 91f; of Individual 102, 260–66, 261f; Lesley and,

123; Magician's, 15f, 15t, 17–23, 18f, 20f; of Neolithic Nomad at Dakhleh Oasis, 106–8, 107f; Plaza G woman and, 249–50; at Polis Chrysochous, 152, 154–55; of seamstress at Polis, 154–55; shells in, 15, 19, 20f, 22, 86, 106, 162, 168–69, 171, 172f; at Tell Abraq, 123; Viking, 38; of Vulcan, 182, 183f, 184

Guam, 45, 46f, 49, 52, 55

Guaman Poma de Ayala, F., 86

Guma' latte (latte house): capstones, 45, 48f; construction, 54, 54t, 59–60; foundation columns, 45, 48f; House of Taga, 45, 48f, 60

Gum disease, 186

Gunnlaug Serpent-Tongue, Saga of, 37

Hale, John R., 129–31

Haligi (latte house foundation columns), 45, 48f

Hallucinogenic snuff, 92

Harvie Cemetery: historical background of, 219; location of, 217, 221f–222f; SC and JC at, 217–23, 221f–222f; stable isotope data for, 224t

Heel spurs, 105, 105f

Height: of Axed Man of Mosfell, 31–32; of Burials 56 and 57, 174; of Chamorros, 50–51, 51t; of Magician, 16–17; of Neolithic Nomad at Dakhleh Oasis, 103; of Taotao Tagga', 50–51, 51t; of Vulcan, 185

Heleno, Manuel, 127, 129, 143

Hematite disks, 261, 261f, 264

Herdade de Torre de Palma, 128, 143

Heterarchy, 181

Historic period, Maya, 69, 71t, 72, 74, 77

Hohman, John, 22

Hohokam society, 23

Homicide, of Axed Man of Mosfell, 35–37

Hopi: continuity among ancestral and contemporary, 21; NAGPRA and, 23; sleight-of-hand ceremony of, 12, 22. *See also* Sinagua

Hornbostel, Hans, 44–45

House of Taga, 45, 48f, 60

Hrísbrú: Axed Man of Mosfell at, 26–32,

28f–29f, 38–40; settlement of, 31; sickness at, 39

HSRI-2. *See* Humeral shaft index

Hubert, Virgil, 16f

Huehueteotl (Old Fire God) incense burner, 165, 169–71, 170f

Human remains: focus on, 3; justification of study of, 2

Humeral shaft index (HSRI-2), 56–57, 57f, 58t

Hypercementosis, 198

Hypoplasia. *See* Enamel hypoplasia

Icelandic sagas: Egil's, 27–28, 31, 36; of Gunnlaug Serpent-Tongue, 37; historicity of, 27; violence in, 36–37, 39–40

Ignacio de Loyola, Martin, 49

Illugi the Black, 37

Immigrants, Scottish, 5, 226. *See also* JC; RC; SC

Incense burner, Huehueteotl, 165, 169–71, 170f

Incisors, shovel-shaped, 16, 75, 75f, 79, 186

Individual 101, 262

Individual 102: at Bajo Hill, 255, 258, 259f; burial of, 255, 258–66, 260f–261f; death of, 255; grave goods of, 260–66, 261f; individual profile of, 255; osteobiography of, 262; skeleton of, 262

Individual 4769 v.2. *See* Skeletal Individual 4769 v.2

Infant, at Nuvakwewtaqa: burial of, 229–33, 232f; death of, 5–6, 238–39; individual profile of, 229; mother of, 239; radiography and, 229, 233, 235f; ribs of, 233–36, 234f–235f, 239; skeleton of, 229–30, 232–36, 234f–235f

Infanticide, 250

Infant mortality, Pueblo, 234–36, 238–39, 246

Isotopic analysis: of Axed Man of Mosfell, 30; breast-feeding and, 5, 223–24; Chau Hiix and, 68, 80; *curandero* of Yaral and, 85, 92; diet and, 30, 188, 222–23, 226; Harvie Cemetery data and, 224t; migration and, 3, 92; SC, JC and, 217,

219, 223–24, 224t; Skeletal Individual 4769 v.2 and, 127, 143; of Vulcan, 177, 187–88; weaning and, 5, 223–24. *See also* Nitrogen isotope analysis; Stable carbon isotope analysis; Strontium isotopes

Jamison, Paul, 140

JC: breast-feeding and, 5, 223–24; burial of, 217; death of, 217–19, 225–26; at Harvie Cemetery, 217–23, 221f–222f; historical background of, 219, 223; individual profile of, 229; nitrogen isotopes and, 223, 226; skeleton of, 224f, 225; stable carbon isotope analysis and, 217, 219, 223–24, 224t

Jernigan, Wesley, 18f

JH, 224, 224t

Joya de Cerén, 263

Kellis, cemetery at, 97

Kewanwytewa, James, 13, 17, 21

Kiribati, 60–61

Kirkjuhóll: cemetery at, 28, 29f, 30; location of, 26, 28; map of, 29f

Krogman, Wilton, 16, 132

Kunen, Julie, 258

Lacandon Maya, 264

Lamanai, 69, 71t, 77–80

La Milpa, 255, 258

Late Bronze Age (LBA), 194–96

Late Classic Maya, of Lowlands, 257–62

Late Intermediate Period, of Peru, 87

Latte house. *See Guma' latte*

Lazenby, Richard, 217–18

LBA. *See* Late Bronze Age

Leprosy, 122

Lesley: burial of, 113, 116–18, 123–24; clubfoot of, 118, 122; death of, 113, 118; differential diagnosis of, 120–22; grave goods and, 123; illness of, 118; individual profile, 113; osteoarthritis and, 118, 121; poliomyelitis and, 118, 120–23; radiography and, 113, 118; skeleton of, 116–24, 117f, 119f–120f; teeth of, 120, 120f; at Tell Abraq, 4, 113

Taotao Tagga': burial of, 44–45; death of, 44; facial reconstruction of, 45, 47f; height of, 50–51, 51t; HSRI-2 of, 56–57, 57f, 58t; as iconic culture hero, 4, 47; individual profile of, 44; infracranial skeletal changes of, 55; OSS and, 51, 51t, 52f–53f, 53–54, 54t; skeletal robusticity and, 44, 55–59, 57f, 58t; skeleton of, 44–45, 53, 53f, 55–61, 57f, 58t; strength of, 45, 47–49, 53, 55–56, 59–61; at Taga, 44–45, 56

Taphonomy, 3

Tasa (latte house capstones), 45, 48f

Teeth: ancestry and, 16, 75, 79, 137–38, 138f; ASUDAS and, 75; Carabelli's cusp, 137; shovel-shaped incisors, 16, 75, 75f, 79, 186. *See also* Dental modification

Tell Abraq: collective tomb at, 114–15, 116f; disability at, 123–24; grave goods at, 123; Lesley discovered at, 4, 113; location of, 114, 115f; map, 115f; secondary burial at, 118

Tell Atchana: biocultural context, 195–97, 196f; chronological framework, 194, 194t; political context, 195–97, 196f; S04-4 from, 5, 193–206

Teotihuacán, 5, 163, 165, 173, 175. *See also* Tlajinga

Tepetate bedrock, 165, 168–69

Textile production: in Alalakh, 202–3; in Cyprus, 139, 159

Thai Fine Arts Department, 177–78

Thermal ionization mass spectrometry, 26

Tinian, 44–45, 46f, 49, 52. *See also* Taotao Tagga'

Tipu: animal taxonomic diversity at, 80; long bone measurements of, 74, 74t; porotic hyperostosis and, 79; religious syncretism of, 69, 77–78; teeth of, 75, 79

Tlajinga, 33; Burial 56 at, 165, 167f, 168–69; Burial 57 at, 5, 162–71, 167f; Feature 18 at, 165, 166f–167f, 169, 169f–170f; location of, 162–63, 164f; maps, 163f, 166f; Room 66 at, 165, 167f; stature in, 174

Tlajinga 33 Project, 162

Tobacco snuff, 265

Tombs: collective, 114–15, 116f; symbolism of, 87

Tools: adze, 182, 184, 185f, 187; prehistoric, on Cyprus, 158–59; of Vulcan, 5, 182, 184, 185f, 187

Torre de Palma: church at, 4, 128–29, 141–42; continuity of cemetery space at, 143; cranial metrics, 130–31, 132t–133t; discovery of, 128; location of, 127, 129; Monte at, 128, 128f; Skeletal Individual 4769 v.2 at, 4, 127–29

TOT. *See* Occipital torus tubercles

Trade, with Sinagua, 22–23

Trauma: accidental, 236; childbirth, 236–38; craniofacial, 200; injury from, 3

Tringham, Ruth, 256

TSP. *See* Posterior supramastoid tubercles

Tuberculosis, 39, 122

Turkey, Republic of, 193. *See also* Tell Atchana

Two Horn sodality, 22

Typhus, 225

Ulnar fracture, 200, 201f

UNESCO World Heritage Site, 179

University of Chicago, 16, 193

University of Pennsylvania Museum, 177–78

Valdez, Fred, Jr., 255

Vertebral fracture, 55, 96, 104

VG Prism II mass spectrometer, 223

Viking Age: Axed Man of Mosfell in, 27–41; grave goods, 38; outlaws, 37; sickness, 39; violence, 36–37, 39–40; weapons, 35–37, 35f–36f; women, 36–37

Violence, in Viking Age, 36–37, 39–40

Visita missions, 69, 77

Vitamin D deficiency, 246–48

Vulcan: adze of, 182, 184, 185f, 187; at Ban Chiang, 5, 177–90; burial of, 177, 181–84, 183f, 189; death of, 177, 187–88; discovery of, 181; grave goods of, 182,

183f, 184; height of, 185; individual profile of, 177; isotopic analysis of, 177, 187–88; osteoarthritis of, 187; osteobiography of, 184–88, 185f–187f; pulmonary infection and, 187–88; radiography and, 177; skeleton of, 184–88, 185f–187f; strontium isotopes and, 177, 188; teeth of, 185–86, 186f; tools of, 5, 182, 184, 185f, 187

War axes, Viking Age, 35–37, 35f–36f
Ward, Rick, 140
Wassén, Henry, 86

Weaning, 5, 223–24
Weapons, Viking Age, 35–37, 35f–36f
Western Desert, 99
Wetherill, Milton, 12–13, 17, 21
White, Joyce, 178
Women, in Viking Age, 36–37
Woolley, Leonard, 194
Works Projects Administration (WPA), 12

Yaral, *curandero* of. See *Curandero*, of Yaral
Yarn spinning, 202
Yener, K. Aslıhan, 193

BIOARCHAEOLOGICAL INTERPRETATIONS OF THE HUMAN PAST:
LOCAL, REGIONAL, AND GLOBAL PERSPECTIVES
Edited by Clark Spencer Larsen

This series examines the field of bioarchaeology, the study of human biological remains from archaeological settings. Focusing on the intersection between biology and behavior in the past, each volume will highlight important issues, such as biocultural perspectives on health, lifestyle and behavioral adaptation, biomechanical responses to key adaptive shifts in human history, dietary reconstruction and foodways, biodistance and population history, warfare and conflict, demography, social inequality, and environmental impacts on population.

Ancient Health: Skeletal Indicators of Agricultural and Economic Intensification, edited by Mark Nathan Cohen and Gillian M. M. Crane-Kramer (2007; first paperback edition, 2012)
Bioarchaeology and Identity in the Americas, edited by Kelly J. Knudson and Christopher M. Stojanowski (2009; first paperback edition, 2010)
Island Shores, Distant Pasts: Archaeological and Biological Approaches to the Pre-Columbian Settlement of the Caribbean, edited by Scott M. Fitzpatrick and Ann H. Ross (2010)
The Bioarchaeology of the Human Head: Decapitation, Decoration, and Deformation, edited by Michelle Bonogofsky (2011)
Bioarchaeology and Climate Change: A View from South Asian Prehistory, by Gwen Robbins Schug (2011)
Violence, Ritual, and the Wari Empire: A Social Bioarchaeology of Imperialism in the Ancient Andes, by Tiffiny A. Tung (2012; first paperback edition, 2013)
The Bioarchaeology of Individuals, edited by Ann L. W. Stodder and Ann M. Palkovich (2012; first paperback edition, 2014)
The Bioarchaeology of Violence, edited by Debra L. Martin, Ryan P. Harrod, and Ventura R. Pérez (2012; first paperback edition, 2013)
Bioarchaeology and Behavior: The People of the Ancient Near East, edited by Megan A. Perry (2012)
Paleopathology at the Origins of Agriculture, edited by Mark Nathan Cohen and George J. Armelagos (2013)

Bioarchaeology of East Asia: Movement, Contact, Health, edited by Kate Pechenkina and Marc Oxenham (2013)

Mission Cemeteries, Mission Peoples: Historical and Evolutionary Dimensions of Intracemetery Bioarchaeology in Spanish Florida, by Christopher M. Stojanowski (2013)

Tracing Childhood: Bioarchaeological Investigations Of Early Lives In Antiquity, edited by Jennifer L. Thompson, Marta P. Alfonso-Durruty, and John J. Crandall (2014)

www.ingramcontent.com/pod-product-compliance
Lightning Source LLC
Chambersburg PA
CBHW020830270326
41928CB00006B/480